When Culture Impacts Health

When Culture Impacts Health
Global Lessons for Effective Health Research

Edited by

Cathy Banwell
National Centre for Epidemiology
and Population Health (NCEPH),
Australian National University,
Canberra, Australia

Stanley Ulijaszek
Institute of Social and Cultural Anthropology,
University of Oxford,
United Kingdom

Jane Dixon
National Centre for Epidemiology
and Population Health (NCEPH),
Australian National University,
Canberra, Australia

ELSEVIER

AMSTERDAM • BOSTON • HEIDELBERG • LONDON
NEW YORK • OXFORD • PARIS • SAN DIEGO
SAN FRANCISCO • SINGAPORE • SYDNEY • TOKYO

Academic Press is an Imprint of Elsevier

Academic Press is an imprint of Elsevier
32 Jamestown Road, London NW1 7BY, UK
225 Wyman Street, Waltham, MA 02451, USA
525 B Street, Suite 1800, San Diego, CA 92101-4495, USA

First edition 2013

British Library Cataloguing-in-Publication Data
A catalogue record for this book is available from the British Library

Library of Congress Cataloging-in-Publication Data
A catalog record for this book is available from the Library of Congress

ISBN: 978-0-12-415921-1

For information on all Academic Press publications
visit our website at elsevierdirect.com

Typeset by TNQ Books and Journals Pvt Ltd.
www.tnq.co.in

Printed and bound in United States of America

13 14 15 16   10 9 8 7 6 5 4 3 2 1

Contents

Part C
Methodological Lessons   237

Conclusion

Contributors

Shaila Arman, International Centre for Diarrheal Disease Research, Bangladesh (ICDDR,B), Dhaka, Bangladesh

Polly Atatoa-Carr, University of Auckland, New Zealand

Robert Attenborough, The Australian National University, Canberra, Australia

Phillip Baker, National Centre for Epidemiology and Population Health, Australian National University

Cathy Banwell, National Centre for Epidemiology and Population Health, Australian National University, Canberra, Australia

Juliet Bedford, Director, Anthrologica, www.anthrologica.com and Research Associate, School of Anthropology, University of Oxford

Dorothy Broom, The Australian National University, Canberra, Australia

Mark Brough, Queensland University of Technology, Brisbane, Australia

Don Byrne, Department of Psychology, The Australian National University, Canberra, Australia

Paul Callister, Victoria University, Wellington, New Zealand

Kate Crosbie, University of New South Wales, Sydney, Australia

Jane Dixon, National Centre for Epidemiology and Population Health, Australian National University, Canberra, Australia

Rebecca Fanany, School of Humanities and Social Sciences, Deakin University, Burwood, Victoria, Australia

Ismet Fanany, School of Humanities and Social Sciences, Deakin University, Burwood, Victoria, Australia

Matthew Freeman, University of Adelaide, Australia

Judith Galtry, Victoria University, Wellington, New Zealand

Don Gardner, Universitaet Luzern/University of Lucerne, Switzerland and The Australian National University, Canberra, Australia

Sandra M. Gifford, The Swinburne Institute for Social Research, Swinburne University of Technology, Victoria, Australia

Marewa Glover, University of Auckland, New Zealand

John D. Glover, University of Adelaide, Australia

Emily S. Gurley, International Centre for Diarrheal Diseases Research, Bangladesh (ICDDR,B), Dhaka, Bangladesh

Jill Guthrie, National Centre for Indigenous Studies, Australia National University, Canberra, Australia

Anthony Hogan, School of Sociology, The Australian National University, Canberra, Australia

Claire Hooker, University of New South Wales, Sydney, Australia

M. Saiful Islam, International Centre for Diarrheal Disease Research, Bangladesh (ICDDR,B), Dhaka, Bangladesh

Vivienne Ivory, University of Otago, Wellington, New Zealand

Helen Keane, The Australian National University, Canberra, Australia

Matthew Kelly, The Australian National University, Canberra, Australia

Te Kani Kingi, Massey University, Wellington, New Zealand

Julie Leask, University of New South Wales, Sydney, Australia

Judith Littleton, Department of Anthropology, The University of Auckland, New Zealand

Stephen P. Luby, Director, Centre for Communicable Diseases, International Centre for Diarrheal Disease Research, Bangladesh (ICDDR,B), Dhaka, Bangladesh and Director of Research, Center for Innovation and Global Health, Stanford University, USA

Ian Maddocks, Flinders University of South Australia, Bedford Park, Australia

Susan Morton, University of Auckland, New Zealand

Anna Olsen, The University of New South Wales, Sydney, Australia

Julie Park, Department of Anthropology, The University of Auckland, New Zealand

Shahana Parveen, International Centre for Diarrheal Diseases Research, Bangladesh (ICDDR,B), Dhaka, Bangladesh

Katherine J. Reynolds, Department of Psychology, The Australian National University, Canberra, Australia

Juliet Richters, University of New South Wales, Sydney, Australia

Johanna Schmidt, University of Auckland, New Zealand

Daniel Schwekendiek, Sungkyunkwan University, Jongno-gu, Seoul, Republic of Korea

Sam-ang Seubsman, The Australian National University, Canberra, Australia

Adrian Sleigh, The Australian National University, Canberra, Australia

Rebeca Sultana, International Centre for Diarrheal Diseases Research, Bangladesh (ICDDR,B), Dhaka, Bangladesh

Sarah Tennant, University of Adelaide, Australia

Stanley Ulijaszek, Institute of Social and Cultural Anthropology, University of Oxford, UK

Leanne Unicomb, International Centre for Diarrheal Disease Research, Bangladesh (ICDDR,B), Dhaka, Bangladesh

Maggie Walter, School of Sociology and Social Work, University of Tasmania, Tasmania, Australia

Minhee Yeo, Institute of Social and Cultural Anthropology, University of Oxford, UK

Chapter 1

When Culture Impacts Health

Jane Dixon,[1] Cathy Banwell,[1] and Stanley Ulijaszek[2]

[1]*The Australian National University, Canberra, Australia,* [2]*Institute of Social and Cultural Anthropology, University of Oxford, UK*

More complete understanding of the range of cultural influences on disease patterning will come as more frequent and profound interactions take place between the disciplines of medical anthropology and epidemiology, among others.

Trostle, 2005, p. 8

RATIONALE

In a context of growing populations, aging populations, and the rise of diseases of affluence, governments are increasingly concerned that future health care expenditures will be unsustainable. Thus, it is not surprising that disease prevention is high on national agendas. Making the job more difficult is the inevitability that disease control will always be a moving target. Infectious and chronic diseases emerge with changing ecologies, and the latter is an outcome to some extent of interactions between ever-evolving human genes and ever-changing environments. In this dynamic scenario public health leaders are questioning both the adequacy of population health research and the relevance of much of that research for developing effective interventions. As one of the pioneers of social epidemiology, Leonard Syme (2005, p. xi), said:

[In the last twenty years], we epidemiologists have suffered a whole series of embarrassing failures. ... Our model is to identify the risk factors and share that information with a waiting public so that they will then rush home and, in the interests of good health, change their behaviours to lower their risk. It is a reasonable model, but it hasn't worked. In intervention study after intervention study, people have been informed about the things they need to do, and they have failed to follow our advice.

He noted that the exigencies of daily life often hijacked intentions to behave more healthily; and in order to rectify epidemiology's neglect of the fact that people have priorities in life beyond pursuing good health, Syme called on anthropologists and epidemiologists to collaborate more closely. In a context of the sedimentation of health risks among certain populations—inevitably the least powerful in society—another leading epidemiologist, Nancy Krieger (2001), called on social epidemiology to broaden its focus beyond identifying who is sick, and expend energy on examining "who and what is responsible for population patterns of health, disease and well-being." She shared Syme's concern about the need to understand and act on the pressure points that generate health behaviors.

One such pressure point concerns the genesis of cultural factors: ranging from individual biological traits, social group practices and rules, to globally circulating ideas and discourses. Thus it is timely that renewed attention is being paid to the proposition that culture can be causal, contributory, or protective in relation to ill health (Helman, 2007; Trostle, 2007; Hruschka and Hadley, 2008; Hahn and Inhorn, 2009).

We say "renewed" because in the mid-1800s, Rudolf Virchow, doctor, statesman, and anthropologist, proclaimed disease to accompany cultural loss (Virchow, 1848/2006). He argued that epidemics are warning signs against which the progress of states can be judged. More than a century later, and with many of the infectious disease epidemics of Virchow's time remaining unconquered, lifestyle diseases (obesity, diabetes, lung and diet-related cancers) have joined a lengthy list contributing to the global burden of disease. Disconcertingly, less economically and socially powerful groups are more likely to experience multiple behavioral and disease risk factors (Lynch et al., 1997)—smoking, alcohol and drug abuse, poor nutrition—demanding investments in understanding the determinants that underpin the risks. In the absence of resource redistribution, including cultural capacity, their risk of unequal and unjust health status is also likely to persist across generations (Mackenbach, 2012).

There is widespread agreement that the reasons for inferior health outcomes are complex, involving socioeconomic factors (income, education, occupation), area-based factors (quality of water, sanitation, shelter, transport, nutrition), sociopolitical factors (gender, race, ethnicity), and sociocultural factors (values, rules, beliefs, behaviors). Culture forms part of the multifactorial etiology of disease operating in concert with social, economic, and political factors.

The primary aim of this book is then to encourage more sophisticated research designs, based on the inclusion of culture, however framed, in a range of public health research and intervention approaches in order to better explain and address contextual influences over population health behaviors. We provide researchers with conceptual and measurement tools to gain a more thorough understanding of the way culture helps "to produce asymmetries in the abilities of individuals and social groups to define and realise their [health] needs" (Johnson, 1986/1987, p. 39). At the same time, we want to avoid the situation where cultural explanations can be misused to blame people for their action or inaction. This situation arises when outsiders consider cultural matters to reflect ignorance or irrationality, rather than trying to understand local rationalities in relation to health and sickness.

Health behavior choices are shaped by belief and action systems, which arise in two ways. In part, they are based on local and historical understandings of disease, as well as the health systems available (e.g., Chinese complementary medicine, Ayurveda). They also result from interactions with environmental, economic, and political conditions, including government policies. Often over-looked are ways in which health policies can provide people with social status and material rewards for adopting certain behaviors (Farmer, 1999). For example, women who are the major food provisioners in many societies are enticed into labor markets through child-care subsidies and lowered benefits for stay-at-home women. While we might personally approve such initiatives, it must be recognized that the government's actions are not simply economic in nature but also have significant repercussions for many facets of cultural life, whether they involve food, parenting, or gender relationships.

So what are we talking about when we refer to culture? Chapter 2 describes in greater detail how contested the term is within the field of anthropology, and other contributors to this book refer to their own struggles with the term.

Drawing from anthropology and sociology, we understand culture as operating like a blueprint guiding but not dictating what is imaginable, moral, and possible. Ideas, knowledge, language, discourses, and practices constitute a significant part of social activity. This array of different forms of culture does not arise from the ether but is promulgated by a variety of societal institutions, including religious and research bodies; government departments; the legal system; the system of production, exchange, and consumption; the kin, gender, and ethnic systems of authority; and the "world of commerce." Individuals and communities also generate culture through initiating and practicing dialects, folk wisdom, and customary approaches to decision making, among other things. The resulting institutions, ideas, and practices that are generated change over time and are variable in their reach and effect depending on a people's historical experience of new ideas as well as existing belief and local power systems. In short, culture is an ever-evolving guidance system, where the major actors may be in dispute about the legitimacy of what is being said and done.

Second, we understand culture as described above (sets of meaning-laden behaviors, beliefs, artifacts) to produce "cultures," or groups of people who carry a common culture. Cultures are found at multiple levels: global, nation state, village/community, social, group, family, and individual levels. At the global level, there are adherents to the global rule of law, trade rules, financial system rules, and environmental treaties along with ideas shared through migration, technology, and the media. At the national level, governments enact societal level laws and policies that are intended to encourage particular behaviors and not others. At the same time, a nation's citizenry inherits and adapts practices from their forebears while reproducing and incrementally altering their culture through embracing new ideas, practices, and technologies.

At the level of the social group, cultural systems may legitimize/encourage or rule out/constrain decisions about how, when, where, and what health-related actions to take and equally what happens at this level can also change the cultural system. Forty years ago, for example, violence against women was tolerated in many nations. Then the second wave of the women's movement emerged to demand that the perpetrators of violence become subject to legal and community sanctions. Nevertheless, long-standing cultural norms and values leave women subjected to subtler forms of symbolic violence, such as the portrayal of women in pornography.

At the level of the individual, there is growing interest in the idea of human adaptability, or the ability of populations to adjust biologically, culturally, and behaviorally to environmental conditions. Biocultural anthropology of health and disease acknowledges different cultural models of disease, and although these are influenced by environmental conditions they operate independently as Chapters 16 and 19 in this book make clear. This strand of research has been particularly vibrant in small-scale and sometimes premodern societies that are deeply embedded in, and reliant upon, their physical environment (Maddocks, 1978).

Culture's importance as a determinant of individual health lies in the way that ideas, discourses, and ways of acting become embodied—a part of the taken-for-granted habitus or "the right way of doing things." Until there is a big jolt—an epidemic, or change in life circumstances like marriage breakdown—socialized routines dominate reflexive (self-conscious) approaches. The extent of routinized and novel behaviors typically varies depending on the socioeconomic circumstances of people. Traditional or relatively rigid thoughts and actions may persist among often less powerful groups, those less exposed to novelty, and those who are under threat from ecological collapse or resource scarcity (Gelfand et al., 2011), but this may not be a bad thing because some traditions can protect against health risks (many traditional diets are preferable to the industrial diets implicated in so many chronic diseases). However, the adoption of new ideas and practices can also be health protective, and it is important to identify under what conditions traditional and new behaviors are beneficial.

As important as it is to identify relevant cultural "risk factors" (ideas, knowledge, or traditions) (operating at each level), it is also important to identify the sociocultural processes that facilitate the transmission of the ideas, discourses, practices, and other material effects of people acting together. So our third understanding of culture is as a process, consisting of a variety of mechanisms to transmit cultural factors, which exposes some in the population and not others. Anthropologists and sociologists have identified key processes of social transmission, including emulation, mimesis, magic, socialization, diffusion of innovations, social network effects, and social status distinction (Rogers, 1962; Bourdieu, 1984; Taussig, 1993; Gerbauer and Wulf, 1995; Bell, 1999; Borch, 2005). Global cultures are becoming more common, enabled by global media, mass migrations, and technologies, which facilitate flows of ideas, norms, and practices from one society to another (Appadurai, 1996).

A primary task for culture-in-health researchers is to identify the pathways by which ideas and practices arise, circulate, and are adopted, transformed, and repudiated.

For example, the logic of infectious disease contagion is now being applied to the spread of chronic disease. In studies of lung cancer, obesity, illicit drug use, and alcohol-related illness there is growing acceptance that health-compromising ideas, emotions, and consumption practices are highly contagious and constitute relevant risk factors (Ferrence, 2001; Pampel, 2005; Christakis and Fowler, 2007; Cockerham, 2007).

With our three-part understanding of culture, we echo Susser's (2004) call for the development of an "eco-epidemiology," which considers multiple levels of causation and risks and exposures across time and space. Figure 1 summarizes our understanding of culture as shared systems of ideas, rules, language, and practices generated and transmitted within and across various levels of social organization, interacting with physical environments and biological status, and along the way influencing health experiences and outcomes.

A second aim of this book is to provide greater insight into how public health might more effectively influence culture to diffuse or spread healthy lifestyles. Against a backdrop of policy failures to eradicate major health risks and to "close the gap" in health disadvantage and inequity, there is a growing push to incorporate insights from all the disciplines critical to understanding complex public health issues, such as epidemiology, anthropology, sociology, history, economics, biology, geography, and the policy sciences (Macintyre, 1994; Porter, 1999; Gesler and Kearns, 2002; Graham, 2002; Williams, 2003; Navarro and Muntaner, 2004; Commission on the Social Determinants of Health, 2008; Fairchild et al., 2010). The smoking epidemic is the most studied of the recent

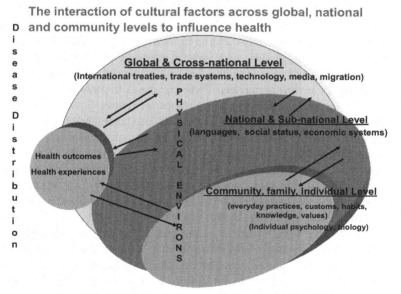

FIGURE 1.1   The levels at which culture impacts health.

noncommunicable disease risk factors; yet, despite thousands of academic papers on the etiology of smoking and 40 years of state activity to halt cigarette smoking behavior, approximately one in five males continue to smoke in most Organization for Economic Cooperation and Development countries, and in Europe, is at historically high levels (Australian Institute of Health and Welfare, 2008; Gallet et al., 2009; Glover, 2012). There has also been a steady rise in obesity rates, and predictions about obesity-related premature death have been made (Peeters et al., 2003). In many of the world's poorer countries infectious diseases coexist with growing prevalence of these noncommunicable diseases.

While we can predict different subpopulation's relative vulnerability in terms of socioeconomic factors, these factors do not completely account for or explain people's health behaviors. According to Thomas et al. (2004, p. 2050), "[t]here is credible evidence suggesting that cultural norms within Western societies contribute to lifestyles and behaviours associated with risk factors of chronic diseases." This also applies to non-Western societies.

If cultural norms are contributing to the rise in health risks such as obesity and the persistence of smoking, then it follows that cultural forces need to be unleashed to counteract their present trajectories. Cultural processes are observable in the here and now as well as through the historical record. Understanding the history of the evolution of ideas and practices shows culture to be a battleground of contestations over what is imaginable and possible, with some societies having more mutable systems of belief and actions than others. Cultural history analysis provide valuable insights into cultural pressure points, including which groups will resist change.

It is important to recognize that producing evidence of cultural pressure points is often not a sufficient reason for action. The problem with cultural interventions is their propensity to become highly politicized; think the Nanny State discourse. While citizens rarely question the need for government to shape the economy, even if they disagree over specific interventions, many feel governments should not intervene in culture because matters of taste, religion, and everyday values are private matters. These arguments overlook the ways that, historically, the economic and cultural spheres intertwine. Governments cannot avoid intervening in culture when they introduce labor market policies, for example. Elaborating on this example we would argue that under the pressures of global economic agencies, national governments profoundly affect household cultural activities through their labor market policies. Different employment policies require different allocations of time and temporal rhythms, which then influence who is working, when and where, which in turn influences the cultural realm of eating. With long work hours or unsociable shifts, solo eating and eating convenience foods on the run become normalized or the new eating routine for busy working people. This particular style of eating is often framed as a modern social trend; however, equally it can be viewed as a modern instance of Virchow's cultural disturbance that is contributing to weight gain because there is some evidence suggesting that eating together has health protective effects

(Fischler, 2011). The disturbance in shared eating practices is an unintended outcome of government labor market policy, but is becoming part of the contemporary cultural context into which new generations are socialized.

Just as governments can unwittingly contribute to chronic disease risks, they can mitigate risks through regulations that foster a cultural change in attitudes and practices. In Australia bans on public smoking have contributed to an attitudinal change where most people (including smokers) find smoking in enclosed public spaces unthinkable. In another instance of the positive cultural shifts that can be unleashed by governments, we can point to equal opportunity legislation that regulates the most extreme forms of discriminatory practice toward women and ethnic minorities. In addition to governments, commercial firms, political parties, religious institutions, and social movements all contribute to the ideas and practices that constitute the cultural environment that individuals inhabit. In a previous book, *The Seven Deadly Sins of Obesity*, we reported on public health successes that have involved cultural shifts beginning in civil society prior to government intervention (Dixon and Broom, 2007). Examples include the gay community's leadership on safe sex in response to HIV and AIDS, Mothers Against Drunk Driving and road rules in the United States, and the health community's actions to the SIDS epidemiology. In each instance these groups intervened in the cultural realm to reinstate earlier safe health behaviors or to encourage the adoption of new behaviors.

THE BOOK'S ORIENTATION

This book is animated by a desire for greater public health effectiveness in relation to chronic and infectious disease risks, which are engulfing all nations. We hope to demonstrate how cultural perspectives enrich and inform understandings of intractable public health problems. In this way, we anticipate that there are lessons for nongovernment and government agencies as they grapple to design effective interventions to improve public health. In particular, the book reinforces the argument that understanding the complex array of social forces responsible for health and illness requires a true collaboration between disciplines to be successful (Janes et al., 1986; DiGiacomo, 1999; Weiss, 2001; Trostle, 2005; Hahn and Inhorn, 2009). The range of material in this book will be useful for expanding the repertoire of both medical anthropologists and social epidemiologists. Indeed, it has great potential to provide the theoretical background linking medical anthropology to social epidemiology and public health.

In particular, this book offers a companion text or reader for those keen to go beyond risk factor epidemiology, sometimes known as "black box" epidemiology with its narrow interpretation of what constitutes good research based on an understanding of causality. One of the critics of this type of epidemiology, E. Susser (2004), has called on health researchers "to adopt a wider and richer framework." Part of the richer framework involves generating detailed insights into the contextual determinants of risk behaviors. Traditionally the terrain of

medical anthropology and social medicine, a wider group of disciplines has
been contributing to this endeavor of late, including social epidemiology, life
course epidemiology, medical geography, health sociology, bio-anthropology,
and public health history. Since the late 1980s, this multidisciplinary cast has:

- Greatly enhanced insights into the embodiment of social structure: how social
  status hierarchies, for example, create psychosocial stresses that are unhealthy
- Shown how risks can accumulate due to repeated and successive physical and
  social environmental exposures, and how risks change according to life stages
- Indicated the genetic influence over behavioral dispositions, and the disso-
  nance between behavioral dispositions acquired over millennia and contemporary human environments
- Widened the appreciation of the transmission of culture through the application of social network theories
- Revealed how public health interventions can fail because the incentives for
  behavior change are at odds with prevailing cultural systems

THE BOOK'S STRUCTURE

Section A, Research Approaches, contains four chapters from leading international authorities in their respective fields: health sociology, medical and
bio-anthropology, cultural anthropology, and field-based epidemiology. They
set out their perspectives on the history and role of culture-in-health research,
pointing to a century's worth of attempts to bring the hard-to-quantify aspects
of lived experience to the analysis of health and illness. They also reveal what is
lost in interventions if cultural insights are absent.

Section B, Local Tales, contains 15 chapters that bring together elements of
one or more of the intellectual currents described above. Each case study articulates its methods and many reflect critically on any deficits. Part 1 provides
examples from industrial and postindustrial societies, which are among the more
wealthy nations on earth: Australia, New Zealand, and South Korea. These case
studies focus on marginalized and disadvantaged populations and attribute part
of the marginal status and poor health outcomes to culturally insensitive medical and social systems. Part 2 focuses on economically transitioning societies
in South East Asia and the Pacific: Indonesia, Malaysia, Bangladesh, Papua
New Guinea, the Cook Islands, and Tuvalu. These case studies shine a particular focus on human society—physical environment interactions and cultural
struggles around long-standing versus "modern ways of living." The chapters in
Parts 1 and 2 highlight the effects of the ongoing process of the medicalization
of societies, and detail the effects of maintaining lay knowledge in the face of
dominant medical knowledge. The chapters in this section reveal a diversity of
cultural factors, actors, and processes.

Several chapters showcase the importance of anthropological approaches to
improving the efficacy of interventions. Again a critical approach is adopted,

where failures as well as successes are noted. This section advances the intellectual rationale for teams of epidemiologists and social researchers, including anthropologists, to work together from the beginning on any public health research.

Section C, Methodological Lessons, contains eight chapters that address in greater detail the methods used by Section B authors as well as introduce some additional tools. Among the research approaches included are the interrogation of epidemiology datasets by relevant sociocultural theories, cultural economy audits of social trends that are plausibly linked to health trends, ethnographic approaches to longitudinal studies of health and well-being, cultural consensus modeling to determine the extent of common values, and elite interviewing as a basis for social network mapping and for gathering the cultural history of a health policy or intervention. Two chapters detail the highly important and sensitive issues of ethnic identification and respect for alternative practices that arise when research is conducted among first people in postcolonial western societies such as Australia and New Zealand. The section concludes with a chapter describing multidisciplinary team work.

The Conclusion section provides a synthesis of the conceptual, methodological, and intervention lessons that emerge across the book. These are lessons that apply to a vast array of settings in which culture-in-health research is required.

REFERENCES

Appadurai, A., 1986. Introduction: Commodities and the politics of value. In: Appadurai, A. (Ed.), The social life of things, Cambridge University Press, Cambridge, pp. 3–63.

Australian Institute of Health and Welfare (AIHW), 2008. Australia's health 2008. Cat. No. AUS 99. AIHW, Canberra.

Bell, V., 1999. Mimesis as cultural survival. Theory, Culture and Society 16, 133–161.

Borch, C., 2005. Urban imitations. Tarde's sociology revisited. Theory, Culture and Society 22, 81–100.

Bourdieu, P., 1984. Distinction: A Social Critique of the Judgement of Taste. Routledge, London.

Christakis, N., Fowler, J., 2007. The spread of obesity in a large social network over 32 years. The New England Journal of Medicine 357, 370–379.

Cockerham, W.C., 2007. Health lifestyles and the absence of the Russian middle class. Sociology of Health and Illness 29, 457–473.

Commission on the Social Determinants of Health, 2008. Closing the gap in a generation: Health equity through action on the social determinants of health. World Health Organization, Geneva.

DiGiacomo, S, 1999. Can there be a "cultural epidemiology"? Medical anthropology quarterly 13 436–457.

Dixon, J., Broom, D., 2007. The Seven Deadly Sins of Obesity. University of New South Wales Press, Sydney.

Fairchild, A., Rosner, D., Colgrove, J., Bayer, R., Fried, L., 2010. The exodus of public health. What history can tell us about the future. American Journal of Public Health 100, 54–63.

Farmer, P., 1999. Infections and Inequalities: The Modern Plagues. University of California Press, Berkeley.

Ferrence, R., 2001. Diffusion theory and drug use. Addiction 96, 165–173.

Fischler, C., 2011. Commensality, society and culture. Social Science Information 50, 1–21.

Gallet, C.A., Hoover, G.A., Lee, J., 2009. The determinants of laws restricting youth access to tobacco. Contemporary Economic Policy 27, 16–27.

Gelfand, M., Raver, J., Nishii, L., Leslie, L., Lun, L., Lim, B., Duan, L., Almaliach, A., Ang, S., Arnodottir, J., Aycan, Z., Boehnke, K., Plus 33 other authors, 2011. Differences between tight and loose cultures: a 33-nation study. Science 332, 1100–1104.

Gerbauer, G., Wulf, C., 1995. Mimesis: Culture, Art, Society. University of California Press, Berkeley and Los Angeles.

Gesler, W., Kearns, R., 2002. Culture/place/health. Routledge, London.

Glover, M., 2012. When Culture Impacts Health: Global Lessons for Effective Health Research, Chap 11. Elsevier, UK.

Graham, H., 2002. Building an interdisciplinary science of health inequalities: the example of life-course research. Social Science & Medicine 55, 2005–2016.

Hahn, R., Inhorn, M. (Eds.), 2009. Anthropology and public health: Bridging differences in culture and society, second ed. Oxford University Press, Oxford.

Helman, C., 2007. Culture, health and illness, fifth ed. Hodder Arnold, London.

Hruschka, D., Hadley, C., 2008. A glossary of culture in epidemiology. Journal of Epidemiology and Community Health 62, 947–951.

Janes, C.R., Stall, R., Gifford, S. (Eds.), 1986. Anthropology and epidemiology, Reidel Publishing Company, Dordrecht.

Johnson, R., 1986/87. What Is Cultural Studies Anyway? Social Text 16, 38–80.

Krieger, N., 2001. Theories for social epidemiology in the 21st century: an ecosocial perspective. International Journal of Epidemiology 30, 668–677.

Lynch, J.W., Kaplan, G.A., Salonen, J., 1997. Why do poor people behave poorly? Variation in adult health behaviours and psychosocial characteristics by stages of the socioeconomic lifecourse. Social Science and Medicine 44, 809–819.

Mackenbach, J., 2012. The persistence of health inequalities in modern welfare states: the explanation of a paradox. Social Science & Medicine 75, 761–769.

Macintyre, S., 1994. Understanding the social patterning of health: the role of the social sciences. Journal of Public Health Medicine 16, 53–59.

Maddocks, I., 1978. Pari Village. In: Hetzel, B. (Ed.), Basic Health Care in Developing Countries; an Epidemiological Perspective, Oxford University Press, Oxford, England, pp. 403–415.

Navarro, V., Muntaner, C., 2004. Political and Economic Determinants of Population Health and Well-Being: controversies and Developments. Baywood Publishing Company, New York.

Pampel, F., 2005. Diffusion, cohort change, and social patterns of smoking. Social Science Research 34, 117–139.

Peeters, A., Barendregt, J., Willekens, F., Mackenbach, J., Al Mamum, A., Bonneux, L., 2003. Obesity in adulthood and its consequences for life expectancy: a life-table analysis. Annals of Internal Medicine 138, 24–32.

Porter, D., 1999. Health, civilization and the state. Routledge, London.

Rogers, E., 1962. Diffusion of innovations. Free Press, New York.

Susser, E., 2004. Eco-epidemiology: thinking outside the black box. Epidemiology 15, 519–520.

Syme, S., 2005. Foreword. In: Trostle, J. (Ed.), Epidemiology and culture, Cambridge University Press, New York.

Taussig, M., 1993. Mimesis and Alterity. Routledge. Chapman and Hall, New York.

Thomas, S., Fine, M., Ibrahim, S., 2004. Health disparities: the importance of culture and health communication. American Journal of Public Health 94, 2050.

Trostle, J., 2005. Epidemiology and culture. Cambridge University Press, New York.

Virchow, R., 1848/2006. Report on the typhus epidemic in Upper Silesia. American Journal of Public Health 96, 2102–2105.

Weiss, M., 2001. Cultural epidemiology: an introduction and overview. Anthropology & Medicine 8 (1), 5–29.

Williams, G., 2003. The determinants of health: structure, context and agency. Sociology of Health & Illness 25, 131–154.

Research Approaches

Chapter 2

Antecedents of Culture-in-Health Research

Dorothy Broom,[1] Cathy Banwell,[1] and Don Gardner[1,2]

[1]The Australian National University, Canberra, Australia, [2]Universitaet Luzern/University of Lucerne, Switzerland

INTRODUCTION

Scholarly and practical interest in the relationship between the health of populations, variously defined and contested, and the sociocultural realm has a long and distinguished history, under such headings as social medicine, community health, medical anthropology, medical sociology, sociology of health and illness, and social and cultural epidemiology. The boundaries between these various categories are blurred at many points, and observers often use the terms interchangeably. This brief discussion is designed to highlight the characteristic emphasis of each rather than to define clear distinctions. The comments that follow sketch activity during the twentieth century, although theoretical and applied origins could be traced across hundreds of years.

SOCIAL MEDICINE

The origins of this enterprise are often attributed to Rudolf Virchow, a nineteenth century Prussian pathologist and clinical researcher who famously stated that

Medicine is a social science, and politics is nothing else but medicine on a large scale. Medicine, as a social science, as the science of human beings, has the obligation to point out problems and to attempt their theoretical solution: the politician, the practical anthropologist, must find the means for their actual solution.

Virchow, nd

Virchow's clarion call to doctors to become "the natural attorneys of the poor" was taken up with great commitment in the early decades of the twentieth century by doctors in southern Africa, several of whom founded the Pholela Health Centre in KwaZulu Natal in 1940. Emily and Sidney Kark, Sidney and Gwen Sax (later significant influences on the Australian community health movement), John Cassel, and Mervyn Susser played a range of roles in the foundation and development of the visionary "holistic" service for southern Africa's

When Culture Impacts Health. http://dx.doi.org/10.1016/B978-0-12-415921-1.00002-6

most vulnerable population, combining primary medical and a wide range of other health and social services under one roof.

The distinctive focus on the links between society and health were articulated by the UK Society for Social Medicine (founded in 1950) who define social medicine on their Web site as

... the study of health in its widest sense. It recognizes the broad determinants of health—income and poverty, education, environmental factors such as housing and transport—as well as health care and genetic influences.

... The nature of social medicine requires a multi-disciplinary approach to the development of scientific knowledge. The disciplines involved include medicine, epidemiology, statistics, economics, social science and many others.

Much like the World Health Organization (WHO) Commission on the Social Determinants of Health decades later, social medicine is positioned at the intersection between scholarly research and practical application, and makes no claim to value neutrality or disciplinary separation. Instead, it articulates fundamental principles:

- Social and economic conditions profoundly impact health, disease, and the practice of medicine.
- The health of the population is a matter of social concern.
- Society should promote health through both individual and social means (Rosen, 1974).

These perspectives continue to be expressed in the work of famous institutions and researchers, including the Department of Global Health and Social Medicine in the Harvard Medical School whose Web page explains that it "applies social science and humanities research to constantly improve the practice of medicine, the delivery of treatment, and the development of health care policies locally and worldwide."

MEDICAL ANTHROPOLOGY

Contributing substantially to social medicine, medical anthropology emerged initially from ethnographic research, often in less developed nations or among aboriginal inhabitants of colonized nations. The American Anthropological Association's Society for Medical Anthropology Web page defines their enterprise (in 2010) as:

... a subfield of anthropology that draws upon social, cultural, biological, and linguistic anthropology to better understand those factors which influence health and well being, ... the experience and distribution of illness, the prevention and treatment of sickness, healing processes, the social relations of therapy management, and the cultural importance and utilization of pluralistic medical systems.

As part of this enterprise, medical anthropology includes, among other things, the study of health disorders that may be self-defined or community-defined, including those not validated as "real" by biomedical epistemology. This often raises questions about biomedicine's claim to ultimate authority on the nature of disease. It also critiques medical research and practice for being largely free of theoretical commitments, and often turns its research gaze back onto medicine itself.

In responding to questions about the health of populations, medical anthropologists now draw upon many disciplines including epidemiology, psychology, sociology, history, politics, and economics. This contemporary broadening of approach is in part related to the expansion of their field study sites to include western and westernizing societies.

SOCIOLOGY OF HEALTH

Like their cousins in anthropology, sociologists have sometimes had uneasy relationships with clinicians. Their connection has taken a number of forms, signaled in part by tension between "medical sociology" and "health sociology," sometimes glossed as a contrast between sociology *in* medicine as opposed to sociology *of* medicine (Straus, 1957). The former represents work that has often involved collaborations between sociologists and clinicians, occasionally placing the social scientist in the service of the clinician, potentially risking the distinctive social science perspective. Nevertheless, social science entered medicine because of the conviction that the sociological imagination had essential contributions to make to medical practice, training, and research. Health sociology (or the sociology of health and illness) has tended to focus on, and validate, the experiences of laypeople as well as medical professionals, and to turn its research attention onto the conduct of professionals (Becker et al., 1961) rather than restricting itself to the investigation of "noncompliant" or difficult patients.

Whatever the label, the trademark concept of medical sociology is *society*, especially social structures (social roles and social institutions). The *Oxford Dictionary of Sociology* defines it as a field concerned with the social dimensions of health and illness covering three main areas such as the:

1. Conceptualization of health and illness
2. Study of their measurement and social distribution
3. Explanation of patterns of health and illness

Like anthropological investigations of medical epistemologies and practices, those of health sociologists have critiqued the notion that official (including vital) statistics are unproblematic representations of the real world. Instead, sociologists have argued that bureaucracies and professionals are engaged in "claims-making" and "rates-making" and hence in generating social and medical problems through the definitions they employ and the assumptions on which they rely. First expressed in research on crime and deviant behavior (Spector and Kitsuse, 1977), a similar logic has been applied to the understanding of various forms of ill health, including mental illness (Szasz, 1960) and more recently obesity (Gard and Wright, 2005), elaborated theoretically in the concept of "medicalization" (Conrad, 1992). When applied to a specific condition, such as obesity, contestations about definitions and assumptions from the perspectives of biomedicine and the critical social sciences can last for decades.

Again, health sociology is similar to medical anthropology in interrogating the assumptions and operational definitions of epidemiology (DiGiacomo, 1999), while ambivalently relying on epidemiological facts about the distribution of disease. However, epidemiology and the social sciences share a common focus on ill health in populations, as opposed to the clinical focus on individuals. Health and medical sociology remain among the largest sections in the sociological associations of the UK, United States, and Australia, testimony to the continuing appeal of these perspectives.

SOCIAL EPIDEMIOLOGY

Interaction between early epidemiologists and exponents of social medicine could lead to the conclusion that all epidemiology is social epidemiology. However, over the twentieth century growing attention to clinical epidemiology, which aims to identify risks that can be modified in a clinical setting, has led to the recent growth of a distinct variant, defined as the study of the social determinants of health (Berkman and Kawachi, 2000). A more detailed definition suggests that social epidemiology investigates "how social interactions—social norms, laws, institutions, conventions, social conditions, and behavior—affect the health of populations" (Oakes and Kaufman, 2006). If the difference between clinical and social epidemiology is comparatively clear, there is perhaps more difficulty knowing where social epidemiology leaves off and the health social sciences begin. To an extent, this is a matter of emphasis, in which epidemiology has been particularly focused on "gradients" in health or health inequalities. An uncharitable observer with a social science background might suggest that it merely represents a discovery by epidemiologists of what social medicine, anthropologists, and sociologists have been doing for decades. The WHO Commission on the Social Determinants of Health (2008) has, for the moment anyway, placed health inequalities higher on the international policy and research agenda than they had been for many decades. However, the community or public health movement at the time of the Alma Alta Declaration (1978) had a similar agenda.

CULTURE IN ANTHROPOLOGY, THE SOCIAL SCIENCES, AND EPIDEMIOLOGY

The trademark concept in (medical) anthropology is culture, although as Park and Littleton in Chapter 14 note, the discipline is not reducible to the study of culture alone. Furthermore, as Attenborough and Gardner observe in Chapter 16, the concept of culture is highly contested among contemporary anthropologists.

Despite strong resistance from some quarters, the paradigmatic conception of culture from the 1980s increasingly criticized in the name of concepts such as *power, practice, agency,* or *history,* all of which tended to be sensitive to local patterns of difference within the broader domain. At the same time, a growing number of scholars from other disciplines began to write enthusiastically of the liberation from "positivistic" orthodoxies offered by anthropological conceptions of cultural meanings (Sewell, 1997). Despite contrasts among scholars, all contemporary anthropologists and their colleagues in neighboring disciplines stress that variations in cultural *meanings* are both important and observable, and that these constitute differences that make a difference to all dimensions of human life. The effect of the critique of older notions of culture has led anthropologists to focus on the analysis of specific cultural settings and their historical trajectories, including differences within social formations. Culture has come to be seen as a matter of what happens at a *local* level; it attends to life as lived and experienced by socio-historically located people. The theoretical pressure from within anthropology has lent greater significance to its unique method, long-term fieldwork. In an increasingly globalized world, an anthropological perspective means attending to what people do on a day-to-day basis, and not just to what they say about what they do, or to official or media representations of people's lives. As Brightman (1995) observed and Sahlins lamented (1999), this local focus has led to a stress on the *cultural* and evasion of the noun *culture* while less (or at least differently) freighted terms like "hegemony" or "discourse" took its place in many anthropological texts.

Ambiguities and tensions continue to characterize the theoretical status of the concept of culture and its relationships with other master concepts of contemporary anthropological analysis. Accordingly, there are also difficulties about which sense of "cultural" applies to the concept of epidemiology, if it is defined as "… a methodologically exacting discipline … devoted to the discovery of disease prevalence and incidence rates and to the statistical assessment of causal associations between risk factors and disease outcomes in human populations" (Hahn and Inhorn, 2009, p. 169). Adopting the epidemiological focus on individual risk behavior makes it theoretically difficult to retain the ideas of systematicity and holism, which have always been integral to an understanding of culture. In relation to epidemiology, the concept of culture has been important for those wishing to identify otherwise hidden risk factors and patterns of disease, or seeking to explain why medically available options for mitigating risk are not available to some members of a population.

Regarding the pairing of the cultural with epidemiology, one might well ask what room is there for yet another subdiscipline, and what is achieved by introducing yet another distinction. However, much epidemiology might benefit from interdisciplinary collaboration and a greater reflexivity regarding its own thinking and practice, some of those who have sought to engage in such collaboration have raised the unsettling prospect that it may only result in "… the medicalization of culture understood as difference" (DiGiacomo, 1999).

When "culture" is reduced to a simple (often dichotomous) variable (Kaufert, 1990) on which to categorize patients or survey respondents, it is unlikely to bear much fruit, either for social theory or health improvement. On the other hand, the cultural might be construed as a more nuanced way of investigating and describing the context of health (including the context of epidemiological careers and research) rather than as a single causal agent, list of "traits," or a "risk factor." Recent examples of research labeled "cultural epidemiology" are provided by Weiss (2001), who used the term to describe a specific methodology that is called an Explanatory Model Interview Catalogue (EMIC), thus referencing the notion of the "emic" insider's view. They concentrate on clinically based research and community surveys about the experience of tropical infectious diseases and psychiatric conditions to align cultural understandings with "the WHO's International Classification of Disease (ICD) and the American Psychiatric Association's Diagnostic and Statistics Manual (DSM)" (Weiss, 2001, p. 24).

To consider the rough border between social epidemiology and cultural epidemiology (which may run parallel to the border between sociology and anthropology), Trostle (2005) briefly explored how each might approach an understanding of mortality on the Titanic. Social epidemiology focuses its attention chiefly on social structure, documenting class differences in mortality rates (controlled for gender). On the other hand, a cultural approach described by Trostle draws attention to the underlying rules and norms shaping access to survival opportunities: specifically, rules and norms regarding gender, age, and the particular obligations of passengers *versus* crew (Trostle, 2005) from the perspective of each. Social scientists of a variety of persuasions may prefer to attend to differences in the practices of crew and passengers.

CULTURE-IN-HEALTH

In summary, many anthropologists and epidemiologists strenuously resist the use of the term cultural epidemiology. Anthropologists mainly object to the connotations of this formulation, given that "culture" is disputed within the discipline. Epidemiologists argue that having newly and only recently accepted the notion of social epidemiology, there is no need to further subdivide the discipline. Those on both sides are concerned with an undue emphasis on measurement; anthropologists fear the misrepresentation of culture as a set of measurable variables, while epidemiologists are bothered by the difficulty of measuring it effectively. These differences stem from the centrality of allegedly objective measures of epidemiology in contrast to the supposedly subjective nature of some social science studies of public health issues. The famous epidemiologist Rothman (2002) claimed that epidemiology is the core discipline of public health. However, others are now arguing that a more inclusive disciplinary approach is required. As another epidemiologist put it "[i]t is high time that public health stopped behaving as if one single dominant paradigm was enough"

(McPherson, 1998). The push for culture-in-health research exemplified in this volume aims to extend the epistemological foundation of public health research beyond epidemiology alone and to upset previously rigid boundaries.

Anthropology and sociology (and political science via political economy) have typically insisted on the pertinence to health of *power*, a concept often neglected by mainstream epidemiology. Will this significant concept be given more prominence in culture-in-health research? The health social sciences have also raised concerns about the definition and measurement of socioeconomic and racial categories (Nazroo, 1998) and even the superficially unproblematic dichotomy of "gender" (Broom, 2008). If taken seriously, these questions raise critical issues for epidemiological measurement and research, quite apart from the potential relevance of the distinction between true groups (people who interact with one another) and statistical categories (aggregates of individuals).

Ultimately, the value of a still nascent approach in public or population health may be a question of questions: What research questions and methods come to the fore under the banner of culture-in-health research? How much should epidemiological research be driven by health policy imperatives? How and where should answers be sought? What counts as evidence? What are the units of analysis? What is brought into focus that is otherwise neglected? Is the aim of studying culture to understand disease, or is it studying disease to understand culture? Which will be the dominant discourse? Or is it a true hybrid, a new discipline that can genuinely consolidate the many strengths of this rich heritage?

This book seeks to add to three decades of writing that has explored the interface between anthropologically and epidemiologically informed studies that see public health outcomes as always already cultural. The contributing authors have sometimes used cultural epidemiology in a generic sense to describe the many ways in which they study both patterns and experiences of ill health among diverse social groups in poor and rich nations, and they illustrate the richness that is generated in these interstitial research spaces. In acknowledging the difficulties that many have with the term, we have instead employed the more laborious phrase "culture impacting on health" in the book's title. By partnering culture with (public) health rather than epidemiology we embrace a broader epistemological focus. Nevertheless, this book provides examples of, and reflections on, the practical and theoretical complexities and value of combining culturally informed approaches and understandings with epidemiology in public health.

REFERENCES

Becker, H.S., Geer, B., Hughes, E.C., Strauss, A.L., 1961. Boys in White: Student Culture in Medical School. University of Chicago Press, Chicago.

Berkman, L.F., Kawachi, I. (Eds.), 2000. Social Epidemiology, Oxford University Press, Oxford.

Brightman, R., 1995. Forget culture: replacement, transcendence, relexification. Cultural Anthropology 10, 509–546.

Broom, D.H., 2008. Gender in/and/of health inequalities. Australian Journal of Social Issues 34, 11–28.

Commission on the Social Determinants of Health, 2008. Closing the Gap in a Generation. Technical.

Conrad, P., 1992. Medicalization and social control. Annual Review of Sociology 18, 209–232.

DiGiacomo, S.M., 1999. Can there be a 'cultural epidemiology'? Medical Anthropology Quarterly 13, 436–457.

Gard, M., Wright, J., 2005. The Obesity Epidemic: Science, Morality and Ideology. Routledge, London.

Hahn, R., Inhorn, M. (Eds.), 2009. Anthropology and Public Health: Bridging Differences in Culture and Society, Oxford University Press, New York.

Kaufert, P., 1990. The 'Box-Ification' of Culture: the Role of the Social Scientist. Santé, Cutlure, Health 7, 139–148.

McPherson, K., 1998. Wider causal thinking in the health sciences. Journal of Epidemiology and Population Health 52, 612–618.

Nazroo, J.Y., 1998. Genetic, Cultural or Socio-Economic Vulnerability? Explaining Ethnic Inequalities in Health. In: Bartley, M., Blane, D., Davey Smith, G. (Eds.), The Sociology of Health Inequalities, Oxford, Blackwell.

Oakes, J.M., Kaufman, J.S. (Eds.), 2006. Methods in Social Epidemiology, Jossey Bass, San Francisco.

Rosen, G., 1974. From Medical Police to Social Medicine: Essays on the History of Health Care. Science History Publications, New York.

Rothman, K., 2002. Epidemiology: An Introduction. Oxford University Press.

Sahlins, M., 1999. Two or Three Things That I Know About Culture. The Journal of the Royal Anthropological Institute 5, 399–421.

Sewell, W., 1997. Geertz, cultural systems, and history: from synchrony to transformation. Representations 59, 35–55.

Spector, M., Kitsuse, J.I., 1977. Constructing Social Problems. Cummings Publications, Menlo Park.

Straus, R., 1957. The nature and status of medical sociology. American Sociological Review 22, 200–204.

Szasz, T., 1960. The myth of mental Illness. American Psychologist 15, 113–118.

Trostle, J., 2005. Epidemiology and Culture. Cambridge University Press.

Virchow, R. (nd). "Rudoph Virchow on Pathology Education," http://www.pathguy.com/virchow.htm.

Weiss, M., 2001. Cultural epidemiology: an Introduction and overview. Anthropology and Medicine 8, 5–29.

Chapter 3

Biological and Biocultural Anthropology

Stanley Ulijaszek

Institute of Social and Cultural Anthropology, University of Oxford, UK

INTRODUCTION

Biological anthropology deals with human evolution and human biological variation. The place of disease in this framework is as an environmental stressor that can shape human population structure and variation through differential mortality and fertility. The emphasis on human–environmental interactions in the production of disease has obvious synergies with epidemiology, and it is no surprise that there are many biological anthropologists working with epidemiologists and in public health. Human ecology is a subfield of biological anthropology that deals with human adaptability, or the ability of populations to adjust, biologically and behaviorally, to environmental conditions. These are the processes that lead to human population variation. Humans inevitably change their environments while adapting, and this leads to new stresses. Understanding the interactions between humans and their increasingly complex environments, especially with economic modernization and change across the past 50 years, has also become part of the remit of human ecology and therefore also of biological anthropology (Ulijaszek and Huss-Ashmore, 1997). Since society and culture construct the environments that humans negotiate and the behavioral responses to them, the incorporation of social and societal factors into studies of human adaptability is essential (Thomas, 1997). Biocultural anthropology is a subdiscipline of biological anthropology that considers this. With respect to health and disease, biocultural anthropology acknowledges different cultural models of disease (including biomedicine) and examines how society, culture, and behavior shape patterns of disease (Wiley and Allen, 2009). This chapter will describe the ways in which biological anthropology and biocultural anthropology study disease.

When Culture Impacts Health. http://dx.doi.org/10.1016/B978-0-12-415921-1.00003-8

BIOLOGICAL ANTHROPOLOGY AND CONSTRUCTIONS OF DISEASE

Adaptation and adaptability have been defined as processes in which beneficial relationships between humans and their environments are established and maintained, making individuals better suited to survive and reproduce in given environments (Lasker, 1969). They have also been viewed as the processes that allow human populations to change in response to changing or changed environments (Ellen, 1982). In this frame, Disease is seen as a marker of maladaptation, which at its extremes, can lead to death. Differential mortality is one mechanism in which natural selection operates, and understanding disease and mortality helps biological anthropologists understand how human populations are shaped biologically.

The question of what constitutes successful human adaptation remains elusive. Since the measure of success is usually taken to be straightforwardly Darwinian, it is necessary to demonstrate that specific biological alterations favor survival and reproduction. This has proved difficult to demonstrate in human populations, and Darwinian selection is more often inferred in relation to genetic and physiological traits that might confer selective advantage. For example, the genetic ability to resist malaria can be framed in adaptive terms and inferred from trait biology and empirical study of distributions of genes and gene products. Generally, the study of trait biology involves examination of morphological and physiological factors that show marked geographical variation in their distributions; the task is to show that variants are each adapted to their own environmental circumstances (Smith, 1993). The empirical study of distributions of genes and gene products involves their spatial mapping, and relating these maps to potential selective pressures such as nutrition and infectious disease. This is easier to demonstrate for malaria than any other disease, largely because of the intense selection that it imposed on prehistoric and historic human populations, and its relative lack of pathogenic diversity. With respect to nutritional adaptation, it is easiest to infer natural selection having taken place for the consumption of milk, because lactose intolerance among past populations would have carried high mortality.

Physiological adaptation involves shorter-term changes that individuals show in response to environmental stressors. They can be observed as both processes and states, and include immunological responses to infection and chronic disease, as well as nutritional state. Behaviors that can confer some advantage, ultimately reproductive, can also be termed adaptive. Such behaviors may include proximate determinants of reproductive success (such as mating and marriage patterns), types and patterns of parental investment, including ones that may be protective against infection such as breastfeeding, or patterns of resource acquisition, including food acquisition.

Culture is also an adaptive force (Laland and Kendall, 2007). Cultural similarities emerged from common proximity, history, language, and identification of groups of people (Brumann, 1999), as well as shared and socially

transmitted normative ideas and beliefs (Alexrod, 1997). Shifts in social structure and cultural practices can drive the evolution of genetic and phenotypic
novelties through the promotion of some allele frequencies but not others; this
is known as gene-culture co-evolution (Odling-Smee et al., 2003). Culture is
not primarily adaptive, however, and adaptation should not be read into all
aspects of culture (Morphy, 1993). Behavior may buffer against environmental stress, but environmental changes induced by such buffering often bring
new stresses and adaptive challenges. In Wiley's (1992) terms, adaptation is
"tracking a moving target." Such tracking is nowhere more evident than with
immunological adaptation to infectious disease.

Adaptation to infection has been studied most successfully in relation to
malaria. Mortality due to the *Plasmodium falciparum* parasite is by far the
greatest among the four species of *Plasmodia* that can infect humans, and it
continues to be a major cause of mortality in the contemporary world. Genetic
analyses have shown that *P. falciparum* crossed the species barrier from gorillas
to humans long before the origins of agriculture (Liu et al., 2010), a time when
humans became exposed to a range of new adaptive challenges. The human
subsistence transition from hunting and gathering to agriculture and animal
husbandry resulted in changes to nutritional and infectious disease ecologies,
exposing mothers and their children to nutritional stresses and new pathogenic
environments. Agriculture originated independently in several parts of the
world, around 10,000 years ago in the Near East and New Guinea, and around
8,000 years ago in China and the Americas (Ulijaszek et al., 2012). Genetic
analyses of the *P. falciparum* genome sequence and of the speciation of human
malaria vectors (Coluzzi, 1999) suggest an expansion of this *Plasmodium* species within the last 6,000 years from Africa. *Plasmodium vivax*, on the other
hand, is thought to have emerged as a primate malaria in Asia between 46,000
and 82,000 years ago, initially colonizing hominoids via a macaque parasite
lineage that later became *P. vivax* (Escalante et al., 2005), affecting humans as
they migrated out of Africa.

The adoption of agriculture led to increased population density, planting
seasons associated with rainfall, and in subsequent millennia, irrigation. This
would have brought humans engaged in agricultural work, the *Plasmodium*
parasite, and its mosquito vector together on a regular if not continuous basis.
With the emergence of towns and cities, water storage would have facilitated
the breeding of the mosquito vectors of malaria. These conditions would have
permitted runaway malarial infection among humans. Intense positive selection of malaria-protective genes among populations exposed to this disease took
place (Kwiatkowski, 2005), with the emergence of a range of malaria-protective
genotypes and phenotypes independently in different parts of the world. These
include glucose-6 phosphate dehydrogenase (G6PD) deficiency, alpha and beta
thalassemias, hemoglobins S and C, and the Duffy blood group antigen. In
any population exposed to malaria, adaptation has involved alleles of multiple
genes, often giving rise to multiple resistant traits (e.g., G6PD deficiency and

alpha thalassemia sometimes occurring in the same individual) (Sabeti et al., 2006). These resistance alleles continue to shape the patterns of malarial infection to the present day. It has been argued that natural selection in response to HIV/AIDS is under way and is of similar amplitude to natural selection against malaria (Galvani and Novembre, 2005). The genes associated with resistance to HIV/AIDS are related in their phenotypic functions, which are immunological (Galvani and Novembre, 2005), although existing genetic variation in susceptibility to HIV/AIDS is not explained by natural selection in recent times (Gonzales et al., 2001).

The physical development of the immune system is another adaptation, as are immune responses and immunological memory that come with exposure to pathogens. Developmentally, a human neonate is immunologically immature, but is largely protected from pathogens at birth by antibodies from the mother. Breastfeeding supplies an infant with maternal immunoglobulin A, which is protective against a wide range of infections. Most aspects of the immune system are close to fully mature by the age of five years, making early childhood the time when susceptibility to infection is usually the greatest. The ability to digest lactose in milk by the enzyme lactase is another physiological adaptation. This is high in all human infants, but declines rapidly after weaning in most populations, but not in many of those that traditionally consume dairy foods. For many people, as the origins of agriculture allowed continued consumption of milk beyond infancy, this would have led to malabsorption, diarrhea, and possibly death. For others, genetically inherited lactase persistence would have been selected for. The lactase persistence allele $LCT*P$ arose specifically in humans (and not among ancestral primates) and is most common among populations that are either northern European or of northern European origin (Swallow, 2003). The mini-chromosome maintenance protein 6 gene ($MCM6$) is upstream of the LCT gene and regulates its expression. The $C-14010$ allele of $MCM6$ was positively selected for around 7,000 years ago in Africa, around the time that pastoralism was adopted and milk consumption became a principal part of the diet (Tishkoff et al., 2007), permitting lactose tolerance beyond infancy among those that had this gene variant.

Another type of physiological adaptation involves phenotypic plasticity, which permits exploitation of changing and changeable environments. For example, human children can undergo growth faltering due to poor food availability and exposure to infection, and show catch-up growth when these stresses are removed. This was probably an adaptation acquired in human evolution in response to seasonal environments, by tuning body size to food availability (Ulijaszek et al., 2012). This remains a fundamental phenotypic response to poor food security, whether seasonal or not, across the less-developed world in the present day. At the extreme, growth faltering is associated with protein energy malnutrition and increased susceptibility to infectious disease, at least in early childhood. Growth faltering is therefore also associated with suppressed immunological sufficiency that comes with undernutrition and the greater likelihood of becoming infected and potentially dying. For the biological anthropologist, this represents an adaptation that both permits survivorship under difficult circumstances and can shape future genetic adaptation. For epidemiologists, this represents a biomedical and public health problem.

BIOCULTURAL ANTHROPOLOGY AND DISEASE

Biocultural approaches in anthropology are those that explicitly recognize the dynamic interactions between humans as biological beings and the social, cultural, and physical environments they inhabit. Livingstone (1958) did not use the term "biocultural" to describe his framework, but initiated an important new approach to the study of health and disease. He described the linkages among population growth, subsistence strategy, malaria, and the distribution of the sickle cell gene in West Africa as an interaction between culture and biology. More explicitly biocultural approaches to human adaptation emerged from the 1960s (Bindon, 2007). Current formulations of biotoculturalism, as defined by Wiley (1992) and Goodman and Leatherman (1998), privilege neither culture nor biology, and unlike sociobiology, do not seek to understand the evolutionary basis of human behavior and culture. Rather, localized and measurable human biological outcomes are examined in relation to aspects of history, politics, and economics, while past evolutionary outcomes are viewed as forming the genetic basis for biological responses to interactive physical, social, and biological stresses in the present. Biocultural approaches have come to recognize the pervasiveness and dynamism of interactions between biological and cultural phenomena, past and present, and explicitly work toward integration of biological, sociocultural, environmental, and other kinds of observation.

Livingstone's (1958) landmark study shows the complexity of adaptive processes when culture, behavior, and society are invoked in understanding disease processes. Both malaria and tuberculosis emerged as human diseases before the origins of agriculture, but only became very prevalent after it, with increased transmission rates as population densities grew (Armelagos and Harper, 2005). At the origins of agriculture in Africa, forest clearing would have constructed niches that increased the potential for mosquito breeding and increased the spread of malaria (Laland and Kendal, 2007), while population growth and crowding in houses in new urban centers would have helped the spread of tuberculosis. With the organization of human populations into the complex societies that followed the origins of agriculture, disease ecology changed such that density-dependent pathogens became more important than sylvatic infections (ones that exist in animals and infect humans directly). Sedentism, clearing land for agriculture and animal husbandry, along with increased human contact with human and animal feces, provided ideal conditions for the transmission and fixation of novel pathogens in human populations. The emergence of towns and cities would have made crowd infections dominant in those places. The nutritional stresses that came after the origins of agriculture would have further facilitated the spread of infectious diseases because of impaired immunological responses and the now well-documented synergies between infection and nutrition (Suskind and Tontisirin, 2001). In particular, weaning and dietary supplementation at the origins of agriculture would have offered a new vehicle for infection by the newly emergent human gastrointestinal pathogens associated with higher-density living.

Infant delivery, breastfeeding, supplementation of an infant's diet, exposure to infection, and illness management practices are culturally variant behaviors that also influence morbidity and mortality, thus making physiological, and ultimately genetic, adaptations biocultural. Breastfeeding, and the behavioral patterns that go with it, help to buffer an infant against exposure to the pathogenic environment. Dietary supplementation, however, increases exposure of infants to pathogenic agents, while cessation of breastfeeding both increases pathogenic exposure and removes the maternal antibody contribution from the infants' immune system. Breastfeeding therefore has a number of traits that favor infant growth and survivorship, including balanced nutrition and immunological protection.

Resistance to infection can be shaped non-immunologically by diet as well. Katz and Schall (1979) elaborated a biocultural model for the development of genetic resistance to malaria in the Mediterranean region that involves fava bean consumption, one of the founder crops of the Fertile Crescent, from approximately 9,000 years ago. According to Katz and Schall, consumption of this legume favored natural selection of the Mediterranean variant of the G6PD deficiency malaria-resistance genotype. When G6PD-deficient individuals are oxidant-challenged, they experience hemolysis (Greene, 1993); malarial infection imposes a particularly high oxidant challenge to red blood cells. Fava beans contain oxidants, including divicine and isouramil, which contribute to the low antioxidant capacity of red blood cells in people with G6PD deficiency, and increase the likelihood of hemolysis when exposed to oxidant challenge such as that imposed by malarial infection. Although such hemolysis results in significant morbidity and mortality in some G6PD-deficient individuals, increased vulnerability of G6PD-deficient erythrocytes to oxidant stress confers protection against *P. falciparum* (Greene, 1993), because it breaks the cycle of infection by denying the parasite a red blood cell host. In the Mediterranean region, experience and cultural knowledge of the use of fava beans would have facilitated the emergence of red blood cell G6PD deficiency. This adaptation still remains important. Fava beans continue to be a major part of Middle Eastern diet, being consumed in stews, salads, and as pastes with unleavened bread. Oxidant stress only has a selective advantage when malarial infection is a threat to survival, however, and malaria has largely been eradicated in the Mediterranean region. While public health nutrition now might promote the consumption of antioxidant-rich foods to potentially reduce risk of developing atherosclerosis, some cancers, some inflammatory conditions, and aging (Young and Woodside, 2001), this is potentially harmful in populations with both high rates of G6PD deficiency and fava bean consumption (Ulijaszek et al., 2012).

The adaptations that humans carry constantly shape their experience of health and disease, and the most commonly known genetic adaptations to disease and diet were selected for, across prehistoric time. However, adaptation is an ongoing process. Political, economic, and social processes continue to operate on human biology and in the production of health disease to the present day. Biocultural anthropologists aim to understand human biological responses to social structures and processes. Some of them examine ways in which politics and globalization, which are involved in the production of economic inequality and uncertainty, impact nutritional state, health, and disease. To this end, there have been biocultural studies of human biological responses to uncertainty (Huss-Ashmore and Thomas, 1988), health outcomes associated with poverty and pollution (Schell, 1991), the political economy of physical growth (Bogin and Loucky, 1997), the social production of stress and cardiovascular disease (Dressler, 1995), and obesity (Ulijaszek and Lofink, 2006; Brewis, 2011). Other biocultural anthropologists examine social and cultural processes in shaping normative biology, such as breastfeeding (Stuart-Macadam and Dettwyler, 1995), mental and physical developmental plasticity (Li, 2003), reproductive ecology, and infant health (Wiley, 2004). The gap between biocultural anthropology and epidemiology is created by differences in theory and practice. Young (1994) proposed that culture should be systematically incorporated into epidemiological study. There are many operational and intellectual reasons that make this difficult (Dufour, 2006), but it is important, not least because for humans, that disease is never totally biological.

REFERENCES

Armelagos, G.J., Harper, K.N., 2005. Genomics at the origins of agriculture, part two. Evolutionaly Anthropology 14, 109–121.

Axelrod, R., 1997. The complexity of cooperation: Agent-based models of competition and collaboration. Princeton University Press, Princeton.

Bindon, J., 2007. Biocultural linkages—cultural consensus, cultural constructs, and human biological research. Collegium Anthropologicum 31, 3–10.

Bogin, B., Loucky, J., 1997. Plasticity, political economy, and physical growth status of Guatemala Maya children living in the United States. American Journal of Physical Anthropology 102, 17–32.

Brewis, A.A., 2011. Obesity. Cultural and Biocultural Perspectives. Rutgers University Press, New Brunswick.

Brumann, C., 1999. Why a successful concept should not be discarded. Current Anthropology (special issue) 40, S1–S14.

Coluzzi, M., 1999. Malaria genetics. The clay feet of the malaria giant and its African roots: hypotheses and inferences about origin, spread and control of *Plasmodium falciparum*. Parassitologia 41, 277–283.

Dressler, W.W., 1995. Modeling biocultural interactions: examples from studies of stress and cardiovascular disease. Yearbook of Physical Anthropology 38, 27–56.

Dufour, D.L., 2006. Biocultural approaches in human biology. American Journal of Human Biology: the official Journal of the Human Biology Council 18, 1–9.

Ellen, R., 1982. Environment subsistence and system. Cambridge University Press, Cambridge, UK.

Escalante, A.A., Cornejo, O.E., Freeland, D.E., Poe, A.C., Durrego, E., Collins, W.E., Lal, A.A., 2005. A monkey's tale: the origin of *plasmodium vivax* as a human malaria parasite. Proceedings of the National Academy of Sciences 102, 1980–1985.

Galvani, A.P., Novembre, J., 2005. The evolutionary history of the CCR5-Δ32 HIV-resistance mutation. Microbes and Infection 7, 302–309.

Gonzalez, E., Dhanda, R., Bamshad, M., Mummidi, S., Geevarghese, R., Catano, G., Anderson, S.A., Walter, E.A., Stephan, K.T., Hammer, M.F., Mangano, A., Sen, L., Clark, R.A., Ahuja, S.S., Dolan, M.J., Ahuja, S.K., 2001. Global survey of genetic variation in CCR5, Rantes, and MIP-1: impact on the epidemiology of the HIV-1 pandemic. Proceedings of the National Academy of Sciences 98, 5199–5204.

Goodman, A.H., Leatherman, T.L., 1998. Building a New Biocultural Synthesis. Political-Economic Perspectives on Human Biology. University of Michigan Press, Ann Arbor.

Greene, L.S., 1993. G6PD Deficiency as protection against Falciparum malaria: an epidemiologic critique of population and experimental studies. Yearbook of Physical Anthropology 36, 153–178.

Huss-Ashmore, R.A., Thomas, R.B., 1988. A framework for analyzing uncertainty in highland areas. In: de Garine, I., Harrison, G.A. (Eds.), Coping with Uncertainty in Food Supply, Clarendon Press, Oxford, pp. 452–468.

Katz, S.H., Schall, J., 1979. Fava bean consumption and biocultural evolution. Medical Anthropology 3, 459–476.

Kwiatkowski, D.P., 2005. How malaria has affected the human genome and what human genetics can teach us about malaria. American Journal of Human Genetics 77, 171–192.

Laland, K.N., Kendal, B., 2007. The niche construction perspective. Journal of Evolutionary Psychology 5, 51–66.

Lasker, G.W., 1969. Human biological adaptability. Science 166, 1480–1486.

Li, S.-C., 2003. The biocultural orchestration of developmental plasticity across levels: the interplay of biology and culture in shaping the mind and behavior across the life span. Psychological Bulletin 129, 171–194.

Liu, W., Li, Y., Learn, G.H., Rudicell, R.S., Robertson, J.D., Keele, B.F., Ndjango, J.-B.N., Sanz, C.M., et al., 2010. Origin of the human malaria parasite *Plasmodium falciparum* in gorillas. Nature 467, 420–425.

Livingstone, F.B., 1958. Anthropological implications of sickle cell gene distribution in West Africa. American Anthropology 60, 533–562.

Morphy, H., 1993. Cultural adaptation. In: Harrison, G.A. (Ed.), Human Adaptation, Oxford University Press, Oxford, pp. 99–150.

Odling-Smee, J., Laland, K.N., Feldman, M.W., 2003. Niche Construction: the Neglected Process in Evolution. Princeton University Press, Princeton.

Sabeti, P.C., Schaffner, S.F., Fry, B., Lohmueller, J., Varilly, P., Shamovsky, O., Palma, A., Mikkelsen, T.S., Altshuler, D., Lander, E.S., 2006. Positive natural selection in the human lineage. Science 312, 1614–1620.

Schell, L.M., 1991. Risk focusing: an example of biocultural interaction. In: Huss-Ashmore, R., Schall, J., Hediger, M. (Eds.), Health and Lifestyle Change, MASCA Research Papers in Science and Archaeology Number 9, Philadelphia, pp. 137–144.

Smith, M.T., 1993. Genetic adaptation. In: Harrison, G.A. (Ed.), Human Adaptation, Oxford University Press, Oxford, pp. 1–54.

Stuart-Macadam, P., Dettwyler, K.A., 1995. Breastfeeding: Biocultural Perspectives. Aldine de Gruyter, Chicago.

Suskind, R.M., Tontisirin, K., 2001. Nutrition, immunity and infection in infants and children. Lippincott Williams and Wilkins, Philadelphia.

Swallow, D.M., 2003. Genetics of lactase persistence and lactose intolerance. Annals Reviews Genetics 37, 197–219.

Thomas, R.B., 1997. Wondering to the age of adaptability: adjustments of and then people to change. In: Ulijaszek, S.J., Huss-Ashmore, R.A. (Eds.), Human Adaptability: Past, Present and Future, Oxford University Press, Oxford, pp. 183–232.

Tishkoff, S.A., Reed, F.A., Ranciaro, A., Voight, B.F., Babbit, C.C., et al., 2007. Convergent adaptation of human lactase persistence in Africa and Europe. Nature genetics 39, 31–40.

Ulijaszek, S.J., Huss-Ashmore, R.A. (Eds.), 1997. Human Adaptability: Past, Present and Future, Oxford University Press, Oxford.

Ulijaszek, S.J., Lofink, H., 2006. Obesity in biocultural perspective. Annual review anthropology 35, 337–360.

Ulijaszek, S.J., Mann, N., Elton, S., 2012. Evolving Human Diet. Its Implications for Public Health Nutrition. Cambridge University Press, Cambridge.

Wiley, A., 1992. Adaptation and the biocultural paradigm in medical anthropology: a critical review. Medical anthropology Quarterly 6, 216–236.

Wiley, A.S., 2004. An ecology of high-altitude infancy. Cambridge University Press, Cambridge.

Wiley, A., Allen, J.S., 2009. Medical anthropology. A biocultural approach. Oxford University Press, New York.

Young, T.K., 1994. The Health of Native Americans: Toward a Biocultural Epidemiology. Oxford University press, Oxford.

Young, I.S., Woodside, J.V., 2001. Antioxidants in health and disease. Journal of clinical pathology 54, 176–186.

Chapter 4

Toward Cultural Epidemiology: Beyond Epistemological Hegemony

Mark Brough

Queensland University of Technology, Brisbane, Australia

INTRODUCTION

It is more than 10 years since the anthropologist DiGiacomo (1999) answered the question "Can there be a cultural epidemiology?" with disappointment, concluding that ethnographic and epidemiological narratives are divergent not complementary. In the same year, the epidemiologist Krieger (1999, p. 1151) asked related questions about the epistemological foundations of epidemiology: "Epidemiology is—or is not—the basic science of public health. Epidemiology is—or is not—an objective science. Science and advocacy are—or are not—distinct and contrary endeavours." Again in the same year the Indigenous researcher in New Zealand, Tuhiwai Smith (1999, p. 1), wrote, "From the vantage point of the colonized, a position from which I write, and choose to privilege, the term 'research' is inextricably linked to European imperialism and colonialism." The act of conceptualizing and practicing cultural epidemiology thus brings with it a series of deep epistemological questions about the nature of knowledge production. The Western academy of health research assumes an intellectual and moral privilege to fill gaps in knowledge aimed at yielding improvements in health status. With such privilege comes responsibility, since the power to conceptualize health problems and their solutions deserves considerable critical, historical, and political reflexivity, particularly at the boundaries between dominant and oppressed cultural spaces.

In this chapter, some of the forces at work that produce epistemological hegemony in relation to the emerging field of cultural epidemiology are considered. This chapter also considers the ways in which this epistemological hegemony privileges certain forms of knowledge, drawing potentially on the same dynamics of power that underpin the privileging of one cultural space over another more broadly. Thus, cultural epidemiology sits squarely within the academic contradiction identified by Rigney (2001, p. 8) as both a site for

When Culture Impacts Health. http://dx.doi.org/10.1016/B978-0-12-415921-1.00004-X

raising consciousness about oppression (and the health inequalities stemming from that oppression) and a site for the continued production of that oppression. The latter possibility remains an "inconvenient truth" of health science research. Without epistemological self-awareness, the act of investigating and intervening in the health of cultural "others" is in danger of being not just insensitive or using research tools that may be culturally invalid but unreflexively part of the social apparatus of cultural and political domination. Drawing on observations of the epidemiology of Aboriginal and Torres Strait Islander health as well as the epidemiology of asylum seeker and refugee health within the Australian context, the implications of this hegemony for the politics of knowledge are also explored.

EPISTEMOLOGICAL HEGEMONY

Epistemology is essentially concerned with the philosophy of knowledge, provoking us to ask: What is knowledge and how should it be produced? Within the field of public health, much rides on how this question is answered. At an epistemological level, this is a question about the frameworks we use to think about knowledge. Epistemological self-awareness, like cultural self-awareness, is not always easy to find in a health system created by and for a dominant cultural group. As Lincoln and Guba (1985, pp. 8–9) remind us: "We are so imbued with the tenets of science that we take its assumptions utterly for granted, so much so that we almost cannot comprehend the possibility that there may be other ways of thinking." It is not surprising then, that many critical observers of health research have noted the dominance of a singular, universalist logic of practice (e.g., Saunders et al., 2010). Drawing on the Gramscian notion of hegemony, which focuses our attention on the ideological domination achieved through the institutions of civil society (Bocock, 1986), I am concerned here with the power of dominant ideas. Bocock (1986, p. 37) summarized the hegemonic project as involving the development of intellectual, moral, and philosophical consent. Raymond Williams (1977, p. 109) defined hegemony in relation to "dominant meanings and values." Epistemological hegemony represents a concern for the domination of one view of knowledge and the subordination of all other forms. Hegemony is never complete, however, and as the three quotes at the beginning of this chapter suggest, there are multiple sites of contestation. Such acts of reflexivity ought to form part of the intellectual accountability of cultural epidemiology, as important as the explication and defense of specific methods. The project of constructing a vibrant cultural epidemiology capable of meaningfully informing collaborative, culturally safe partnerships with communities is thus laden with the need for critical epistemological reflexivity.

Cultural epidemiology contains two broad areas of epistemological challenge. First, there is the challenge of attempting to understand and act on health improvement across different cultural spaces. Second, there is a more deeply reflexive epistemological challenge concerned with making visible the cultural workings of dominant forms of knowledge production. By definition, cultural epidemiology is such a producer of knowledge. Asking how such knowledge is (or should be) produced involves much more than an account of the technicalities of method. Rather there is also *discipline* in critical reflection about the underpinnings of the act of legitimating knowledge. This act will always be contested, since by definition if some knowledge is legitimated, inevitably some knowledge will be de-legitimated. De-legitimating the knowledge of cultural "others" is one of the foundation stones of cultural domination; hence the stakes are particularly high in cultural epidemiology.

The Sources of Epistemological Hegemony

Cultural epidemiology represents a set of research practices that acknowledges the culturally diverse ways in which communities of people think about and manage health. These research practices are culture bound; hence, epidemiology is as legitimate a site for cultural reflection as any study of "ethnomedicine" (Brough, 2001; Trostle, 2005, p. 7). The whiteness of the academy generally and of health research in particular has been a trigger for much "talking back," "writing back," and "researching back" within the postcolonial and anti-colonial literature (Smith, 1999, p. 7). The intellectual agency of colonized peoples to make the whiteness of the academy visible and the consequent subject of critical cultural scrutiny have provided a powerful catalyst for examining the neo-colonial dynamics of the contemporary academy (Denzin et al., 2008). At the core of this neo-colonial dynamic lies the western Hegelian premise, which assumes an accessibility and knowability; thus within the western academy the "not known" is predominantly framed as the "still-to-be-known," an epistemological notion that strongly underscored historical forces of discovery, exploration, and colonization (Jones and Jenkins, 2008, p. 481).

Next I consider the drivers of epistemological hegemony as I observe them. I do not expect that these are definitive. I suggest them merely as a contribution to a shared responsibility for contesting the privileging of a singular logic of knowledge and consequent practice in the health of culturally diverse peoples.

DRIVERS OF EPISTEMOLOGICAL HEGEMONY

Positivism

The dominance of positivist epistemology draws on a view of the universe as "'endowed with an essential reality prior to and autonomous from the meanings human subjectivity may project upon it" (DiGiacomo, 1999, p. 439). Moreover, positivist epistemology applies itself in the logic of research via reductionism; hence, the emphasis is on the relationships between the parts (variables), and for statements about these relationships (most importantly cause–effect) to demonstrate rigor they must be verifiable or falsifiable (Howe, 2009, p. 428). This epistemological cornerstone and all that flows from it dominates health research

(Buchanan, 1998, p. 439). While there has been a proliferation of methods in public health research including various takes on both qualitative and quantitative methods, it remains questionable whether such growing diversity of method is paralleled by recognition of diverse epistemologies. Instead, it seems to have become an accepted wisdom that all "useful" knowledge in public health is about the causal chain. Consider, for example, the attempt by Brownson (1999) (cited in Rychetnik et al., 2004, p. 538) to conceptualize the range of evidence that contributes to public health as either:

1. Research that describes risk–disease relations
2. Evidence that identifies the effectiveness of interventions aimed at addressing the risk problem

There is no facilitation of critical epistemological reflection here because the boundaries of knowledge have been locked in as givens. It is not that identifying risk–disease relations, or finding ways to effectively intervene in those relations, is not valuable. The concern here is that it is not the only way to imagine or respond to health. Outside of this assumed universalism there are other conceptualizations which, for example, understand health inequality and disease as a form of violence in which the social hierarchy becomes written on the body (Nguyen and Peschard, 2003, p. 447). There are alternative views of health practice that emphasize values and relationships rather than causal chains and intervention (McCarthy and Rose, 2010). There are frameworks for research that reflexively acknowledge the potential ethical tensions involved within "close the gap" strategies of health improvement (Altman, 2009). There are non-pathologizing forms of community-based public health practice that emphasize strengths rather than deficits (Brough et al., 2004). There are approaches to research concerned with contextual understanding rather than explanation of linear causation (Chapman and Berggren, 2005). There are Indigenous methodological frameworks that reject the colonizing assumptions of positivism (Denzin et al., 2008). The multiplicity of understanding and practice alluded to here is invisible within the intellectual poverty produced by the "one size fits all" hegemony of positivism.

Counting Culture

With its explicit identification of "culture," *cultural* epidemiology necessarily raises issues of reflexivity in connection with the "measurement" of culture. This is perhaps the most "obvious" area for epistemological reflexivity for a *cultural* epidemiology. Consider then a recent report concerned with Indigenous health released by the Australian Bureau of Statistics titled The City and the Bush: Indigenous Wellbeing Across Remoteness Areas (2010), which attempted to measure the level of cultural attachment via indicators of speaking an Indigenous language at home; participation in cultural events in the last 12 months; and identification with clan, tribal, or language group. I will not repeat the many criticisms that have been made of the stereotypical construction of "authentic" Aboriginality as it has been imagined in the public health discourses surrounding the health of Aboriginal and Torres Strait Islander people in Australia (e.g., see Bond, 2005). Suffice it to say that implied within such culture counting is often an unsophisticated view of culture premised on a concern for determining how "cultural" one individual or community is compared with another. The positivist assumptions are clear given the level of reductionism required to sustain such an enterprise.

The continued capacity of an unreflexive white academy to make determinations of authentic versus nonauthentic cultural spaces in regards to Aboriginal and Torres Strait Islander people tells us more about the white cultural underpinnings of colonization than it does about the "cultural others" it purports to "know." In terms of migrant and refugee health the parallel strand of research has been a concern to measure the level of "acculturation" again on a presumed linear pathway between "ethnic" culture and "mainstream" culture. In Hunt et al.'s (2004) critical review of this area of research as it has played out in regard to the United States Hispanic community, there was found to be little attempt by most researchers to conceptualize the culture concept despite its supposed centrality to the research. Most revealing was the "strangely absent" definition of "mainstream" (Hunt et al., 2004, p. 977) and the required assumption of a homogenous "invented majority" (Ponce and Comer, 2003, p. 4; quoted in Hunt et al., 2004, p. 977). While the Australian historical context of a white invasion of Aboriginal land later followed by a long period of a white Australia policy governing immigration, as well as a contemporary moral and political panic concerning the "influx" of asylum seekers, tells us something about the "invented majority" of Australia—it is unlikely that the study of acculturation ever had these markers of "whiteness" in mind.

This is not the place to engage with the long-standing and complex debates related to defining the culture concept. It is, however, at least pertinent to acknowledge the fundamental epistemological differences between a common public health assumption of culture as "an ensemble of measurable 'factors' with deterministic power over specific aspects of illness" (DiGiacomo, 1999, p. 443) versus, for example, Geertz's (1973, p. 5) notion of culture as "webs of significance" and the consequent analysis of those webs requiring "not an experimental science in search of law but an interpretative one in search of meaning." Slicing culture into components for measurement also holds a powerful synergy with the neo-liberal temptation to then begin to confuse culture with lifestyle as DiGiacomo implies above. Thus as Rock (2003, p. 156) has also forcefully argued "lifestyle" in health research has become conceptually no more than "an assemblage of bodily practices amenable to quantification."

Evidence-Based Practice

The central contemporary logic of the nexus between research, policy, and practice is no doubt the tantalizing specter of "evidence-based practice" (EBP). EBP applies its logic to an ever-expanding set of possibilities for improvements in evidence. Positivist research is the prime source of this evidence. The EBP mantra is particularly apparent within public health research where it has provided not only an intellectual logic for knowledge translation into practice but also a moral privilege to do so. Traynor's (2000) analysis of the discourse of evidence-based medicine, the forerunner to EBP, demonstrates a rhetorical strategy that parallels styles of evangelical religious argument. Both forms of discourse discredit those who do not join the cause, and both assume the hegemonic position of "norm" against which the inferiority of the "other" is normalized (2000, p. 142).

Thomas et al. (2010, p. 15) have identified an increasing recognition of values-based health care in the last decade and see it in part as a response to an over-reliance on EBP. Values-based care is based on a blending of the values of the service user and the health and social care professional and is an equally valid premise from which to think about professional practice in health. However, tension between EBP and values-based practice (see McCarthy and Rose, 2010, for vignettes of a variety of practice tensions in this area) remains a somewhat ambiguous area of scholarship, since EBP as the dominant narrative in health research assumes it is the only "logic in town." Thus as Van de Luitgaarden (2009) points out there is little guidance to the practitioner whose experience suggests a course of action in contravention of "best evidence."

For the many practitioners who are members of their client communities (a relatively common occurrence in many areas of "transcultural" health practice), and for whom either by lack of available evidence, inability to enact "interventions" because of lack of resources, or most important through choice to privilege other forms of knowledge such as lived experience within a particular cultural context, EBP remains a problematic foundation on which to build a universal premise for best practice. In short, the privileging of certain kinds of knowledge assumes an epistemological advantage that may not be present (Fox, 2003, p. 86).

The Questions We Ask

In a recent review of cancer epidemiology among Indigenous people in Australia, New Zealand, Canada, and the United States, Shahid and Thompson (2009, p. 110) were able to identify 119 papers, yet only 6 papers were concerned with Indigenous beliefs about the disease. So while we know a lot about the risk factors for various forms of cancer, we know little of the Indigenous experience. Research questions tend to be predominantly "investigator driven" rather than driven by the communities they seek to understand and are an important area for reflexivity (Street et al., 2007). Research questions can thus reflect the political hegemony.

Indeed the shift in the 1980s to questions of health inequality between Indigenous and non-Indigenous Australians was initially actively discredited at both a political and methodological level (Brough, 2001). Equally in the 2000s political attempts to discredit research findings regarding the health status of refugee communities (Steel et al., 2004) remind us that research questions about the health of vulnerable communities remain deeply political. Such a reflection might provoke us to juxtapose key epidemiological questions regarding the health of immigrant, refugee, and Indigenous Australians and reflect on the political inconveniences attached to the framing of those questions. For example, it is very commonplace in refugee health studies to be concerned with the impacts of past traumas (Miller et al., 2006). This focus is not surprising given the common experience of torture and trauma among this group. However, this focus also contains a synergy with dominant host country political narratives where the "host" country becomes positioned as "savior." The dominance of trauma-based epidemiology reinforces this position, lessening questions of the present and obscuring the importance of a growing understanding that *post*-migration living difficulties are also important to understanding the well-being of refugee communities. On the other hand, asking questions of the past in Aboriginal health reveals different politics in which it is acknowledgement of the past that is inconvenient, while focus on the present sits more comfortably with the neo-liberal/neo-colonial concern for ahistorical individual behavior and the capacity to construct an agenda of blame removed from systemic structures of inequality. Here the political narrative works more conveniently if the past is avoided and the focus is on the present. Hence, while an understanding of past human rights violations is an accepted part of understanding refugee health, it has taken a remarkably long time to introduce this lens into the production of knowledge about Indigenous health. Some potentially important lines of research have recently opened up in this area including, for example, smoking research indicating the impact of being a member of the stolen generations potentially has on tobacco use (Thomas et al., 2008). This sort of historical acknowledgement begins to shift attention away from a set of neo-liberal questions about lifestyle, which have emphasized the agency of individuals as the source of their own health problems.

CONCLUSION

Returning to the three moments of reflexivity described briefly at the beginning of this chapter, it is appropriate to consider how such moments problematize but also potentially invigorate cultural epidemiology. DiGiacomo's (1999) paper was in part inspired by her experience as an anthropologist working in an epidemiology department, in which she faced constant resistance to any attempt to acknowledge culture rather than measure cultural "factors." At the heart of this resistance was a variety of epistemological differences. Krieger (1999, p. 1152) as the epidemiologist answered her questions emphatically that epidemiology is just *one* (not *the*) basic science in public health, that it is both objective *and* partisan, and that science and advocacy "mutually require critical assessment of competing theoretical and ideological explanatory frameworks and of the evidence they generate." Finally, Smith (1999, p. 8) as the Indigenous researcher reminds us that research has been an encounter between "the West and the Other" and that such encounters contain codes and rules that speak to the management of the colonial encounter. Thus while important debates need to play out between and within the disciplinary epistemologies informing cultural epidemiology, a larger debate needs to play out in relation to *both* qualitative and quantitative methodologies, *both* of which have been used in the name of colonization (Denzin and Lincoln, 2008, p. 4). Denzin and Lincoln (2008, p. 12) thus advocated for change within the academy along the following lines:

A decolonized academy is interdisciplinary and politically proactive. It respects indigenous epistemologies and encourages interpretive, first-person methodologies. It honors different versions of science and empirical activity, as well as values cultural criticism in the name of social justice. It seeks models of human subject research that are not constrained by biomedical, positivist assumptions.

There is no neat solution to the epistemological challenges outlined here. They are challenges of history and of social, economic, political, and cultural position. They are challenges of the contradiction of being both concerned with addressing health inequality but are also aware that even "well-meaning" pursuits of health research bring responsibilities of reflexivity. This is not then an argument about either conspiracy or a naive counter-hegemonic argument that "nothing is possible." Cultural epidemiology as an applied health science is important because it *can* address issues of social justice in health. Its ability to do so will rest though as much on what it can learn about itself as anything it might learn about any sociocultural *other*.

REFERENCES

Altman, J., 2009. Beyond Closing the Gap: Valuing Diversity in Indigenous Australia Centre for Aboriginal Economic Policy Research. Australian National University.

Australian Bureau of Statistics, 2010. The city and the bush: Indigenous wellbeing across remoteness areas. Australian Social Trends 4102.0 Canberra: ABS.

Bocock, R., 1986. Hegemony. Tavistock, London.

Bond, C., 2005. A culture of ill health: public health or Aboriginality. Medical Journal of Australia 183 (1), 39–41.

Brough, M., 2001. Healthy imaginations: a social history of the epidemiology of aboriginal and torres strait islander health. Medical Anthropology 20, 65–90.

Brough, M., Bond, C., Hunt, J., 2004. Strong in the city: towards a strength-based approach in indigenous health promotion. Health Promotion Journal of Australia 15 (3), 215–220.

Brownson, R., Gurney, J., Land, G., 1999. Evidence-based decision making in public health. Journal of Public Health Management Practice 5, 86–97.

Buchanan, D., 1998. Beyond positivism: humanistic perspectives on theory and research in health education. Health Education Research 13 (3) 439–450.

Chapman, R., Berggren, J., 2005. Radical Contextualization: contributions to an anthropology of racial/ethnic health disparities health. An Interdisciplinary Journal for the Social Study of Health, Illness and Medicine 9 (2), 145–167.

Denzin, N., Lincoln, Y., Smith, L. (Eds.), 2008. Handbook of Critical and Indigenous Methodologies, Sage, Los Angeles.

Denzin, N., Lincoln, Y., 2008. Introduction: Critical Methodologies and Indigenous Inquiry. pp. 1–20 In: Denzin, N., Lincoln, Y., Tuhiwai-Smith, L. (Eds.), Handbook of Critical and Indigenous Methodologies, Sage, Los Angeles.

DiGiacomo, S., 1999. Can there be a "Cultural Epidemiology"? Medical Anthropology Quarterly 13 (4), 436–457.

Fox, N., 2003. Practice-based evidence: towards collaborative and transgressive research. Sociology 37 (1), 81–102.

Geertz, C., 1973. The Interpretation of Cultures: Selected Essays. Basic Books, New York.

Howe, K., 2009. Epistemology. Methodology, and education sciences: positivist dogmas, rhetoric, and the education science question. Educational Researcher 38 (6), 428–440.

Hunt, L., Schneider, S., Comer, B., 2004. Should "acculturation" be a variable in health research? A critical review of research on US Hispanics. Social Science & Medicine 59, 973–986.

Jones, A., Jenkins, K., 2008. Rethinking Collaboration: Working the Indigine-Colonizer Hyphen. In: Denzin, N., Lincoln, Y., Tuhiwai-Smith, L. (Eds.), Handbook of Critical and Indigenous Methodologies, Sage, Los Angeles, pp. 471–485.

Krieger, N., 1999. Questioning epidemiology: objectivity, advocacy, and socially responsible science. American Journal of Public Health 89 (8), 1151–1153.

Lincoln, Y., Guba, E., 1985. Naturalistic Inquiry, Sage, Beverley Hills.

McCarthy, J., Rose, P. (Eds.), 2010. Values-Based Health and Social Care: Beyond Evidence-Based Practice, Sage, London.

Miller, K., Kulkarni, M., Kushner, H., 2006. Beyond trauma-focused psychiatric epidemiology: bridging research and practice with war-affected populations. American Journal of Orthopsychiatry 76 (4), 409–422.

Nguyen, V.-K., Peschard, K., 2003. Anthropology, inequality, and disease: a review. Annual Review of Anthropology 32, 447–474.

Ponce, C., Comer, B., 2003. Is acculturation in Hispanic health research a flawed concept? JSRI Working Paper 60, .

Rigney, L., 2001. A first perspective of Indigenous Australian participation in science: framing indigenous research towards indigenous Australian intellectual sovereignty. Kaurna Higher Education Journal 7, 1–13.

Rock, M., 2003. Sweet blood and social suffering: rethinking cause-effect relationships in diabetes, distress, and duress. Medical Anthropology 22 (2), 131–174.

Rychetnik, L., Hawe, P., Waters, E., Baratt, A., Frommer, M., 2004. A glossary for evidence based public health. Journal of Epidemiology and Community Health 58, 538–545.

Saunders, V., West, R., Usher, K., 2010. Applying indigenist research methodologies in health research: experiences in the borderlands. Australian Journal of Indigenous Education 39S, 1–7.

Shahid, S., Thompson, S., 2009. An overview of cancer and beliefs about the disease in indigenous people of Australia, Canada, New Zealand and the US. Australian and New Zealand Journal of Public Health 33 (2), 109–117.

Smith, L., 1999. Decolonizing Methodologies: Research and Indigenous Peoples. Zed Books, London.

Steel, Z., Momartin, S., Bateman, C., Hafshejani, A., Silove, D., Everson, N., Roy, K., Dudley, M., Newman, L., Blick, B., Mares, S., 2004. Psychiatric status of asylum seeker families held for a protracted period in a remote detention centre in Australia. Australian and New Zealand Journal of Public Health 28 (6), 527–536.

Street, J., Baum, F., Anderson, I., 2007. Developing a collaborative research system for aboriginal health. Australian and New Zealand Journal of Public Health 31 (4), 372–378.

Thomas, D., Briggs, V., Anderson, I., Cunningham, J., 2008. The social determinants of being an indigenous non-smoker. Australian and New Zealand Journal of Public Health 32 (2), 110–116.

Thomas, M., Burt, M., Parkes, J., 2010. The Emergence of Evidence-Based Practice, pp. 3–24. In: McCarthy, J., Rose, P. (Eds.), Values-Based Health and Social Care: Beyond Evidence-Based Practice, Sage, London.

Traynor, M., 2000. Purity, conversion and evidence based movements. Health 4, 139–158.

Trostle, J., 2005. Epidemiology and Culture. Cambridge: University Press, Cambridge.

Van de Luitgaarden, G., 2009. Evidence-based practice in social work: lessons from judgement and decision-making theory. British Journal of Social Work 39, 243–260.

Williams, R., 1977. Marxism and Literature. Oxford University Press, Oxford.

Chapter 5

The Cultural Anthropological Contribution to Communicable Disease Epidemiology

Stephen P. Luby

*Director, Centre for Communicable Diseases, International Centre for Diarrheal Disease
Research, Bangladesh (ICDDR,B), Dhaka, Bangladesh and Director of Research, Centre for
Innovation and Global Health, Stanford University, USA*

INTRODUCTION

A number of anthropologists have articulated benefits and barriers to
collaboration between epidemiology and anthropology (Inhorn, 1995; Trostle,
2005). The objective of this chapter is to contribute to the smaller literature from
epidemiologists on these issues (Porter, 2006; Behague et al., 2008) and explain
how cultural anthropology has helped this communicable disease epidemiologist
lead a multidisciplinary research group in Bangladesh.

CRITIQUE OF THE BIOMEDICAL PARADIGM

Cultural anthropology articulates the underlying conflict between the
biomedical paradigm invoked by communicable disease epidemiology and the
cultural understanding of target communities. The biomedical paradigm asserts
that our physical environment is filled with invisibly small living organisms,
and that some of these invisible organisms are dangerous and can move from
an infected animal or person sometimes through air, food, water, or personal
contact to reach another person where they can produce serious disease. Public
health professionals use the methods of communicable disease epidemiology to
identify exposures that increase the risk of disease, and then develop interventions aimed at reducing these exposures, preventing illness, and producing a
healthier community.

Most Bangladeshi mothers' perspective on health is quite different, viewing
supernatural forces as the primary cause of unexpected serious illness and death
(Blum et al., 2009). A child contracts a serious disease and dies because of

When Culture Impacts Health. http://dx.doi.org/10.1016/B978-0-12-415921-1.00005-1

43

exposure to an evil spirit or the evil eye of a neighbor. Moreover, the time of death is preordained by Allah, and no human action can change this (Blum et al., 2009). The epidemiologist's causal assessment of death and the use of this knowledge to prevent future mortality in Bangladesh are fundamentally countercultural.

Anthropology assists epidemiology by providing ideas and language to understand these differing perspectives. Anthropological investigation clarifies that while explanations for serious disease by Bangladeshi villagers often invoke supernatural causes, a supernatural paradigm is not universally applied. Villagers often experience some benefits from biomedicine. They take a commercially packaged biomedicine, ibuprofen, and have their knee pain reduced sufficiently so that they are able to work. People hold a diversity of conceptual models to understand and interpret their world (Joel et al., 2003), conceptual models that if fully articulated and analyzed in a western academy may be judged contradictory (Choi and Nisbett, 2000), but absence of contradiction is more highly valued in biomedicine than in most cultures. This mix of indigenous cultural understanding with biomedical understanding is particularly striking among scientifically educated Bangladeshi professionals. They were born into a culture where the truth of an assertion is assessed by appeals to authority, either a senior expert or an authoritative text, yet in their professional lives truth is less fixed; appeals to truth are resolved by evaluating objectively verifiable data. Public health interventions often urge indigenous communities to replace their local conceptualization of disease with a biomedical conceptualization. When a child has a serious respiratory infection, public health authorities urge mothers to have their child evaluated by an allopathic health care provider who can assess whether the child has pneumonia and needs antibiotics. Among most Bangladeshi villagers respiratory infections are believed to arise from too much exposure to cold and are best treated with a massage of garlic and mustard oil (Rashid et al., 2001). Biomedically trained scientists are often the strongest advocates for this conversion in explanatory models, to urge their fellow citizens to follow the cognitive pathway of their own intellectual journey.

Cultural anthropology urges caution in preaching the biomedical paradigm to target communities. Indeed, many anthropologists question the very project of applied epidemiology and institutional public health. An epidemiologist investigates a typical low-income community and sees problems, such as malnutrition, disability, and premature mortality. In the anthropological critique, epidemiology problematizes community life (Gaines, 2011). Anthropology reminds us that humans have lived in food-scarce high-mortality communities for most of our history (Coale, 1974; Davis, 1986). For over a thousand generations our ancestors raised their children, worked to secure food and shelter, shared hardships and joys, and lived lives filled with meaning—lives that less threatened the global ecosystem compared with the current population explosion fueled by the industrial and technological revolutions and spread of global capitalism. When a communicable disease epidemiologist enters a Bangladeshi village and sees children, chickens, and ducks sharing the same courtyard he sees a risk of new deadly strains of influenza being transmitted from poultry to children. The children's mother, on the other hand, sees raising poultry as a practice that has been passed on for centuries, a cornerstone of household welfare and nutrition.

Should epidemiologists so respect existing cultural practices that they accept high child mortality and periodic famine? If epidemiology and institutional public health rejects this critique, what is the role of anthropology within public health? Does anthropology so compromise its commitment to cultural relativism that it cannot both critique and be a part of public health (Scheper-Hughes, 1990)? Within my experience the anthropological perspective encourages a constructive conversation within the public health scientific team. Anthropologists, unique among all of the disciplines working within public health, are keenly aware of alternative cultural constructs, and so are uniquely placed to identify the conflicts between the biomedical public health perspective and a local perspective. At each stage of the scientific process identifying which issues merit scientific attention, the development of concept notes, funding proposals, and scientific protocols as well as the analysis and interpretation of data, anthropologists provide an essential perspective.

Epidemiologists often assume an underlying model that the community is ignorant of certain vital information, and that if we identify this lack of knowledge and develop an educational intervention to improve knowledge, then community practices and health will improve. Epidemiologists often initiate this approach by assessing community knowledge of a particular issue. Epidemiologists within my group exploring the knowledge of communities regarding the H1N1 influenza pandemic reported, "only 21% of respondents had heard of the term swine flu." Anthropology provides a critique of such studies that compare local residents' ideas to a biomedical construct. When pressed, the epidemiology team explained that there was no Bengali translation for the English term "swine flu." Therefore, they asked the question using the English phrase. So an anthropological interpretation is that 21% of the population recognized a term from a foreign language. Not surprisingly, those with the most education and the most media access were more likely to recognize this foreign term. While an epidemiologist might conclude that the community lacks important knowledge, an anthropological critique is that this episode is an example of how people from different cultures often talk past each other. The epidemiological report went on to note, "Of those respondents who had heard of the word 'pandemic' in 2010, none correctly reported the year in which the last influenza pandemic occurred (2009–2010)." Anthropology helps to avoid such meaningless assessment of villagers' understanding cast in terms of an unexamined hegemonic biomedical construct. In this case the anthropological critique resulted in a decision not to submit the epidemiological findings for scientific presentation and publication. More broadly this type of anthropological critique has led our group to avoid pursuing some projects of interest to biomedicine when we have judged that communities would neither be interested nor assisted.

FRAMING PUBLIC HEALTH ISSUES COMPREHENSIVELY

Epidemiology describes patterns of disease in a community. A primary tool of a quantitative epidemiologist is the structured interview. Their classical questions posed to study participants probe who, where, when, and how. An interviewer asks a question, and the respondent replies with one of several pre-coded responses. For such questionnaires to generate useful information, the person being interviewed has to share a common understanding of the meaning of the question with the epidemiologist who wrote the question. Each closed-ended question is an exercise in cross-cultural communication. Simply down-loading questions from a Web site and translating them into the local language risks substantial miscommunication. For example, to frame meaningful questions on exposure to poultry that might be associated with avian influenza, epidemiologists need to understand the context of how poultry is raised, sold, and slaughtered. In our experience anthropologists, using an in-depth discussion guide developed with input from the many scientists who constitute the study team and administered either to key informants or in group discussions and complemented by informal observations, can efficiently explore exposures of interest and gather rich information both on village context and the local categories that residents use to understand and describe their experience.

So, on a practical level, anthropologists help epidemiologists construct questions that are meaningful to respondents, and help understand who is exposed to poultry, and where, when, and how this exposure occurs. In addition anthropologists characteristically ask study participants "why." Why do you raise poultry? Why do you keep the poultry under the bed at night? Why do you raise chickens and ducks together? The anthropological method actively seeks to understand issues from the study subject's perspective, to generate subjective knowledge. Using open-ended in-depth questions they generate narrative that broadens the epidemiological understanding of what occurs in the community to a nuanced understanding of why it occurs. Such understanding is often cru-cial for developing interventions that are sufficiently relevant to the community to reduce disease risk.

Anthropology and epidemiology frame public health situations differently. Applied communicable disease epidemiology favors linear causal models and employs a sophisticated portfolio of tools to identify proximate causes of dis-ease (McMichael, 1999). When epidemiologists review questionnaires we ask ourselves: Will these questions help explicate our causal model? Will we iden-tify the transmission pathways or the opportunities to interrupt these transmis-sion pathways appropriately through these questions? When communicable disease epidemiologists in our group recently considered maternal mortality in Bangladesh, we focused on those deaths that were associated with jaundice and assessed what proportion resulted from infection with hepatitis E virus (Gurley et al., 2012). Epidemiological investigations of outbreaks of hepatitis E virus conclude that outbreaks are usually associated with sewage contamination of drinking water supplies (Emerson and Purcell, 2004). Reviewing population-based descriptions of maternal deaths in Bangladesh identified a substantial proportion consistent with hepatitis E virus infection. So from a biomedical epidemiological perspective pregnant women who are infected with hepatitis E virus are predisposed to a catastrophic immune response to the virus that progresses to acute liver failure and death. Epidemiology provides the important insight that hepatitis E infection is responsible for substantial maternal mortality. This suggests that either reducing the exposure to or improving maternal immunity against hepatitis E virus could reduce the risk of maternal death. Epidemiologists, then, are interested in exploring the potential for contaminated drinking water exposure at home, at work, when visiting family, when water is used in their food, and when the primary water source is unavailable.

Anthropology strives to frame public health issues comprehensively. Anthropology favors broad models of disease ecology that consider the limits to individual human agency and account for economic forces, social hierarchies, and power structure (Finerman, 1995). When presented with epidemiological findings of increased risk of illness from drinking contaminated water anthropology will naturally ask: What is the community's attitude about their water? How important are concerns with water quality compared with other concerns in this community? Why is the water contaminated? Why does water run intermittently in affected communities? Why is the water not routinely chlorinated by municipal authorities? Who has the capacity to change this? What is their perspective? What social and political forces prevent change? Practicing epidemiologists may raise similar questions as they strive to translate the insights of their studies into public health action, but anthropology adds disciplinary approaches and tools to articulate a broader causal model. Focusing primarily on the proximate cause, epidemiologists might urge a behavior change program to encourage pregnant women to treat their drinking water at home with chlorine bleach to deactivate the hepatitis E virus. A more comprehensive assessment may direct attention to current political and social forces that contribute to thousands of low-income communities throughout Bangladesh having access only to sewage-contaminated drinking water and developing broader interventions to address it.

The epidemiological approach has been famously characterized as a prisoner of the proximate (McMichael, 1999); it efficiently identifies proximate causes along the biomedical pathway, but risks ignoring the broader social context of disease. The anthropological approach can be caricatured as years of observation identifying deeply entrenched social forces wedded to a power structure that has little interest in improving community welfare. The disciplines are productive collaborators because anthropology encourages epidemiologists to frame their understanding of the problem and potential interventions with a broader appreciation of local choice; local constraints; and cultural, social, and political factors. Epidemiology, in turn, encourages anthropologists who are interested in public health and who have a broad array of concerns regarding power structure and justice in communities to focus efforts in a particular area that can substantively reduce community disease burden.

COMMUNICATES THE VOICE OF THE COMMUNITY

When public health professionals work to improve the health of communities, there is a risk that their aspirations and values will conflict with the aspiration and values of the community. Expatriate public health professionals often assume that national public health professionals can provide the local community's perspective, but professionals arise from a different social class than the typical target community. Indeed, the cultural difference that separates educated Bangladeshi scientists from low-income community residents is often larger than the cultural difference between expatriate and Bangladeshi scientists. Bangladeshi professionals who succeed as physicians and scientists master the essential elements of the biomedical paradigm, and come to accept its worldview, but the more that they think, live, and socialize within this world, the more estranged they become from the worldview of villagers.

Anthropologists are the one group of scientists well placed to communicate the voice of the community to the public health team. They can use their discipline's techniques to build rapport with and come to understand the community perspective, and then, they can serve as a cultural conduit between the community and the biomedically trained scientific team. They provide the voice of the community in a way that biomedical scientists can understand. During a Nipah virus outbreak in the Faridpur District, Bangladesh, an anthropologist quoted the husband of a woman who died:

The doctor said that this illness could go to others if anyone comes in close contact with patients, touches the patient or the vomit of patients . . . But I have no faith in it. I think it is a curse from Allah as he is angry with people's sins . . . If the illness is contagious then I must get the disease. As I did not, it cannot be contagious."

Blum et al., 2009

This direct quotation elegantly contrasts the biomedical conceptualization of this outbreak shared by public health professionals with the local understanding of the outbreak among those whom it affects. This voice from the community reminds public health professionals that our conceptualization is not accepted by the affected community, and suggests that prevention messages based solely on this contentious conceptualization are unlikely to be persuasive.

Anthropology is attuned to differences in social power between groups and how these differences affect communication. Anthropologists are skilled at analyzing underlying communication strategies, for example, when the words of a government official assert the speaker's authority instead of substantively addressing the community's problem. At a local scientific conference one of our young female anthropologists presented comments from a community affected by an anthrax outbreak. Several villagers reported that when one of their cattle appeared moribund, a local veterinarian recommended that the animal be slaughtered and the meat sold so that the owner could recoup at least part of their investment. Senior male professional veterinarians interrupted the speaker during her formal presentation and insisted that these results were impossible, that no veterinarian would ever make such a recommendation. The anthropologist explained that she was quoting the villagers. She noted that it was quite possible that villagers might confuse qualified veterinarians from unqualified practitioners who provide veterinary advice, but that people in this community turned to the local experts, and this is what they reported hearing. By providing a clear voice from the community anthropology challenges authoritarian conceptualizations of an event and its cause. They articulate the range of experiences and perspectives among a heterogeneous population including those with less social power and visibility.

The standard presentation of epidemiological findings is a number-filled table that describes the population's characteristics. In a study to estimate the burden of Japanese encephalitis in Bangladesh, the epidemiological analysis concluded with a table of rates, "The estimated JE [*Japanese encephalitis*] incidence was 2.7/100,000 population in Rajshahi" (Paul et al., 2011). In contrast, the archetypal presentation of the anthropologist is a direct (translated) quotation from a person within the community, that is, literally a voice from the community. An anthropological assessment of the burden of Japanese encephalitis quoted a father of a four-year-old boy:

We borrowed forty thousand Taka (US$ 578) from a local NGO for the treatment of my son. The monthly interest rate was 100 Taka per 1000 (US$ 1.44). We could not pay this rate that accumulated up to 70,000 (US$ 1012). We will have to forfeit our house and land to repay the loan. Besides we have to spend at least 2 to 3 thousand Taka for his treatment per month, but he is not getting cured. We live from hand to mouth. We get scared if any other family member gets sick. Every single Taka is burdensome for us and we now cannot even eat three meals a day."

Nadia Ishrat Alamgir, personal communication.

The epidemiological summary provides key data on the number of people involved and on how large the problem is, which helps to provide a rational basis to plan prevention activities. The anthropological perspectives remind public health professionals and policy makers of the human cost of this illness.

ASSISTS IN DEVELOPING AND EVALUATING INTERVENTIONS

Epidemiologists are skilled at characterizing public health problem within communities. Epidemiology offers fewer tools for translating this understanding into interventions that produce healthier communities. Indeed, although evaluating interventions is part of epidemiology, developing interventions is outside of its disciplinary boundaries. However as experts on the public health problem, epidemiologists are routinely asked how to translate these findings into strategies for prevention. Indeed, a central justification for my group's engagement with low-income communities in Bangladesh is the prospect of developing feasible prevention strategies. While there are topic experts on specific types of interventions within public health, for example, experts on behavior change, there is less critical capacity within any single discipline to ask whether behavior change is the most appropriate intervention in this particular setting, or should a vaccine be used, or should changes in government policy or a broader environmental intervention be made. As part of our engagement with communities in Bangladesh, my group strives to identify potential interventions. Although development of interventions is not taught to cultural anthropologists trained in Bangladesh, we find that our anthropologists are so attuned to the context of low-income communities that they consistently provide practical suggestions and input.

The scientific research team is an urban-educated elite whose worldview, attitudes, and perspectives are quite different from the low-income populations who bear the greatest health burden. It is all too easy in our planning to consider ideas and approaches that appear sound to educated public health professionals, but are not relevant to the concerns of the communities most in need. Arsenic commonly contaminates shallow ground water, which is the primary source of drinking water among most communities in Bangladesh. This contamination contributes to a wide range of health problems including high infant mortality, elevated rates of malignancy, and impaired cognitive development (Kapaj et al., 2006; Rahman et al., 2010). My group receives numerous inquiries from scientists and commercial firms who have developed strategies in their laboratories to remove arsenic from water, but however remarkable the laboratory efficacy of these approaches, none has sufficiently addressed the practical constraints of the affected communities, and none has been developed with a central focus on the perspective of the community.

My group has taken a more community-oriented approach in our efforts to increase handwashing with soap. Washing hands with soap reduces the risk of diarrhea and respiratory disease (Luby et al., 2005), the two leading causes of childhood death globally, but in communities with high burden of child deaths, handwashing with soap is rare (Curtis et al., 2009). An important barrier to handwashing in low-income communities is the cost of soap. We adapted an approach developed in Kenya that mixed low-cost detergent with water in discarded plastic bottles to make a low-cost liquid soap. In Bangladesh this was an adaptation of an already common practice of occasionally using detergent powder to wash hands. Our anthropological team illustrated the technique to communities and initiated a small trial. Within a few weeks it was apparent that this intervention was popular and successfully addressed an important cost barrier for many households. Anthropologists also identified concerns with the responsibilities of refilling the soapy water bottle and the deterioration of the bottle over time, issues that would have to be addressed for a larger scale rollout. Epidemiologists on our team are still working to understand the microbiological effectiveness of soapy water and to evaluate its uptake and impact on health.

The advantage of involving the anthropologists early is that they focused the public health team on an intervention that the community is interested in so it has an increased probability of eventual success.

Interdisciplinary collaboration is not a panacea. Practical affordable interventions that improve community health remain incredibly difficult to identify, develop, and implement, but epidemiologists are skilled at evaluating uptake and effectiveness of interventions. Anthropologists complement this skill set by asking key why questions. Why didn't you take up the intervention? Why did you stop using the intervention? What makes this difficult to use? What would be an ideal intervention? Working together, epidemiologists and anthropologists are much more likely to be able to identify and iteratively optimize promising interventions. In short, the public health problems that applied epidemiology in high disease communities face are difficult, but the potential contributions of anthropology to the epidemiological/public health enterprise are so substantial that epidemiologists would be shortsighted not to engage.

REFERENCES

Behague, D.P., Goncalves, H., Victora, C.G., 2008. Anthropology and Epidemiology: learning epistemological lessons through a collaborative venture. Ciencia & Saude Coletiva 13, 1701–1710.

Blum, L.S., Khan, R., Nahar, N., Breiman, R.F., 2009. In-depth assessment of an outbreak of Nipah encephalitis with person-to-person transmission in Bangladesh: implications for prevention and control strategies. The American Journal of Tropical Medicine and Hygiene 80, 96–102.

Choi, I., Nisbett, R.E., 2000. Cultural psychology of surprise: Holistic theories and recognition of contradiction. Journal of Personality and Social Psychology 79, 890.

Coale, A.J., 1974. The history of the human population. Scientific American 231, 40–51.

Curtis, V.A., Danquah, L.O., Aunger, R.V., 2009. Planned, motivated and habitual hygiene behaviour: an eleven country review. Health Education Research 24, 655–673.

Davis, K., 1986. The history of birth and death. Bulletin of the Atomic Scientists 42, 20–23.

Emerson, S.U., Purcell, R.H., 2004. Running like water—the omnipresence of hepatitis E. The New England Journal of Medicine 351, 2367–2368.

Finerman, R., 1995. 'Parental incompetence' and 'selective neglect': blaming the victim in child survival. Social Science & Medicine 40, 5–13.

Gaines, A.D., 2011. Millennial medical anthropology: from there to here and beyond, or the problem of global health. Culture, Medicine and Psychiatry 35, 83–89.

Gurley, E.S., Halder, A.K., Streatfield, P.K., Sazzad, HMS, Huda, TMN, Hossain, M.J., Luby, S., 2012. Estimating the burden of maternal and neonatal deaths associated with jaundice in Bangladesh: the possible role of hepatitis E infection. American Journal of Public Health, Dec;102(12):2248–2254.

Inhorn, M.C., 1995. Medical anthropology and epidemiology: divergences or convergences? Social Science & Medicine 40, 285–290.

Joel, D., Sathyaseelan, M., Jayakaran, R., Vijayakumar, C., Muthurathnam, S., Jacob, K.S., 2003. Explanatory models of psychosis among community health workers in South India. Acta Psychiatrica Scandinavica 108, 66–69.

Kapaj, S., Peterson, H., Liber, K., Bhattacharya, P., 2006. Human health effects from chronic arsenic poisoning—a review. Journal of Environmental Science and Health. Part A, Toxic/Hazardous Substances and Environmental Engineering 41 (10), 2399–2428.

Luby, S.P., Agboatwalla, M., Feikin, D.R., Painter, J., Billhimer, W., Altaf, A., Hoekstra, R.M., 2005. Effect of handwashing on child health: a randomised controlled trial. Lancet 366, 225–233.

McMichael, A.J., 1999. Prisoners of the proximate: loosening the constraints on epidemiology in an age of change. American Journal of Epidemiology 149, 887–897.

Paul, R.C., Rahman, M., ES G, Hossain, M.J., Diorditsa, S., Hasan, A.S.M.M., S.S.B., Alamgir, A.S.M., Rahman, M.A., Sandhu, H., Fischer, M., Luby, S.P., 2011. A novel low-cost approach to estimate the incidence of Japanese encephalitis in the catchment area of three hospitals in Bangladesh. The American Journal of Tropical Medicine and Hygiene 85, 379–385.

Porter, J.D., 2006. Epidemiological reflections of the contribution of anthropology to public health policy and practice. Journal of Biosocial Science 38, 133–144.

Rahman, A., Persson, L.A., Nermell, B., Arifeen, S.E., Ekstrom, E.C., Smith, A.H., Vahter, M., 2010 Nov. Arsenic exposure and risk of spontaneous abortion, stillbirth, and infant mortality. Epidemiology 21 (6), 797–804.

Rashid, S.F., Hadi, A., Afsana, K., Begum, S.A., 2001. Acute respiratory infections in rural Bangladesh: cultural understandings, practices and the role of mothers and community health volunteers. Tropical Medicine & International Health 6, 249–255.

Scheper-Hughes, N., 1990. Three propositions for a critically applied medical anthropology. Social Science & Medicine 30, 189–197.

Trostle, J.A., 2005. Epidemiology and culture. Cambridge University Press.

Local Tales

Industrial and Post-Industrial Societies

Medicalization or Medicine as Culture? The Case of Attention Deficit Hyperactivity Disorder

Helen Keane

The Australian National University, Canberra, Australia

INTRODUCTION

There is a growing field of literature within population health that demonstrates the many ways cultural practices and beliefs impact health and disease in given populations. But in these accounts, medicine and its systems of classification and diagnosis are frequently placed in opposition to, or imagined to exist outside of, culture. Medical knowledge and practice is taken to represent a coherent, universal, and objective account of health and disease, in contrast to the localized and socially embedded nature of cultural systems. While medical sociology has a long tradition of addressing medicine as a social institution and a practice inseparable from the exercise of power, the analysis of medicine as itself a cultural influence on health outcomes and disease prevalence remains underexplored outside of specific ethnographic studies.

This chapter therefore approaches medicine as a cultural practice shaped by particular "styles of thought" and technical practices (Rose, 2007b). Like other cultural systems, it guides what is imaginable, possible, and moral. More specifically, this chapter compares two theoretical approaches that produce different perspectives on the relationship between medical discourse, cultural beliefs, and the condition of attention deficit hyperactivity disorder (ADHD). The first framework is that of medicalization, a sociological theory that developed in the 1970s to describe and criticize the expansion of medical authority into everyday life. In its earlier iterations, medicalization was understood as a process of social control and medical imperialism. Current medicalization theory is less focused on the power of the medical profession than earlier models, in particular, it has expanded its scope to include the role of pharmaceutical and biotechnology companies, insurers, and health consumers in shaping the "medical marketplace" (Ballard and Elston, 2005; Conrad and Leiter, 2004). Nevertheless, as Stefan Beck has observed, medicalization still tends

When Culture Impacts Health. http://dx.doi.org/10.1016/B978-0-12-415921-1.00006-3

to be conceptualized as a linear and cumulative process that unfolds as part of modernity (Beck, 2007, p. 20). By adopting a linear model of the transformation of the non-medical into the medical, medicalization also implies that a discernible boundary exists between these two realms of life. In addition, many uses of the concept of medicalization contain the normative claim that medicine is expanding beyond its legitimate terrain, with negative consequences for society (Conrad, 2007).

The second approach is less a single framework than a set of theoretical tools, which I call "medicine as culture." This approach is similarly concerned with the influence of medicine, not only on understandings of health and illness, but also on forms of subjectivity and selfhood. But unlike medicalization theory, thinking about medicine as culture does not begin by positing a category of "normal life events" or "ordinary problems of living," which are outside the medical until they are medicalized. Rather, following the work of Nikolas Rose, it highlights the long history of medicine's involvement in social, political, and ethical matters and suggests that medicine has "made us what we are" as modern subjects (Rose, 2007a). That is, rather than an external mode of explanation that is imposed on our experiences of living, medical styles of thought are internal to our experiences of contemporary selfhood. In addition, my account of medicine as culture adopts some of the insights about medicine found in the field of Science and Technology Studies (STS). Specifically, it draws on the work of Marc Berg and Annemarie Mol who point out that "western medicine" is not a singular or unified entity but rather "a heterogeneous coalition" of bodies, procedures, technologies, conversations, documents, and medications (Berg and Mol, 1998, p. 3). Berg and Mol's emphasis on the differences within medicine challenge the notion of medicalization as a singular process with predictable effects. A medical definition of a condition as a disease does not necessarily mean that the condition will be understood, treated, or experienced the same way in different contexts. Neither does it mean that other modes of understanding or responding to life problems disappear, even if the language of medicine becomes dominant.

This chapter argues that while both perspectives provide useful insights into the rise of ADHD as a common diagnosis of childhood, understanding medicine as culture better captures the heterogeneity and pervasiveness of medical practice and discourse in contemporary social life. It encourages analysis of both the constraints and possibilities of medicalized life and recognizes the divergent perspectives present *within* medicine.

ADHD

ADHD is not only the most common and most researched mental disorder of childhood, it has become a household word and part of cultural consciousness in countries such as the United States, the UK, and Australia. While the dominant medical view is that ADHD is a highly heritable neurobehavioral disease associated with clearly demonstrated cognitive and motor deficits, the validity of the condition continues to be debated (Singh, 2008). ADHD has attracted controversy because its core symptoms of impulsivity, hyperactivity, and inattention are characteristic of children's behavior, thus diagnosis inevitably involves subjective assessment of when such behavior is pathological. As the majority of sufferers are diagnosed at school age, and because difficulties in school are frequently the catalyst for diagnosis, critics have also suggested that the rise in ADHD has been driven by parents and teachers seeking to manage unruly behavior and poor academic performance (Radcliffe and Timimi, 2004). The gender imbalance in diagnosis has led others to argue that ADHD is part of a general cultural pathologization and intolerance of boys (Pollack, 1998). The use of stimulant medications as the first line treatment for ADHD has added a particularly charged ethical dimension to the debate (Mayes, et al., 2009). Rather than directly participating in this debate about the validity, prevalence, and treatment of ADHD, this chapter highlights the insights about ADHD that can be gained through different theoretical perspectives on the relationship between medicine and culture.

Medicalization

Peter Conrad, author of many of the key texts on medicalization, describes it as a process "by which nonmedical problems become defined and treated as medical problems, usually in terms of illnesses and disorders" (1992, p. 209). Much of the critical commentary about ADHD is based on a normative vision of the process of medicalization. The now familiar argument is that troublesome but normal childhood behavior, once understood as naughtiness or rambunctiousness, has been transformed into a treatable disease. Children are being medicated (or in the more polemical critiques "drugged") so that they can succeed within the competitive modern classroom (Breggin, 2001). Parents, teachers, medical professionals, advocacy groups, and the pharmaceutical industry are driving this process, which is a threat to children's autonomy, authenticity, and development (White, 2005; Diller, 2006). While this set of arguments has been important in raising awareness of the social and ethical issues surrounding ADHD, they have also produced some problematic effects. As Iliana Singh (2008) has observed, these arguments can overemphasize the harms of diagnosis and treatment, and promote a reductive and superficial view of the benefits. They may attribute false consciousness to parents and children who express a positive experience with diagnosis and medication, and imply that their often severe difficulties should just be endured as part of everyday life. A moralized discourse of blame can result, with mothers being accused of failing to discipline their badly behaved children and turning to the "quick fix" of medication (Singh, 2004).

However, scholarly and empirically based accounts of the medicalization of hyperactivity have been invaluable in revealing the particular role of medical knowledge and practice in producing ADHD as a treatable condition. Indeed the first book-length empirical study of medicalization was about ADHD. Peter Conrad's (2006) book, *Identifying Hyperactive Children*, originally published in 1976, highlights the social processes required to form the medical entity of hyperactivity out of children's problem behavior. In the United States hyperactivity clinic that Conrad studied, heterogeneous information from school reports, parent questionnaires, and neurodevelopmental screening tests was converted into the medical evidence required to make a diagnosis of disease. Despite the efforts of the clinic staff, uncertainty often remained and other strategies such as invoking the authority of the clinic director and referring to the "typical case" were employed in order to achieve a diagnosis.

In a more recent sociological study, Adam Rafalovich (2004) also emphasizes the negotiation of uncertainty and ambiguity involved in diagnosis and treatment of ADHD. In contrast to Conrad, he also stresses the multiplicity of discourses surrounding ADHD and the agency exercised by clinicians, parents, teachers, and children in their everyday experiences with the condition. As he states "…ADHD is experienced from a variety of personal and professional perspectives that are influenced by myriad factors, including personal evaluation, skepticism, acceptance and ambivalence" (Rafalovich, 2004, p. 178). Thus Rafalovich's work represents the development of medicalization into a multidimensional concept more able to capture the hybridity of contemporary medical categories and practices, especially as they travel outside the institution of medicine.

As seen in the work of Conrad and Rafalovich, the medicalization perspective on ADHD provides insights into the complex social processes in which children's personal and social troubles become framed and legitimated as a disease. The medicalization approach, with its roots in a critical analysis of professional power and social control, is particularly effective in identifying the benefits of medical models of deviant behavior to institutions and interest groups. It reveals the institutional, economic, and social functions fulfilled by the ADHD diagnosis, including the legitimization of special educational support for the child and the conversion of ill-defined "trouble" into an understandable and named condition. The more recent work on ADHD has also illuminated the powerful influence of the pharmaceutical industry as an engine and beneficiary of medicalization. For example, as Conrad (2007, p. 68) has observed, the expansion in the 1990s of ADHD into a "lifespan" disorder, which affects adults as well as children, has dramatically increased the market for ADHD medications.

However, the medicalization perspective on ADHD also has limitations. Firstly, although recent reformulations stress the multidimensional nature of the process, the term itself still suggests a smooth linear trajectory in which all interested groups (teachers, parents, clinicians, and drug companies) are committed to and promote the medical/neurological model of ADHD. But as Rafalovich's (2004) work reveals, the prevalence of ADHD discourse in fact masks significant ambivalence and resistance, as well as struggles between different forms of authority. Many of the clinicians he interviewed were, for example, skeptical of the validity of the *Diagnostic and Statistical Manual of Mental Disorders*, Fourth Edition (DSM-IV), diagnostic criteria for ADHD, and many believed stimulants were overprescribed. They also stressed that it was schools that instigated the ADHD diagnostic process, with some seeing their own role as the *confirmation* of a diagnosis that had already been made, with considerable pressure applied to "solve the problem" by prescribing medication (Rafalovich, 2004, pp. 65–66). While parents might endorse a genetic brain dysfunction model of ADHD, this belief was put into practice in the home through a variety of techniques, which included medication, diet, the regulation of family routine, methods of discipline and reward, and increased tolerance of difference. Rather than a bounded medical category that produced a rigorous application of medical rationality, ADHD was manifested in domestic space as a hybrid set of knowledges, relationships, and practices (see also Malacrida, 2003).

Moreover, there is the risk that by presenting ADHD as an iconic case of medicalization, a hierarchy of diseases based on their presumed realness is reinforced. Medicalization scholarship is based on the sociological understanding of illness and disease as human constructions rather than natural phenomena. As Conrad and Schneider (1992, p. 30) state in their influential text *Deviance and Medicalization*, diseases "do not exist without someone proposing, describing and recognizing them." Following this definition, all diseases, including those with clear physiological symptomology and etiology, are socially constructed by the process of medicalization. On the other hand, the term medicalization is more likely to be applied to behavioral and psychological conditions such as ADHD, which are contested and lack clear-cut pathophysiognomies. In these cases of uncertain and contested disease, medicalization frequently takes on another meaning, that of the invention of an illegitimate or fabricated entity. Medicalization discourse can therefore suggest that some diseases are more socially constructed than others, thus reinforcing a model of disease, which is surprisingly close to the valorization of objective pathophysiology found in biomedicine. The unintended consequence can be the further stigmatization of the sufferers of contested conditions (and their families) whose struggles are dismissed as less worthy of medical care than those whose illnesses are based on irrefutable biological dysfunction.

Medicine as Culture

In contrast to understandings of medicalization, which see medicine as encroaching into the realm of everyday life, sociologist Nikolas Rose argued that since the end of the eighteenth century medicine has played a formative role in *producing* our everyday experiences of life. Under the "regime of the self" produced by modern medicine, we understand ourselves in terms of health or normality, a form of medical thinking that exists independent of any specific episode of illness or diagnosis of disease (Rose, 2006, 2007a). By insisting that medical expertise and knowledge was one of the constitutive elements that formed the modern idea of "the social," Rose (1994) undermines claims about the expansion of medical discourse into non-medical problems.

In his recent work on biopolitics in the twenty-first century, Rose (2007b) provides an updated account of the relationship between medicine and the social, highlighting the shift to a molecular style of thought and a new engagement with technologies of optimization. Rose argued that as a result of advances in fields such as genetics, genomics, neuroscience, and biotechnology, novel forms of citizenship have emerged in which individuals understand their selfhood, their aspirations, and their rights and responsibilities in biological terms. As Rose (2007b, p.25) stated "this is an ethic in which the maximization of lifestyle, potential, health and quality of life become almost obligatory, and where negative judgments are directed toward those who will not, for whatever reason, adopt an active, informed, positive, and prudent relationship to the future." At the same time, a new global bio-economy has developed in which health, disease, and other vital processes become sites of entrepreneurship, capital investment, and sources of wealth. In the resulting medical marketplace, pharma and biotech companies offer new technologies of selfhood that promise to help individuals enhance their capacities and achieve their aspirations as well as treat their illnesses (Rose, 2007b).

The discourses and practices that constitute ADHD are a vivid example of the landscape Rose outlined, a landscape in which individuals' hopes, anxieties, and discontents become expressed in medical and psychiatric terms. In the dominant medical theory, ADHD is the result of brain dysfunction, specifically an impairment in executive function (Barkley, 1997). The ascription of neurological difference as the core of the condition shapes the responses of doctors, educators, parents, and children. Psychopharmaceutical treatments are more readily accepted if they are seen as remedying specific deficits in brain functioning rather than simply modifying difficult behavior, but their wide adoption is not solely attributable to the authority of the disease model of ADHD. Stimulant medications, like many other pharmaceutical products, have become enrolled in the culturally normative project of active and responsible self-invention. For parents, this project includes taking charge of their child's future as well as their present, by realizing his or her potential and optimizing his or her chances of success. Psychopharmaceutical drugs, including stimulant medications, have become meaningful and valuable because of their compatibility with these hopes for the future (Rose, 2006). As Miller and Leger (2003, p. 29) stated, Ritalin can be seen as "one more cosmopolitan investment in human capital, in a risk society that wagers its future on the very people about whom it most panics."

Similarly, the constitution of ADHD as a brain-based learning disability has multiple meanings and effects. In the school setting, the diagnosis can allow for teaching and assessment techniques to be modified according to the perceived needs of the individual child (Mayes et al., 2009). Thus while the medical model places the sufferer in a category in which defines his or her identity, it can also have an individualizing effect within the institution of the school. Moreover, while the label of disability is traditionally seen as a stigma, the disability rights movement has produced a powerful counterdiscourse of disability as a positive identity rather than tragic or shameful defect. In this discourse, the disadvantages faced by the disabled are produced by prejudice and social exclusion rather than inherent incapacity (Mayes et al., 2009). The disability rights discourse cannot be simply defined as medicalized. It provides an interpretation of ADHD that is simultaneously biological, social, and political. It enables those with ADHD to request accommodations in the language of rights, rather than as requests for help.

The neurological model of ADHD can also be deployed to challenge the idea that it is a disease or disorder. The notion that the differences found in the ADHD brain represent a form of neurodiversity rather than pathology has become popular, for instance, in the theory that proposes ADHD represents characteristics that were adaptive in nomadic hunter–gatherer societies (Hartmann, 1997). According to this theory, it is only in evolutionarily novel environments such as the modern school that "the ADHD brain" becomes a liability. Without necessarily adopting the evolutionary explanation, parents do employ the idea of ADHD as part of their child's authentic self when making decisions about medication. For example, Singh (2005, p. 42) found that some mothers withheld medication on weekends because they wanted their sons to have the chance to be themselves. As one mother she interviewed stated, "why should we drug him on the weekend? That's who Stuart is. If he wants to be off the walls, why not?"

The notion of medicalization tends to overlook the diversity of these forms of action and explanation because they use a common medical and neurological language. It is not simply that ordinary troubles are transformed into the disease category of ADHD through a process of medical expansion. Rather, the relationship between normality and pathology and treatment and optimization has been altered by twenty-first century biomedicine (Rose, 2006). Normality and pathology are coexistent and operate on a continuum. Medical understandings and the will to improvement are pervasive in our culture and indeed constitutive of many of our beliefs about how to live a good life and how to be a productive and responsible citizen. ADHD and its treatments are by no means unique in the way they involve medical practice and the use of pharmaceuticals beyond the clear-cut boundaries of disease (Fox and Ward, 2008).

However, a general account of medicine as a constitutive part of modern culture and ideals of citizenship runs the risk of reifying "western medicine" as a coherent and unified entity. Here the work of STS scholars such as Marc Berg and Annemarie Mol (1998) can assist, by focusing attention on the incoherencies and variations contained within medicine. They investigate the way that networks of human and nonhuman actors bring medical entities such as atherosclerosis or asthma into being in laboratories, clinics, hospitals, homes, or any other space where medicine in its broad sense is practiced. Mol (1998, p. 157) calls this "the local performance of objects' to emphasize the specificity, variability and temporality of the entities that are brought into being by medical practice." As she (Mol, 1998, p. 144) states in her ethnographic study of athero-sclerosis and its treatment, the activities that fill hospitals do not just point to a disease, say what it is, where it is or whether it is, they also act on it, transform it and perform it: in fact "they *do* artherosclerosis."

Applying this perspective to ADHD would reveal the different ADHDs brought into being in different contexts: the suburban home in Australia, the UK inner-city community health center, the U.S. neuroscience lab, the Swedish psychiatrist's clinic, the drug company office, the high school staff meeting, and the primary school playground. It would also suggest that the spaces and times where ADHD disappears as a meaningful or at least dominant category are equally worthy of study. Another set of differences worth exploring is those that exist between the diagnosis of ADHD (based on fixed and generic criteria such as those found in the DSM-IV) and the treated condition (based on what can be done for the particular child's most pressing problems, as interpreted by a particular physician). Thinking of ADHD as a phenomenon of local net-works, produced by linkages between medical and educational practice, could also refigure the continuing debates about stimulant therapy. Rather than try-ing to determine whether stimulants are overprescribed or underprescribed in a general sense, this approach would promote assessment of the local value of the effects mobilized by ADHD in specific contexts.

This chapter has argued that medicine itself should be included in exam-inations of culture as a determinant of health and illness. It has highlighted the insights about ADHD, which can be gained through different theoretical perspectives on the styles of thought and intervention that are characteristic of medical discourse. While medicalization offers a valuable account of ADHD as a transformation of children's problem behavior into a treatable disease, it tends to give the entity of ADHD an unwarranted uniformity and stability. Understand-ing medicine as culture (rather than culture as medicalized) promotes a more heterogeneous vision of biopolitics and biomedicine, in which medical thinking is constitutive of normal life and selfhood rather than an incursion into it.

REFERENCES

Ballard, K., Elston, A., 2005. Medicalisation: a multi-dimensional concept. Social Theory & Health 3, 228–241.

Barkley, R., 1997. Behavioral inhibition, sustained attention, and executive functions: constructing a unifying theory of ADHD. Psychological Bulletin 121, 65–94.

Beck, S., 2007. Medicalizing culture(s) or culturalizing medicine(s). In: Burri, R.V., Dumit, J. (Eds.), Biomedicine as culture, Routledge, New York, pp. 17–34.

Berg, M., Mol., A. (Eds.), 1998. Differences in medicine, Duke University Press, Durham.

Breggin, P., 2001. Talking back to Ritalin. Da Capo, New York.

Conrad, P., 1992. Medicalization and social control. Annual Review of Sociology 18, 209–232.

Conrad, P., 2006. Identifying hyperactive children: The medicalization of deviant behavior, expanded edition. Ashgate, Aldershot.

Conrad, P., 2007. The medicalization of society: On the transformation of human conditions into treatable disorders. The Johns Hopkins University Press, Baltimore.

Conrad, P., Leiter, V., 2004. Medicalization, markets and consumers. Journal of Health and Social Behavior 45, 158–176.

Conrad, P., Schneider, J., 1992. Deviance and medicalization: From badness to sickness. Temple University Press, Philadelphia.

Diller, L., 2006. The last normal child. Praeger, New York.

Fox, N., Ward, K., 2008. Pharma in the bedroom … and the kitchen … The pharmaceuticalisation of daily life. Sociology of Health and Illness 30, 856–868.

Hartmann, T., 1997. Attention Deficit Disorder: A different perception, second ed. Underwood Books, Grass Valley, CA.

Malacrida, C., 2003. Cold comfort: Mothers, professionals and Attention Deficit Disorder. University of Toronto Press, Toronto.

Mayes, R., Bagwell, C., Erkulwater, J., 2009. Medicating children: ADHD and pediatric mental health. Harvard University Press, Cambridge.

Miller, T., Leger, C., 2003. A very childish moral panic. Journal of Medical Humanities 24, 9–33.

Mol, A., 1998. Missing links, making links. In: Berg, M., Mol., A. (Eds.), Differences in medicine, Duke University Press, Durham, pp. 144–165.

Pollack, W., 1998. Real boys: Rescuing our sons from the myths of boyhood. Henry Holt, New York.

Radcliffe, N., Timimi, S., 2004. The rise and rise of ADHD. Clinical Psychology 40, 8–13.

Rafalovich, A., 2004. Framing ADHD children. Lexington Books, Lanham.

Rose, N., 1994. Medicine, history and the present. In: Jones, C. (Ed.), Reassessing Foucault: Power, Medicine and the Body, Routledge, London, pp. 48–72.

Rose, N., 2006. Disorders without borders? BioSocieties 1, 465–484.

Rose, N., 2007a. Beyond medicalisation. Lancet 369, 700–702.

Rose, N., 2007b. The Politics of Life Itself. Princeton University Press, New Haven.

Singh, I., 2004. Doing their jobs; mothering with Ritalin in a culture of mother blame. Social Science & Medicine 59, 1193–1205.

Singh, I., 2005. Will the "real boy" please behave: dosing dilemmas for parents of boys with ADHD. American Journal of Bioethics 5, 34–47.

Singh, I., 2008. Beyond polemics: science and ethics of ADHD. Nature Reviews Neuroscience 9, 957–964.

White, G., 2005. Splitting the self. American Journal of Bioethics 5, 57–59.

Chapter 7

Filthy Fingernails and Friendly Germs: Lay Concepts of Contagious Disease Transmission in Developed Countries

Kate Crosbie, Juliet Richters, Claire Hooker, and Julie Leask
University of New South Wales, Sydney, Australia

INTRODUCTION

The rise of cultural epidemiology has been significant for the growing understanding of the gap between official models of disease and what Weiss (2001) refers to as "locally valid representations of illness," that is, lay or folk conceptions of disease. To date, research on contagious disease etiologies has primarily focused on folk beliefs held by inhabitants of developing countries or immigrant and indigenous groups in developed countries and, to a lesser extent, children's etiologies in developed countries. Research on adult etiologies of contagious diseases in developed countries remains limited by comparison. This may be due, in part, to what Mary Douglas (1996) refers to as "cultural innocence," the difficulty in holding up an analytical mirror to the norms of one's own culture and the failure to recognize the contradictions and amalgams in familiar beliefs as opposed to those of the exotic "Other." Despite this, research on adult etiologies of major lifestyle diseases, such as diabetes, cancer, and hypertension, in developed countries is expanding (Pérez-Stable et al., 1992; Maskarinec et al., 2001; Wilson et al., 2002; Lawton et al., 2007). Perhaps the primacy of a fixed biomedical germ model in formal education and health systems has led to the assumption that it is similarly the dominant, fixed etiological model among the adult populace. Certainly most health promotion campaigns for infectious disease prevention depend on the Health Belief Model in some form, as in the following:

1. Rational knowledge of transmission (disease caused by germ)
2. Personal susceptibility and severity (*I* might catch it and it might be severe)

When Culture Impacts Health. http://dx.doi.org/10.1016/B978-0-12-415921-1.00007-5

3. Knowledge of way to avoid catching it

4. Skill/power to employ that knowledge (Strecher and Rosenstock, 1997).

Knowledge, however, is a complex field in which different models of explanation compete and interact (Arce and Long, 1995; Carrier et al., 2005). Individuals can, and do, adopt understandings selectively from a range of models and mold them into their existing framework. Individuals may use different explanatory rationales and behaviors depending on the context (Nemeroff and Rozin, 1994; Adam et al., 2000; Ridge, 2004). It is heartening to note that health researchers are increasingly focusing on the complex and variable nature of knowledge as a way of understanding respondents' rationales, particularly when these may seem to be contradictory. Adam et al. (2000), for example, recognized that individuals may have high levels of knowledge, which are in accord with official medical explanations, yet these authors also explored "the reasoning processes by which people exempt themselves from these messages."

In view of the evident complex understandings of contagion, this chapter reviews the available literature to examine (1) the research that has been conducted on lay understandings of contagious disease transmission in Australia, New Zealand, Canada, the United States, and the UK and (2) to explore the main themes, metaphors, and images arising within these understandings.

METHODOLOGY

We carried out a literature review of studies published between January 1, 1980, and September 30, 2010. Relevant studies referred to, or examined, the beliefs of adolescents and adults from developed Western countries (the UK, Ireland, the United States, Canada, Australia, and New Zealand) concerning the transmission of contagious diseases. Similar data queries were run in three major databases: Medline, Anthropology Plus, and Sociological Abstracts. Search queries were kept broad, and overlapping queries were run in order to capture the full range of literature. Search queries that generated more than 750 results were refined by adding additional search terms; otherwise, titles and abstracts were briefly examined to determine relevance. Queries were run in a snowball fashion. Web of Science was used to search both for articles citing key works (e.g., Douglas, 1966) and for additional works by authors of relevant studies. References from relevant articles were also checked.

We excluded studies which focused on indigenous groups living in isolation or traditionally, recent immigrant populations from developing countries, and self-identified immigrant groups who maintained traditional ideas (e.g., Chinese groups living in the United States); children (except adolescents in high school); intervention studies (e.g., education techniques and/or success); preventive activities, such as condom use and immunization (including predictors of use); risk (including risky behavior and external variables like alcohol consumption); epidemiology, modeling, and prevalence of transmission; social inequalities in transmission populations; attitudes and stigma toward people with contagious diseases and high-risk populations; conspiracy theories; and sexual ethics (e.g., partner notification). Theoretical articles, historical perspectives, and reviews were disregarded, although they were used for snowballing purposes.

We found a large number of quantitative studies that assessed individual knowledge of sexually transmitted infection (STI) transmission against biomedical understandings. Similar transmission pathways were usually explored (e.g., casual contact vs. biomedical germ models); therefore we selected only a few that were representative of the most commonly asked questions. Selected studies also included participant responses that differed from what was deemed biomedically accurate, since these indicated possible alternative understandings of transmission (such as casual or social contact). Otherwise, we concentrated on mixed method and qualitative studies for their ability to provide richer data and in-depth understandings, and to contextualize findings.

FINDINGS

In all, 52 relevant studies were identified. Of these, 27 were conducted in the United States, 15 in Australia, 6 in England, 2 in Canada, 1 in Scotland, and 1 in New Zealand. Twenty-five studies used qualitative methods of data collection (including focus groups, semistructured and in-depth interviews, ethnography, observation, and participant-observation), 17 used quantitative methods (questionnaires), and 10 used mixed methods. Given the rising rates of STIs and the concomitant health promotion focus on their reduction, it is not surprising that the overwhelming majority of papers concentrated on STIs. Twelve studies focused on one or more STIs, 27 exclusively on HIV/AIDS, 3 exclusively on syphilis, and 3 exclusively on hepatitis C. These studies mostly focused on special groups within society: gays and lesbians, drug users, African Americans, and STI clinic patients. Of the non-STI studies, one focused on the common cold, one on influenza, one on tuberculosis, one on methicillin-resistant *Staphylococcus aureus* (MRSA), one on an unidentified contagious germ, and one on hygiene in general (with reference to a range of bacteria and viruses). A final study examined a range of sources of contagion (people and objects), as well as contagious diseases (HIV/AIDS and hepatitis) (Nemeroff and Rozin, 1994).

Several themes emerged from the literature: somatic cues, protective hygiene acts, magical contagion and casual contact, familiarity and trust, symbolic pollution, and special immunity.

Somatic Cues: Sight, Sound, and Smell

Belief that somatic cues, primarily visual, could be used to distinguish healthy from diseased individuals (or those more likely to be diseased) was the most common finding of the research, particularly for STI studies. Of the 52 studies reviewed, 20 involved respondents stating that they could tell by looking at someone whether they were healthy or diseased, or explaining how they used visual cues to judge the likelihood of whether a person carried a disease (Balshem et al., 1992; Sibthorpe, 1992; Lamport and Andre, 1993; LeBlanc, 1993; Lowy and Ross, 1994; Zimet et al., 1995; Peart et al., 1996; Plumridge et al., 1996; Sobo et al., 1997; Hoffman and Cohen, 1999; Adam et al., 2000; Skidmore and Hayter, 2000; Bakopanos and Gifford, 2001; McDonald et al., 2001; Essien et al., 2002; Padgett, 2002; Ridge, 2004; Lambert et al., 2006; Brown et al., 2007; Elam et al., 2008). Even where participants acknowledged the lack of reliability in using visual cues, they continued to refer to them (Sobo et al., 1997; McDonald et al., 2001; Lambert et al., 2006). Rarely did participants refer to the transfer of organisms (bacteria, viruses, etc.) when discussing disease transmission (Balshem et al., 1992; McDonald et al., 2001; Curtis et al., 2003). Instead, in the STI studies, participants usually focused on the appearance, behavior, or beliefs of individuals, or on the participant's relationship with his or her potential partner. Thus, for example, if a person looked healthy or fit, respondents assumed that they were disease-free (Elam et al., 2008). This could be because many diseases have visual symptoms, or it could be linked to a belief that individuals can only spread infection if they are ill, as 46% of adolescents believed to be the case for HIV-positive people in Sobo et al.'s (1997) study.

Frequently, somatic cues were linked with social and moral assumptions. In several studies, cues of social class were important. Higher social classes, identified, for example, by diction, the car driven or a "high-powered job," were usually perceived as safer (Lowy and Ross, 1994; Hoffman and Cohen, 1999; McDonald et al., 2001; Lambert et al., 2006; Jackson et al., 2008). Most studies did not expand on why people thought this was the case, although one participant suggested that people from a higher class were more likely to have completed a higher level of education and thus have a better understanding of the "complexities" associated with HIV, which, it was assumed, would translate into safer sexual health practices (Lowy and Ross, 1994). In contrast, lower social classes were associated with a greater risk of transmission, including contagious diseases other than STIs. In Jackson et al.'s (2008) study, Glaswegian tuberculosis patients and their next of kin were more likely to suggest homeless people, poor people, and "tramps" as the cause of their infection, despite being aware of conventional transmission theory, which requires close, prolonged contact for transmission to occur. In Washer et al.'s (2008) study, respondents associated black cleaners in London hospitals with poor hygienic practices and the spread of MRSA.

Visual cues could be interpreted in contradictory ways. Some participants understood physical attractiveness to be an indicator of a healthy status (Hoffman and Cohen, 1999; McDonald et al., 2001), while others linked attractiveness to likely promiscuity and therefore greater chance of infection

(Lowy and Ross, 1994). Similarly, some participants associated youth with safety (Elam et al., 2008) because of assumed sexual inexperience and hence lower risk of infection (Adam et al., 2000), or because of young men's life-long exposure to safe sex education campaigns (Lowy and Ross, 1994); other participants saw young men as high risk because of possible complacency due to overexposure to safe sex campaigns (Lowy and Ross, 1994).

A second major theme was the emergence of a fuzzy dichotomy, which linked people's understandings of cleanliness with good health and dirtiness with disease. Individuals, locations, or even diseases were described as "clean" and/or "dirty," often through reference to somatic cues (Balshem et al., 1992; Sibthorpe, 1992; Sobo et al., 1997; Hoffman and Cohen, 1999; Skidmore and Hayter, 2000; McDonald et al., 2001; Essien et al., 2002; Padgett, 2002; Flood, 2003; Lambert et al., 2006; Brown et al., 2007). In the case of individuals, dirti-ness was understood in a number of different ways: physical dirt (dirty finger-nails, hands, or clothes) (Hoffman and Cohen, 1999; Padgett, 2002; Lambert et al., 2006; Brown et al., 2007), poor personal hygiene (body odor or greasy hair) (Balshem et al., 1992; Essien et al., 2002; Padgett, 2002; Lambert et al., 2006), or transgressive behaviors (style of clothing was used to intuit promiscu-ity and thus disease; both heterosexual and gay participants also described indi-viduals who "looked" gay as more likely to have or transmit an STI) (Balshem et al., 1992; Lowy and Ross, 1994). Importantly, respondents understood vis-ible features to be reflective of characteristics or behaviors that would have an impact on an individual's health status (Lowy and Ross, 1994; Hoffman and Cohen, 1999; Skidmore and Hayter, 2000; McDonald et al., 2001; Padgett, 2002; Lambert et al., 2006). Thus, for Padgett's (2002) respondents, "dressing well" was "seen as displaying characteristics indicating cleanliness [understood as good hygiene] on the outside as well as on the inside."

When locations were discussed, dirtiness was most commonly associated with poor hygiene, which was understood as a cause of disease. In Curtis et al.'s (2003) study of home childcare workers in Wirral, England, participants under-stood a house to be hygienic if it looked "tidy, bright and ordered." Participants also associated hygiene risks with particular rooms, the kitchen and toilet areas, despite nappy changes occurring in other rooms and microbiological testing finding traces of fecal matter throughout the house. They associated the concept of "hygiene," rather than the biomedical model, with disease transmission. At times, the two concepts overlapped, such as when respondents linked bacteria with a lack of hygiene; at others, they were entirely distinct, as when respon-dents described viruses as "not unhygienic." In Washer et al.'s (2008) hospital study, respondents associated "bad smells" with the threat of MRSA, while the "sterile" smell of disinfectant was understood to indicate good hygiene.

Bodily fluids also played an important role in understandings of disease transmission and were frequently linked with the concept of poor hygiene. Curtis et al.'s (2003) respondents were prompted to wash their hands or clean up by somatic cues, rather than by behaviors that exposed them to infection.

Thus, they cleaned because of the sight of physical dirt, feces or food remains, or bad smells, while they did not wash their hands after 39% of observed nappy changes. The focus on visibility of bodily fluids was particularly important in many of the STI studies, sometimes even at the expense of other somatic indicators that fluid exchange had occurred, such as taste, smell, or touch. Thus, in Richters et al.'s (2003) study, one respondent only feared the possibility of HIV infection when he saw blood on the end of his penis, despite having engaged in unprotected anal intercourse, prompting the authors to note that "emphasis on the visible poses a problem for awareness of the invisible virus as "real." Similarly, several gay respondents recently diagnosed with syphilis suggested that sex was "less risky" if there was "no [visible] mess," such as semen or feces, despite receiving ejaculate in their mouth (Lambert et al., 2006).

In Treloar and Fraser's (2004) study, participants conflated the bodily fluid (blood) with the disease (hepatitis C), and some described the characteristics of blood as changing with transmission: blood became "dirty" if it was infected, stayed "clean" if it was not. However, none of the other reviewed studies investigated the mechanism by which participants understood diseases to be transferred via bodily fluids. Bodily fluids themselves, not the infectious organisms they carried, were often spoken about as the risk. This was particularly prevalent in much of the HIV/AIDS research where not only actual fluid exchange, but the *possibility* of fluid exchange, was associated with disease transmission. Thus, respondents consistently overestimated HIV risks associated with not only saliva transferred during kissing, but also cleaning vomit, being spat on, sharing a toothbrush, nasal/sneeze droplets, urine on toilet seats, sweaty hands, and manual sex (Crawford et al., 1990; Dow and Knox, 1991; Lamport and Andre, 1993; LeBlanc, 1993; Guttman et al., 1998; Hoffman and Cohen, 1999; Herek et al., 2005; Brown et al., 2007). As a result, some participants reported avoiding particular activities associated with fluid transfer, such as kissing and cunnilingus, in order to avoid disease transmission (Hoffman and Cohen, 1999; Brown et al., 2007). Others sought to limit the amount of fluid transferred, such as by withdrawing before ejaculation during fellatio or anal sex, which was deemed to be a "safe" practice despite the sexual encounter being unprotected (Lamport and Andre, 1993; Lowy and Ross, 1994; Adam et al., 2000). In other studies, however, respondents associated different bodily fluids with different levels of danger for transmission of STIs and hepatitis C: vaginal fluids were seen as safer than semen, and the transfer of blood was generally seen as high risk, including *donating* blood[1] (Goodman and Cohall, 1989; Andre and Bormann, 1991; Hoffman and Cohen, 1999; Lamport and Andre, 1993; LeBlanc, 1993; Nemeroff et al., 1994; Zimet et al., 1995; Sobo et al., 1997; Watson et al., 1999;

---

1. Although possible (Donovan, 1988), donating blood is a highly unlikely transmission route given the guidelines around single-use needles in developed countries, where the studies were conducted.

Power et al., 2009). The nature of the act involving fluid transfer also changed the sense of perceived risk associated with STI transmission, so oral and lesbian sex was often identified as safe (Goodman and Cohall, 1989; Downing-Matibag and Geisinger, 2009; Power et al., 2009). However, the danger associated with bodily fluid transfer was frequently mitigated by the relationship between individuals (see the section Familiarity and Trust).

Protective Hygiene Acts

Since respondents often linked the concept of hygiene with disease transmission, many focused on the use of personal hygiene practices—such as showering/bathing, douching, mouth rinsing, toothbrushing, and flossing—as a means of reducing, or ruling out, their chance of contracting STIs (Sibthorpe, 1992; Adam et al., 2000; McDonald et al., 2001; Padgett, 2002; Lambert et al., 2006). Evidence of the critical evaluation and application of different health frameworks—namely, personal hygiene and the biomedical germ model—were apparent. Thus, if protective hygiene acts were undertaken (such as showering), some respondents felt that sexual barriers (such as condoms) were unnecessary (Sibthorpe, 1992; Lambert et al., 2006). While sharing a biomedical understanding of the risk of unprotected sex with a mouth ulcer, one gay sex worker believed that hygiene methods (mouthwashing and flossing) mitigated the risk of HIV infection (Lambert et al., 2006). Importantly, protective hygiene acts took place both before and *after* exposure to transmission. One female sex worker bathed and douched at the end of a night of unprotected sexual encounters with clients in an attempt to avert infection (Padgett, 2002), while another male respondent attributed his contraction of syphilis to "not washing" after a sexual encounter (McDonald et al., 2001). Although some participants did express ambivalence about the reliability of protective hygiene practices, they used them nonetheless (McDonald et al., 2001).

Magical Contagion and Casual Contact

An alternative health framework with considerable traction was the concept of "magical contagion" (Frazer, 1959; Mauss, 1972; Tylor, 1974), which has been most commonly investigated in non-Western countries. The concept "holds that, when two objects touch ... they pass properties to one another" (Rozin et al., 1992). As Nemeroff (1995) described, a striking example of this was the belief that "the contagious entity reflects the essence of its source" and can therefore "result in differential effects, depending on the nature of the relationship between source and recipient." Undergraduate university students expected that, although the likelihood of transmission would remain similar, the virulence of flu germs would differ depending on the source from which they were contracted: least virulent from lovers, more virulent from a stranger, and most virulent from a disliked acquaintance (Nemeroff, 1995). Similarly, junior high school students expected that the severity of an (unspecified) germ and the length of time for which the illness would occur would be longer if it was contracted from a disliked source than from a friend (Sullivan and Terry, 1998).

The magical contagion framework also appears to inform "casual contact" beliefs since brief contact was frequently identified as a transmission route for particular contagious diseases, irrespective of the biomedical possibility or likelihood. In the reviewed literature, "casual contact" was used in a very broad sense, variously referring to physical contact with an infected individual, contact through a shared inanimate object, and even social (nonphysical) contact. Casual contact informed the HIV transmission beliefs of participants in much of the reviewed literature with perceived infection routes between oneself and an infected individual including: kissing, being kissed on the cheek, touching, shaking hands, holding "sweaty hands," sharing a bath, sharing a shower in gym class, sharing objects, sharing a toothbrush or razor, sharing cutlery or a glass, working or attending school together, or living near a home or hospital for AIDS patients (Goodman and Cohall, 1989; Andre and Bormann, 1991; Hobfoll et al., 1993; Lamport and Andre, 1993; LeBlanc, 1993; Nemeroff et al., 1994; Zimet et al., 1995; Sobo et al., 1997; Guttman et al., 1998; Okwumabua et al., 2001; Lim et al., 2007).

Casual contact beliefs are not necessarily the result of ignorance of biomedical explanations, as Guttman et al. (1998) found in their study of individuals as critical consumers of information. Many respondents thought that casual contact was a more likely HIV transmission route than experts suggested. Similarly, Sobo et al. (1997) found that 20 of 98 adolescent respondents agreed that their beliefs differed from those of the experts, although this included both greater and fewer modes of transmission routes than experts outlined. Nemeroff and Rozin's (1994) study was also important for highlighting the way in which individuals may believe in multiple transmission models, critically evaluating them and employing "strategies" to apply them differentially depending on the context. Proposing five contagion models, a germ model (traditional biomedical model), a residue model ("perceptible residues, such as odor, dandruff, body heat, and so forth"), an associative model ("based in the reminding value of the object"), a symbolic interaction model ("the meaning or statement implied by one's interaction with the object"), and a spiritual essence model ("some nonmaterial essence of the source being embodied in the object"), Nemeroff and Rozin (1994) found that some individuals used different models depending on their emotional reaction to the source of contagion (positive or negative), or the nature of the source (physical, interpersonal-moral, etc.), or even their own reasoning approach (articulated or implicit). Similarly, in comparing different scenario responses, Raman and Winer (2002) found that some adults variously employed biological and folkloric reasoning to choose which individuals were more likely to contract a cold first.

Familiarity and Trust

The sense of comparative safety with "friendly" sources can operate within a circular logic, so that familiarity also becomes a basis for selecting "safe" partners. In several of the studies reviewed, respondents explicitly discussed familiarity with the sexual partner as the primary, and sometimes the only, preventive measure against acquiring an STI, since respondents felt that they would not contract disease from familiar partners (Crawford et al., 1990; Sibthorpe, 1992; Abbott-Chapman and Denholm, 1997; Comer and Nemeroff, 2000; Skidmore and Hayter, 2000). Significantly, there were varying degrees of familiarity. This ranged along a spectrum ranging from references to "trust" and "love" with a primary partner (Sibthorpe, 1992; Abbott-Chapman and Denholm, 1997) to previous contact (Sibthorpe, 1992; Hoffman and Cohen, 1999; McDonald et al., 2001) to more symbolic familiarity, including assumptions about the values of particular groups (such as churchgoers) and brief conversations to ascertain a sense of shared or similar values (Balshem et al., 1992; Peart et al., 1996; Plumridge et al., 1996; Hoffman and Cohen, 1999; Skidmore and Hayter, 2000; McDonald et al., 2001; Ridge, 2004).

In Crawford et al.'s (1990) study, 45% of respondents endorsed unprotected vaginal sex with a regular partner as safe. Comer and Nemeroff (2000) found that when faced with a series of scenarios comparing objectively safe, emotionally safe, and casual sexual partners, individuals often made assumptions about HIV status based on emotional security/safety. While the objectively safe scenario specified that the sexual partner had been tested for HIV and was monogamous, these conditions were *not* specified for the "emotionally safe" partner, yet 16% of individuals assumed that an HIV test had been conducted, 32% reported that they were "(somewhat) aware of his or her HIV status," and 61% assumed that the partner was monogamous.[2] Skidmore and Hayter (2000) found that, for heterosexual men, "trust" relied on the knowledge of similarity, which they explained as: "She is like me and I know I am clean [STI free]; therefore, so is she." For their respondents, the length of time allowed for "knowing" or "trusting" a person was often quite limited: an average of 12 days (range 1 day to 4 weeks) for male respondents and within 80 days (range 2 to 18 weeks) for female respondents. Significantly, "knowing" and "trusting" a person as a rationale for unprotected sex can also outweigh known risk factors. In Sibthorpe's (1992) study, injecting drug users felt safe from STI transmission despite having unprotected sex with other injecting drug users and with multiple partners.

---

2. Interestingly, 22% of respondents did not report the objectively safe relationship as monogamous and a small percentage noted that the HIV blood test was fallible, both of which the authors attributed to respondent skepticism.

Previous contact—such as having met through mutual friends, having attended the same school, or having had previous casual sexual encounters—was also used as a protective rationale, which outweighed known risk factors (Balshem et al., 1992; Sibthorpe, 1992; McDonald et al., 2001; Downing-Matibag and Geisinger, 2009). In Sibthorpe's (1992) study, several sex workers did not use condoms with "regular" clients because they considered them STI-free on the basis of repeated contact. A respondent in Balshem et al.'s (1992) study believed one of his sexual contacts to be disease free, despite her high-risk status as a promiscuous crack-cocaine user because he "knew her as she was growing up." In Downing-Matibag and Geisinger's (2009) study, 50% of respondents were not concerned about the possibility of contracting an STI during casual intercourse because of trust in their partners or their community. Symbolic familiarity, or superficial indicators of similarity, which are used to support similarity = safety logic, were also mentioned in several studies. Here, a brief conversation, family background, going to church, (perceived) shared ethnocultural roots, and even assumptions about lower STI rates in people from sexually conservative countries, all played a role in defining potential sexual partners as "safe" (Balshem et al., 1992; Plumridge et al., 1996; Hoffman and Cohen, 1999; McDonald et al., 2001).

Friendship also played a role in perceived disease transmission. Thus, 16% of undergraduate students did not think it was possible to transmit HIV through becoming "blood brothers" (i.e., cutting hands and mingling blood with another individual) (Nemeroff et al., 1994). In Roberts et al.'s (1996) study, young men did not identify their own semen or that of their friends as a potential STI vector, while they did refer to semen from "other men."

Symbolic Pollution and Spontaneous Transmission: Locations, Identities, and Unusual Sexual Acts

"Symbolic pollution" was another key theme to emerge from the studies. Developed by Douglas (1966), the concept refers to the way in which particular forms of contact or actions are understood to upset the social order, and are therefore considered symbolically or ritually polluting. In several of the reviewed studies, *symbolically* polluting occurrences were associated with the *actual* cause and transmission of infection. Locations, individuals, and actions could all be categorized as polluting. The perceived security of "private" versus the dangers of "public" spaces was evident in Jackson et al.'s (2008) study. Most patients rejected conventional medical explanations of the transmission of tuberculosis (close, prolonged social contact, such as in the home). Instead, they focused on their transmission as occurring during "fleeting contact" in public, often in confined or crowded spaces, such as buses, streets, hotels, and restaurants. Polluting individuals were poor, alcoholic, or homeless men, or asylum seekers. In the STI research, polluting individuals were often characterized as "dirty" and included injecting drug users, prostitutes, gay men, and promiscuous individuals (with the greatest focus in the research on the latter two categories) (Crawford et al., 1990; Sibthorpe, 1992; Peart et al., 1996; Roberts et al., 1996; Van de Ven et al., 1996; Abbott-Chapman and Denholm, 1997; Grove et al., 1997; Hoffman and Cohen, 1999; Skidmore and Hayter, 2000; McDonald et al., 2001; Okwumabua et al., 2001; Pryce, 2001; Flood, 2003; Herek et al., 2005; Brown et al., 2007; Downing-Matibag and Geisinger, 2009). Respondents often noted that they would use condoms with people from these polluting categories, whereas they would generally not do so with other sexual partners (Peart et al., 1996; Sibthorpe, 1992; McDonald et al., 2001; Brown et al., 2007). However, factors such as familiarity and emphasis on visual identification of health status played a critical role in individuals excluding sexual partners from "dangerous" categories and placing them into "safe" categories (e.g., Balshem et al., 1992).

The possibility of STI transmission was consistently linked with gay men by heterosexual, gay, and lesbian respondents (Peart et al., 1996; Abbott-Chapman and Denholm, 1997; Grove et al., 1997; Adam et al., 2000; Okwumabua et al., 2001; Flood, 2003; Herek et al., 2005). At the most extreme end of this spectrum, Herek et al.'s (2005) study of 1283 participants across 48 U.S. states found that one-third of male and almost 45% of female respondents believed that HIV could be contracted through unprotected homosexual sex between *uninfected* partners. Even when the scenario included condom use, 25% of male and almost 30% of female respondents still believed infection could occur.[3]

The association of STI transmission with promiscuous individuals was also raised by both heterosexual and gay respondents. In Lambert et al.'s (2006) study, polluting individuals were described as those with "presumed sexual prowess and elaborate sexual repertoire." One man in Elam et al.'s (2008) study went so far as to suggest that "it shouldn't have really been me" who contracted HIV given his sexual reserve and the comparative promiscuity of his friends. Another respondent specifically selected sexual partners who looked "a bit more [sexually] restrained."

Finally, polluting acts were associated with STI transmission. In Lambert et al.'s (2006) study, polluting individuals and polluting acts overlapped as categories associated with the transmission of syphilis. Here "dirty sex" could include sex with "dirty men" and vice versa, but "dirty sex" was also understood to encompass a range of sex acts to which disease transmission was attributed. According to the authors, respondents attributed "esoteric, unusual or adventurous sex" acts, such as fisting or felching, or "rare events," such as sex at sex-on-premises venues, going to "extreme clubs," "unusual pain during anal intercourse," or having sex after "going out" and "getting drunk," as the means

---

3. Interestingly, a smaller, but still significant, percentage of respondents also believed that HIV could be transmitted between *uninfected* heterosexual partners, with and without condom use. This is suggestive of a spontaneous model of transmission, which is perhaps partially an internalization of HIV/AIDS health promotion campaigns, which focus on sexual *encounters* as a risk factor for transmission. For similar findings, see also Hobfoll et al. (1993).

by which they had contracted syphilis. These beliefs were not necessarily a result of ignorance of the biomedical explanation of syphilis transmission. Two individuals consciously selected their explanation of "rare events," instead of the biomedical germ explanation they received during counseling, as the more satisfactory. In Sobo et al.'s study, 14% of respondents identified masturbation as a possible origin of HIV infection (see also Zimet et al., 1995), which the authors suggested could be related to a sense of moral risk (punishment for sin), although this was not clarified with respondents.

Special Immunity

Finally, some individuals expressed a sense of special immunity, which was understood to either reduce the risk of contracting contagious diseases or rule it out altogether. Geographic isolation (Abbott-Chapman and Denholm, 1997; Downing-Matibag and Geisinger, 2009), ethnicity (Bakopanos and Gifford, 2001; Essien et al., 2002), youth (Abbot-Chapman and Denholm, 1997), inexperience (Downing-Matibag and Geisinger, 2009), and being spiritually transcendental (Plumridge et al., 1996) were all identified as either mitigating or exclusionary factors for contracting STIs. Women were variously understood as immune (Grunseit et al., 1995; Essien et al., 2002), or less likely to contract HIV sexually (Sibthorpe, 1992), or as the carriers of STIs (Roberts et al., 1996). Healthy lifestyle habits, a healthy immune system, and previous immunity to infections were also extrapolated to either a reduced risk or immunity to contracting HIV (Lowy and Ross, 1994). Similar reasoning was applied by injecting drug users in relation to hepatitis C in Carrier et al.'s (2005) study, with participants who had not contracted the disease claiming they had a "natural" immunity or their bodies were "stronger" than the hepatitis C virus.

DISCUSSION

A significant finding to emerge from this review is the possibility for individuals to hold a number of competing and ambivalent views outside the biomedical model, which may be applied differently depending on the circumstances. These concepts had contagion as occurring via societal mechanisms such as somatic cues, symbolically protective acts, magical contagion, notions of familiarity, symbolic pollution and spontaneous transmission, and ideas about special immunity conferred through age, geography, ethnicity, and spirituality. As Nemeroff and Rozin (1994) found, an individual may hold a number of models through which he or she perceives different types of contagion or different sources of contagion. Ridge (2004) and Guttman et al. (1998) also established that official discourses may be rejected, interpreted, and/or incorporated into one or more of the models held by an individual. These models were contrasted and conflated with traditional biomedical models of contagion, as the latter are traditionally represented as being static and unchanging. In reality, biomedical models are dynamic with respect to notions of how a particular disease is transmitted, who is at risk, and how that disease is prevented.

Consequently, future research needs to be flexible and expansive enough to adequately capture this diversity. The combination of magical contagion beliefs and biomedical responses to questions in Nemeroff et al.'s (1994) study highlights the importance of using well-designed instruments in quantitative studies. A significant risk is that respondents will be forced to choose from a narrow set of statements, which may not include, or only partially overlap with, their own understandings. Here, qualitative studies such as Padgett's (2002) play an important role. Flexible and innovative approaches, such as Nemeroff's (1995) use of drawings, are also useful methods of accessing implicit beliefs. Similarly, different theoretical approaches such as the use of analytical frameworks normally associated with the study of "traditional" cultures (e.g., "magical contagion") are also valuable for enabling the examination of a familiar culture from new perspectives.

We found very little research regarding lay conceptions about contagious diseases that are not transmitted sexually, although these investigations may be located within studies of the preventive behaviors associated with them, such as vaccination, and hence were less apparent during the literature search. In addition, we did not review books. We cannot assume that the categories in this review are meaningful for all diseases, although some of the findings, such as use of somatic cues and magical contagion, may have broader applications than others. As Nemeroff's (1994, 1995) studies seemed to indicate, casual contact theory to explain transmission may represent an undifferentiated understanding of infection. Alternatively, some types of casual contact (kissing, touching, and sharing drinking glasses) may indicate that individuals conflate the transmission route of one disease (e.g., the common cold) with others (e.g., HIV). More research is needed to understand whether individuals conceptualize different transmission processes for individual diseases or whether they categorize particular groups of diseases as being transmitted in similar ways, and so on. Moreover, future research is required to understand the precise mechanisms by which transmission is thought to occur, if indeed people have any notion of mechanisms. Despite the studies raising a range of factors associated with transmission, such as bodily fluids or poor hygiene, it was largely unclear whether the resulting disease was seen as emerging as a result of spontaneous transmission, the transfer of a physical germ, the host's specific susceptibility, or some other understanding.

Clearly, substantial work remains to be conducted. Several of the most fruitful articles discussed here are now more than a decade old. As can be seen from the research reviewed here, lay perceptions are not limited to marginal or uneducated groups. Nor should these perceptions be dismissed offhand as irrational or superficial. The visual cues used by many to identify illness or good health, for example, are logical considering the physical symptoms that often manifest as indicators of poor immunological function, although as we know this strategy is problematized by the asymptomatic features of some diseases. Respondents

across the studies talked intelligibly and thoughtfully about the logical strategies they employed and how these were often adapted or changed depending
on the specific context. They spoke reflexively about how their beliefs altered
or seemed less convincing in hindsight. As Plough and Krimsky (1987) have
noted, lay concepts of risk (in this case, contagion) may involve "cultural rationality," which is characterized by appeal to folk wisdom, peer groups, and traditions, where risks are personalized, and family and community emphasized.
Cultural rationality stands in contrast to "technical rationality," which rests on
explicitly defined sets of principles and scientific norms and on public health,
which involves aggregate measures of risk.

Understanding lay transmission beliefs is not simply an academic exercise.
The growth of super viruses and pandemics and the rising rates of STIs in
recent decades give lay transmission understandings, particularly those which
inadvertently increase the risk of infection, extra significance. Moreover,
there are social implications when individuals identify a person's riskiness
as occurring in ways that cause social stigma. However, applying normative
("right" or "wrong") logic to participants' responses is unhelpful for improving our understanding of how transmission beliefs operate. If future health
promotion attempts are to have a greater degree of success, policy makers need
to understand that they are dealing with critical consumers of information, whose
attitudes and behaviors are shaped by a range of social, cultural, emotional, and
intellectual factors. It is only once these factors are appreciated that efforts to
communicate with publics will have more relevance and meaning for them.

REFERENCES

Abbott-Chapman, J., Denholm, C., 1997. Adolescent risk taking and the romantic ethic: HIV/AIDS
    awareness among Year 11 and 12 students. Journal of Sociology 33 (3), 306–321.
Andre, T., Bormann, L., 1991. Knowledge of acquired immune deficiency syndrome and sexual
    responsibility among high school students. Youth and Society 22, 339–361.
Adam, B.D., Sears, A., Schellenberg, E.G., 2000. Accounting for unsafe sex: interviews with men
    who have sex with men. Journal of Sex Research 37 (1), 24–36.
Arce, A., Long, N., 1995. The dynamics of knowledge: Interfaces between bureaucrats and peas-
    ants. In: Long, N., Long, A. (Eds.), Battlefields of knowledge: The interlocking of theory and
    practice in social research and development. Routledge, London.
Bakopanos, C., Gifford, S.M., 2001. The changing ties that bind: issues surrounding sexuality and
    health for Greek parents and their Australian-born sons and daughters. Journal of Family Issues
    22 (3), 358–385.
Balshem, M., Oxman, G., van Rooyen, D., Girod, K., 1992. Syphilis, sex and crack cocaine: images
    of risk and morality. Social Science and Medicine 35 (2), 147–160.
Brown, E.J., Smith, F.B., Hill, M.A., 2007. HIV risk reduction in rural African American women
    who use cocaine. Women and Health 46 (2/3), 77–97.
Carrier, N., Laplante, J., Bruneau, J., 2005. Exploring the contingent reality of biomedicine:
    injecting drug users, hepatitis C virus and risk. Health, Risk and Society 7 (2), 123–140.
Comer, L.K., Nemeroff, C.J., 2000. Blurring emotional safety with physical safety in AIDS and
    STD risk estimations: the casual/regular partner distinction. Journal of Applied Social Psy-
    chology 30 (12), 2467–2490.

Crawford, J., Turtle, A., Kippax, S., 1990. Student-favoured strategies for AIDS avoidance. Australian Journal of Psychology 42 (2), 123–137.

Curtis, V., Biran, A., Deverell, K., Hughes, C., Bellamy, K., Drasar, B., 2003. Hygiene in the home: relating bugs and behaviour. Social Science and Medicine 57, 657–672.

Donovan, B., 1988. HIV transmission to a blood donor. Lancet 2 (8608), 452.

Douglas, M., 1996. Thought styles: Critical essays on good taste. Sage, London.

Douglas, M., 1966. Purity and danger: An analysis of concepts of pollution and taboo. Routledge, London.

Dow, M.G., Knox, M.D., 1991. Mental health and substance abuse staff: HIV/AIDS knowledge and attitudes. AIDS Care 3 (1), 75–87.

Downing-Matibag, T.M., Geisinger, B., 2009. Hooking up and sexual risk taking among college students: a health belief model perspective. Qualitative Health Research 19 (9), 1196–1209.

Elam, G., Macdonald, N., Hickson, F.C.I., Imrie, J., Power, R., McGarrigle, C.A., Fenton, K.A., Gilbart, V.L., Ward, H., Evans, B.G., on behalf of the INSIGHT Collaborative Research Team, 2008. Risky sexual behaviour in context: qualitative results from an investigation into risk factors for seroconversion among gay men who test for HIV. Sexually Transmitted Infections 84, 473–477.

Essien, E.J., Meshack, A.F., Ross, M.W., 2002. Misperceptions about HIV transmission among heterosexual African-American and Latino men and women. Journal of the National Medical Association 94 (5), 304–312.

Flood, M., 2003. Lust, trust and latex: why young heterosexual men do not use condoms. Culture, Health and Sexuality 5 (4), 353–369.

Frazer, J., 1959. The golden bough: A study in magic and religion (T.H. Gaster, Ed.). Macmillan, New York (original work published 1890).

Goodman, E., Cohall, A.T., 1989. Acquired immunodeficiency syndrome and adolescents: knowledge, attitudes, beliefs, and behaviors in a New York City adolescent minority population. Pediatrics 84 (1), 36–42.

Grove, K.A., Kelly, D.P., Liu, J., 1997. "But nice girls don't get it": women, symbolic capital, and the social construction of AIDS. Journal of Contemporary Ethnography 26 (3), 317–337.

Grunseit, A.C., Lupton, D., Crawford, J., Kippax, S., Noble, J., 1995. The country versus the city: differences between rural and urban tertiary students on HIV/AIDS knowledge, beliefs and attitudes. Australian Journal of Social Issues 30 (4), 389–404.

Guttman, N., Boccher-Lattimore, D., Salmon, C.T., 1998. Credibility of information from official sources on HIV/AIDS transmission. Public Health Reports 113 (5), 465–471.

Herek, G.M., Widaman, K.F., Capitanio, J.P., 2005. When sex equals AIDS: symbolic stigma and heterosexual adults' inaccurate beliefs about sexual transmission of AIDS. Social Problems 52 (1), 15–37.

Hobfoll, S.E., Jackson, A.P., Lavin, J., Britton, P.J., Shepherd, J.B., 1993. Safer sex knowledge, behaviour, and attitudes of inner-city women. Health Psychology 12 (6), 481–488.

Hoffman, V., Cohen, D., 1999. A night with Venus: partner assessments and high-risk sexual encounters. AIDS Care 11 (5), 555–566.

Jackson, A.D., McMenamin, J., Brewster, N., Ahmed, S., Reid, M.E., 2008. Knowledge of tuberculosis transmission among recently infected patients in Glasgow. Public Health 122, 1004–1012.

Lambert, N.L., Imrie, J., Fisher, M.J., Phillips, A., Watson, R., Dean, G., 2006. Making sense of syphilis: beliefs, behaviours and disclosure among gay men recently diagnosed with infectious syphilis and the implications for prevention. Sexual Health 3, 155–161.

Lamport, L.L., Andre, T., 1993. AIDS knowledge and sexual responsibility. Youth and Society 25 (1), 38–61.

Lawton, J., Ahmad, N., Peel, E., Hallowell, N., 2007. Contextualising accounts of illness: notions of responsibility and blame in white and South Asian respondents' accounts of diabetes causation. Sociology of Health and Illness 29 (6), 891–906.

LeBlanc, A.J., 1993. Examining HIV-related knowledge among adults in the U.S. Journal of Health and Social Behavior 34 (1), 23–36.

Lim, M.S.C., Hellard, M.E., Aitken, C.K., Hocking, J.S., 2007. Sexual-risk behaviour, self-perceived risk and knowledge of sexually transmissible infections among young Australians attending a music festival. Sexual Health 4 (1), 51–56.

Lowy, E., Ross, M.W., 1994. "It'll never happen to me": gay men's beliefs, perceptions and folk constructions of sexual risk. AIDS Education and Prevention 6 (6), 467–482.

Maskarinec, G., Gotay, C.C., Tatsumura, Y., Shumay, D.M., Kakai, H., 2001. Perceived cancer causes: use of complementary and alternative therapy. Cancer Practice 9 (4), 183–190.

Mauss, M. (R. Brain, translation), 1972. A general theory of magic. W. W. Norton, New York (original work published in 1902).

McDonald, M.A., Thomas, J.C., Eng, E., 2001. When is sex safe? Insiders' views on sexually transmitted disease prevention and treatment. Health Education and Behavior 28 (5), 624–642.

Nemeroff, C.J., 1995. Magical thinking about illness virulence: conceptions of germs from "safe" versus "dangerous" others. Health Psychology 14 (2), 147–151.

Nemeroff, C.J., Brinkman, A., Woodward, C.K., 1994. Magical contagion and AIDS risk perception in a college population. AIDS Education and Prevention 6 (3), 249–265.

Nemeroff, C., Rozin, P., 1994. The contagion concept in adult thinking in the United States: transmission of germs and of interpersonal influence. Ethos 22 (2), 158–186.

Okwumabua, J.O., Glover, V., Bolden, D., Edwards, S., 2001. Perspectives of low-income African Americans on syphilis and HIV: implications for prevention. Journal of Health Care for the Poor and Underserved 12 (4), 474–489.

Padgett, P., 2002. Folk constructions of syphilis in an African-American community in Houston, Texas. Culture, Health and Sexuality 4, 409–418.

Peart, R., Rosenthal, D., Moore, S., 1996. The heterosexual singles scene: putting danger into pleasure. AIDS Care 8 (3), 341–350.

Pérez-Stable, E.J., Sabogal, F., Otero-Sabogal, R., Hiatt, R.A., McPhee, S.J., 1992. Misconceptions about cancer among Latinos and Anglos. JAMA 268 (22), 3219–3223.

Plough, A., Krimsky, S., 1987. The emergence of risk communication studies: social and political context. Science, Technology and Human Values 12 (3/4), 4–10.

Plumridge, E.W., Chetwynd, S.J., Reed, A., Gifford, S.J., 1996. Patrons of the sex industry: perceptions of risk. AIDS Care 8, 405–416.

Power, J., McNair, R., Carr, S., 2009. Absent sexual scripts: lesbian and bisexual women's knowledge, attitudes and action regarding safer sex and sexual health information. Culture, Health and Sexuality 11 (1), 67–81.

Pryce, A., 2001. "The first thing I did when I came back from the clinic last week was change the sheets on the bed": contamination, penetration and resistance—Male clients in the VD clinic. Current Sociology 49 (3), 55–78.

Raman, L., Winer, G.A., 2002. Children's and adults' understanding of illness: evidence in support of a coexistence model. Genetic, Social, and General Psychology Monographs 128 (4), 325–355.

Richters, J., Hendry, O., Kippax, S., 2003. When safe sex isn't safe. Culture, Health and Sexuality 5 (1), 37–52.

Ridge, D.T., 2004. "It was an incredible thrill": the social meanings and dynamics of younger gay men's experiences of barebacking in Melbourne. Sexualities 7 (3), 259–279.

Roberts, C., Kippax, S., Spongberg, M., Crawford, J., 1996. "Going down": oral sex, imaginary bodies and HIV. Body and Society 2 (3), 107–124.

Rozin, P., Markwith, M., Nemeroff, C., 1992. Magical contagion beliefs and fear of AIDS. Journal of Applied Social Psychology 22 (14), 1081–1092.

Sibthorpe, B., 1992. The social construction of sexual relationships as a determinant of HIV risk perception and condom use among injection drug users. Medical Anthropology Quarterly 6 (3), 255–270.

Skidmore, D., Hayter, E., 2000. Risk and sex: ego-centricity and sexual behaviour in young adults. Health, Risk and Society 2 (1), 23–32.

Sobo, E.J., Zimet, G.D., Zimmerman, T., Cecil, H., 1997. Doubting the experts: AIDS misconceptions among runaway adolescents. Human Organization 56 (3), 311–320.

Strecher, V.J., Rosenstock, I.M., 1997. The Health Belief Model. In: Glanz, K., Lewis, F.M., Rimer, B.K. (Eds.), Health behavior and health education: Theory, research, and practice. Jossey-Bass, San Francisco.

Sullivan, M.L., Terry, R.L., 1998. Perceived virulence of germs from a liked versus disliked source: evidence of magical contagion. Journal of Adolescent Health 22 (4), 320–325.

Treloar, C., Fraser, S., 2004. Hepatitis C, blood and models of the body: new directions for public health. Critical Public Health 14 (4), 377–389.

Tylor, E.B., 1974. Primitive culture: Researches into the development of mythology, philosophy, religion, art, and custom. Gordon Press, New York (original work published in 1871).

Van de Ven, P., Turtle, A., Kippax, S., Crawford, J., French, J., 1996. Trends in heterosexual tertiary students' knowledge of HIV and intentions to avoid people who might have HIV. AIDS Care 8 (1), 43–54.

Washer, P., Joffe, H., Solberg, C., 2008. Audience readings of media messages about MRSA. Journal of Hospital Infection 70 (1), 42–47.

Watson, R., Crofts, N., Mitchell, C., Aitken, C., Hocking, J., Thompson, S., 1999. Risk factors for hepatitis C transmission in the Victorian population: a telephone survey. Australian and New Zealand Journal of Public Health 23 (6), 622–626.

Weiss, M.G., 2001. Cultural epidemiology: an introduction and overview. Anthropology and Medicine 8 (1), 5–29.

Wilson, R.P., Freeman, A., Kazda, M.J., Andrews, T.C., Berry, L., Vaeth, P.A.C., Victor, R.G., 2002. Lay beliefs about high blood pressure in a low- to middle-income urban African-American community: an opportunity for improving hypertension control. American Journal of Medicine 112 (1), 26–30.

Zimet, G.D., Sobo, E.J., Zimmerman, T., Jackson, J., Mortimer, J., Yanda, C.P., Lazebnik, R., 1995. Sexual behavior, drug use, and AIDS knowledge among midwestern runaways. Youth and Society 26 (4), 450–462.

Chapter 8

Context and Environment: The Value of Considering Lay Epidemiology

Anna Olsen[1] and Cathy Banwell[2]

[1]*The University of New South Wales, Sydney, Australia,* [2]*The Australian National University, Canberra, Australia*

I was angry because we tried to be really good and careful to not catch it ... everybody was warning each other ... it is something that doesn't affect me day to day that I know of. The symptoms are slow, similar to lots of other things. In some ways I am pleased that my body must be so good at dealing with viruses, these things just happen and then go away. I haven't had a hepatitis attack or a herpes attack after that first one ... I've become more aware of what I eat, and exercising and certainly making sure I have enough sleep. And whenever I see stuff about hep C I always try and read it, but nothing much happens. I met a guy who was having Interferon treatment and he looked shocking. He looked so bad. He was almost at the end and I remember ... He was stick thin ... and then when he said he doesn't even know whether it [hep C treatment] is going to be worth it ... But yeah, pretty much everybody I know has got hep C ... But out of all the people I know who have got hep C, none of them are sick. So, I don't know, it's just one of those things.

> Sally [pseudonym], 34 years old, injecting heroin and diagnosed
> with viral hepatitis C infection

Sally has a high school education and no formal biomedical training. She injects drugs and is therefore part of a group marginalized for their behaviors, depicted as irrational in their dependence on drugs, and dangerous to themselves and society. Yet, quite rationally and sensibly Sally describes being aware of the risks of hepatitis C viral (HCV) infection associated with injecting drug use as well as the high infection rates among her peers. She has assembled medical, statistical, and other "legitimate" knowledge along with her personal experiences and observations of the world to develop beliefs about patterns of HCV and related ill health. Most notably, her conclusions about HCV are rather fatalistic; HCV is "just one of those things." Sally observes that none of her friends is sick from HCV infection and that the current treatment with interferon is so difficult that it may not be "worth it."

When Culture Impacts Health. http://dx.doi.org/10.1016/B978-0-12-415921-1.00008-7

From a medical perspective, 3% of the world's population (over 170 million people) is chronically infected with HCV and the World Health Organization recognizes the disease as a global health problem. Approximately 60–70% of those infected will go on to develop chronic liver disease: 5–20% will develop cirrhosis and 1–5% will die from liver cancer or cirrhosis. HCV is currently the leading cause of liver transplant in Australia and the United States. Treatment is 50–80% effective (when the virus is no longer detected in the blood) (Cornberg et al., 2002), although very few Australians are accessing treatment.

There is some congruence between Sally's narrative and that of the biomedical experts. With respect to risk of infection and affected subpopulations, for example, both narratives echo the knowledge that in developed nations HCV predominantly occurs among people who inject drugs. However, the understandings diverge when it comes to the significance and consequence of infection. Sally perceives her risk of ill health from HCV to be relatively small. Her friends are not sick from the virus, which seems to just "sit there" without doing anything, but they get sick if they have treatment. In science and public health, Sally's views about risk of ill health are dealt with as myths that require health education and promotion strategies to increase her "knowledge." Is Sally's perspective founded in ignorance alone? In this chapter we explore the popular culture of HCV among the Australian subpopulation most affected—people who inject drugs—and discuss the interface between lay perspectives and official messages about the risks of contracting this disease and the harms associated with chronic infection. In particular, we elucidate the value of what is often referred to as "lay knowledge" and how it can be integrated into scientific knowledge to improve health care and health promotion.

METHODOLOGY AND METHOD

The quote at the start of this chapter is taken from a qualitative study designed to investigate the "lived experiences" of people with HCV. The emphasis of qualitative research is on the interpretative aspects of knowing and meaning making in human society (Denzin and Lincoln, 2000). Based in methodology that views social life as a complex process, qualitative researchers attempt to work out "how the things that people do make sense from their perspective" (Ezzy, 2002). Naturalistic, rather than experimental, qualitative inquiry is used to search for patterns in meanings, processes, and contexts that help us to explain "how" and "why" individual and social phenomena occur (Creswell, 1998). Qualitative researchers tend not to employ the a priori categories set within methods such as surveys, but investigate participants' narratives, actions, ideas, and histories as a method for inductively testing and building theory. Qualitative research can expose associations between the social, economic, and political aspects of peoples' lives and the contexts in which their experiences occur (Liamputtong and Ezzy, 2005). Data (spoken, written, observed, etc.) are used to build explanations of human behavior and social phenomena at the level of meaning rather than cause.

The qualitative interview research we draw on here is one component of a stream of inquiry that has, over the years, alternated approaches and methods to build a detailed and nuanced picture of the lives of women with HCV. The result of this work is complementary datasets from both qualitative and quantitative methods. The first project was a small in-depth interview-based study of women with HCV. The interview data provided linguistic terms and research categories for a later survey in which 462 women completed a self-administered questionnaire about diagnosis with and symptoms of HCV along with questions about general health and personal relationships. Some of the findings about health and relationships from the survey were not easily interpreted without context and we followed up the survey with another qualitative study designed to explore some of the "why" questions about women's experiences. In-depth, semistructured interviews were conducted with 109 Australian women living with HCV. We were interested in the ways women constructed their narratives about living with HCV infection and how it related to other aspects of their health, relationships, and socioeconomic status. Among other analyses, we examined the ways in which risk of HCV infection and ill health was "socially produced" (Rhodes and Treloar, 2008) by people who use drugs through shared meanings and context. That is, the shared ways in which people who inject drugs perceive HCV risk.

EPIDEMIOLOGY AND RISK

While qualitative research looks for patterns in human narrative, discourse, and behavior in groups of people, epidemiology looks for patterns in disease in populations. Epidemiology, as the study of the distribution and determinants of diseases (Shenker, 1997), has contributed significantly to the development and evolution of the science of risk and the meaning of risk in health discourse. Although epidemiologists stress that the identification of risk factors cannot prove causation, the field has been criticized for turning away from socioenvironmental investigations of population health toward individualized disease causation models (Rothman et al., 1998) and for its focus on behavioral and lifestyle risk factors at the individual level (Pearce, 1996; Shy, 1997). Critics allege that epidemiologists have become hindered by statistical measures and molecular determinants at the individual level rather than underlying and societal determinants of disease (Shy, 1997). Increasingly epidemiologists and, more broadly health science researchers, are being questioned about their focus on isolated risk factors that disconnect individuals from their social context (Popay et al., 1998).

Problematizing Risk

The concept of risk has arguably brought about one of the greatest transformations in twentieth century public health and preventive medicine and the identification of risk factors is now a common method used in the recognition and prevention of disease. Epistemological and ontological criticisms, however, bring into question our reliance on the concept of risk and our assumption that risk is an impartial tool of science (Beck, 1992; Petersen and Lupton, 1996; Shoveller and Johnson, 2006). Before the era of modernity, notes Lupton (1999), risk was a neutral term used to indicate probabilities, with losses and gains. Today, the term risk is interchangeable with danger or hazard and is increasingly ideologically loaded and complex (Lupton, 1993). Beck (1992), one of the most influential thinkers on risk, wrote that risks can be "changed, magnified, dramatised or minimised within knowledge, and to that extent they are particularly *open to social definition and construction.*" These modern critics of risk theory do not necessarily deny the reality of hazards, but draw attention to the role of perception and social context, including the ways in which "experts" also engage in cultural and moral beliefs systems when being scientific about risk (Douglas, 1992).

At its most basic, risk theory assumes a shared rationality with risk avoidance (Rhodes, 2002a). Rational decision making has become synonymous with risk avoidance such that individuals' failure to recognize and respond to "known" risks is often portrayed as ignorance, irrationality, or a cultural failing (Douglas, 1992; Crawford, 1994). If behaving in a way deemed "risky" by the experts, one can then be blamed for this behavior, thereby displacing contextual factors and making socially unacceptable particular ways of living (Lupton, 1993). Attempts to remedy ignorance or modify beliefs have become a ubiquitous public health strategy. Educational initiatives based on biomedicine and the science of risk, it is assumed, will change individual's behaviors once they are made aware of the dangers. The success of individual behavioral change is limited, not in least because it fails to capture the "contradictory and situated pressures of risk decision-making and obscures power inequalities in risk negotiation" (Rhodes, 2002a).

Lay Epidemiology

In contrast to simplistic risk behavior theory there is a long-standing academic tradition in the social sciences "assuming that behavior that may otherwise be difficult to understand is indeed rational within particular cultural contexts" (Lawlor et al., 2003). Often referred to as "lay epidemiology," researchers use real-world examples to show the contextual rationality of many "non-scientific" perceptions of risk (Davison et al., 1989). The study of lay epidemiology looks at the ways "in which individuals interpret health risks through the routine observation and discussion of cases of illness and death in personal networks and the public arena, as well as from formal and informal evidence arising from other sources, such as television and magazines" (Finfgeld-Connett et al., 2012). This research not only highlights the social construction of health terminology and beliefs, it legitimizes nonexpert knowledge about the world.

The Risk: Hepatitis C

In this chapter we are using HCV as a case study through which to examine the intersections of scientific knowledge and cultural attitudes and practices. The association between injecting drug use and HCV transmission is well supported in the epidemiological and biomedical literature. A number of biological factors have contributed to the high prevalence of HCV among people who inject drugs including the high infectivity of the virus, high existing prevalence of HCV infection, and the efficacy of transmission via pierced or open skin (Thomas et al., 2000). Behaviorally, the sharing of needles and syringes as well other drug preparation equipment has been linked to HCV infection (Hagan et al., 2001; Maher et al., 2006). Research also suggests that among people who inject drugs, knowledge about the mechanisms of HCV transmission, biomedical aspects of the disease, and treatment can be poor (Rhodes et al., 2004; Southgate et al., 2005; O'Brien et al., 2008).

Nevertheless, our research and that of others reveal that perceptions of HCV within this group are more closely associated with that of scientists than often assumed. In particular, it is now well known among Australian people who inject drugs that they are at high risk of acquiring HCV (O'Brien et al., 2008) especially when sharing injecting equipment (Maher et al., 1998). This suggests that people who inject drugs have incorporated some medical and epidemiological concepts of HCV status into their understandings of the infection. This knowledge is evident in Sally's narrative at the start of the chapter.

Still, the connotations of what it means to have a high prevalence of HCV in this population are not necessarily shared between lay and expert perspectives. While the mainstream view of HCV advises that it is a serious disease with the potential to disable and kill, recent research suggests that the disease is perceived as relatively "normal" among people who inject drugs across Australia, the UK, and North America (Rhodes et al., 2004; Wozniak et al., 2007). That is, a concept of risk has emerged where HCV infection is acknowledged and accepted as relatively normal or expected. Some people who inject drugs have come to "face the possibility of HCV infection with a complex sense of inevitability" (Davis et al., 2004).

Lay Epidemiology: Providing Context

Undoubtedly useful information in the fight against HCV epidemics, these biological, behavioral, and attitudinal factors gain further validity when interpreted alongside investigations of the complex environmental and social processes involved in population health. Beyond "risk behaviors" (such as illicit drug injecting practices), complex "risk environments" (Rhodes, 2002b) have been documented and described by social researchers as a way of exploring the social, cultural, political, and economic conditions that result in certain groups being more vulnerable to the consequences of risk (Farmer, 1988).

This approach encourages a focus on the interactions between risk factors exogenous to the individual, rather than simply researching endogenous factors (e.g., age, sex, race, or genetic composition), risk practices (e.g., sharing of needles and syringes, or unprotected sex), or pathogenic characteristics (e.g., HCV genetics or infectiousness) (Strathdee et al., 2010). Helping to guide the measurement and interpretation of epidemics and other patterning of disease, an environmental perspective allows for more complex accounts of health and illness across society as well as the investigation of how structural and sociocultural factors act as determinants of health (Marmot, 2000).

One avenue for developing more complex, environmental approaches is to recognize and investigate lay knowledge as a form of "expert" knowledge. The primary conclusion of many investigations of lay epidemiology suggests that the nonexpert perception "is considerably more sophisticated than is generally appreciated by health educators" (Finfgeld-Connett et al., 2012). Part of the inherent sophistication within lay epidemiology comes from the lived experience and insights into the milieu in which people are, to varying degrees, "at risk" of ill health. It reflects the practical knowledge and cultural identity of subpopulations.

In our study sample, for example, most women revealed that they had not only been "at risk" of HCV infection but a whole myriad of health and social issues. They regularly raised topics related to socioeconomic stress including homelessness, unemployment, lack of regular income, mental health, drug dependence, child custody issues, and prison. Their narratives contained important information about complex webs of vulnerability, marginalization, and poverty that suggested a certain lack of control over health and life circumstances. The illegal and stigmatized nature of drug injection including policing, organized crime, concerns about overdose, violence, drug withdrawal, access to money, homelessness, fear, and shame create an environment in which choices are constrained and individuals are disadvantaged (Maher, 2002; Moore and Dietze, 2005). These are all factors that compete with HCV prevention for priority in the lives of people who inject drugs (Harris et al., 2011) and often cannot be well understood without insight into lived experience of the environment.

Considering Context: Lay Building on Expert Knowledge, Expert Building on Lay Knowledge

Epidemiology has enabled a growth in knowledge and understanding of the HCV epidemic including contributing to public health policy and community action. It has not, however, facilitated a full understanding why a particular subpopulation of people report that *"pretty much everybody I know has got hep C"* or how we can stem the epidemic. An overreliance on behavioral and microlevel risk factors in the individual has obscured the contribution of social and environmental conditions, particularly the hard-to-measure effects of social inequality (Israel et al., 1998). The future of HCV prevention among people who inject drugs to a large extent depends upon the degree to which behavioral education is nested within programs aimed at alleviating social and economic inequality (Rhodes et al., 2005).

We have discussed in this chapter one avenue for enhancing our understandings of determinants of health beyond the individual—lay epidemiology. In making use of the knowledge that emerges from lived experience, epidemiologists, and public health researchers more broadly, have the opportunity to create more situated health care responses to diseases like HCV (Busby et al., 1997). This includes challenging the power imbalance within public health where conservative epidemiology is favored over social science or mixed-methods approaches, which can more comprehensively address ecological understandings of the distribution of health and disease (Rhodes, 2002a).

Accessing and synthesizing lay and expert knowledge, however, is not easy or straightforward and requires research inputs and theoretical understandings from epidemiology, anthropology, public health, and other disciplines. Multidisciplinary approaches expand traditional epidemiological notions of risk and vulnerability to construct more nuanced descriptions of human behavior and more contextually situated interventions. These include epidemiological techniques and social science theories and methods that can be used more effectively to investigate the ways in which disease often spreads along lines of social structure (Trostle and Sommerfeld, 1996). Many different interdisciplinary frameworks, including collaborations between the "lay" and the "expert," contribute to developing an understanding of disease patterns as social processes.

REFERENCES

Beck, U., 1992. Risk society: Towards a new modernity. Sage Publications, London.

Busby, H., Williams, G., Rogers, A., 1997. Bodies of knowledge: lay and biomedical understandings of musculoskeletal disorders. Sociology of Health & Illness 19, 79–99.

Cornberg, M., Wedemyer, H., Manns, M., 2002. Treatment of chronic hepatitis C with pegylated interferon and ribavirin. Current Gastroenterology Reports 4, 23–30.

Crawford, R., 1994. The boundaries of the self and the unhealthy other: reflections on health, culture and AIDS. Social Science & Medicine 38, 1347–1365.

Creswell, J.W., 1998. Qualitative inquiry and research design: Choosing among five traditions. Sage, Thousand Oaks, California.

Davis, M., Rhodes, T., Martin, A., 2004. Preventing hepatitis C: 'common sense', 'the bug' and other perspectives from the risk narratives of people who inject drugs. Social Science and Medicine 59, 1807–1818.

Davison, C., Frankel, S., Davey Smith, G., 1989. Inheriting heart trouble: the relevance of common-sense ideas to preventative measures. Health Education Research 4, 329–340.

Denzin, N.K., Lincoln, Y.S., 2000. The discipline and practice of qualitative research. In: Denzin, N.K., Lincoln, Y.S. (Eds.), Handbook of qualitative research, second ed. Sage, Thousand Oaks, California.

Douglas, M., 1992. Risk and blame: Essays in cultural theory. Russell Sage Foundation, New York.

Ezzy, D., 2002. Qualitative analysis: Practice and innovation. Allen & Unwin, Crows Nest.

Farmer, P., 1988. Bad blood, spoiled milk: bodily fluids as moral barometers in rural haiti. American Ethnologist 15, 62–83.

Finfgeld-Connett, D., Bloom, T.L., Johnson, E.D., 2012. Perceived competency and resolution of homelessness among women with substance abuse problems. Qualitative Health Research 22, 416–427.

Hagan, H., Thiede, H., Weiss, N., Hopkins, S., Duchin, J., Alexander, E., 2001. Sharing of drug preparation equipment as a risk factor for hepatitis C. American Journal of Public Health 91, 42–46.

Harris, M., Treloar, C., Maher, L., 2011. Staying Safe From Hepatitis C: engaging with multiple priorities. Qualitative Health Research 21, 31–42.

Israel, B.A., Schulz, A.J., Parker, E.A., Becker, A.B., 1998. Review of community-based research: assessing partnership approaches to improve public health. Annual Review of Public Health 19, 173–202.

Lawlor, D., Frankel, S., Shaw, M., Ebrahim, S., Davey Smith, G., 2003. Smoking and ill health: does lay epidemiology explain the failure of smoking cessation programs among deprived populations? American Journal of Public Health 93, 266–270.

Liamputtong, P., Ezzy, D., 2005. Qualitative research methods. Oxford University Press, Melbourne.

Lupton, D., 1993. Risk as moral danger: the social and political functions of risk discourse in public health. International Journal of Health Services 23, 425–435.

Lupton, D., 1999. Introduction: Risk and sociocultural theory. In: Lupton, D. (Ed.), Risk and sociocultural theory: New directions and perspectives, Cambridge University Press, Cambridge, UK.

Maher, L., 2002. Don't leave us this way: ethnography and injecting drug use in the age of AIDS. International Journal of Drug Policy 13, 311–325.

Maher, L., Dixon, D., Hall, W., Lynskey, M., 1998. Running the risks: Heroin, health and harm in South West Sydney. National Drug and Alcohol Research Centre, University of New South Wales, Sydney, NSW.

Maher, L., Jalaludin, B., Chant, K.G., Jayasuriya, R., Sladden, T., Kaldor, J.M., Sargent, P.L., 2006. Incidence and risk factors for hepatitis C seroconversion in injecting drug users in Australia. Addiction 101, 1499–1508.

Marmot, M., 2000. Social determinants of health: from observation to policy. Medical Journal of Australia 172, 379–382.

Moore, D., Dietze, P., 2005. Enabling environments and the reduction of drug-related harm: re-framing Australian policy and practice. Drug and Alcohol Review 24, 275–284.

O'Brien, S., Day, C., Black, E., Dolan, K., 2008. Injecting drug users' understanding of hepatitis C. Addictive Behaviours 33, 1602–1605.

Pearce, N., 1996. Traditional epidemiology, modern epidemiology, and public health. American Journal of Public Health 86, 678–683.

Petersen, A., Lupton, D., 1996. The new public health: Health and self in the age of risk. Allen & Unwin, St Leonards, New South Wales.

Popay, J., Williams, G., Thomas, C., Gatrell, A., 1998. Theorising inequalities in health: the place of lay knowledge. Sociology of Health and Illness 20, 619–644.

Rhodes, T., 2002a. The 'risk environment': a framework for understanding and reducing drug-related harm. International Journal of Drug Policy 13, 85–94.

Rhodes, T., 2002b. The 'risk environment': a framework for understanding and reducing drug-related harm. International Journal of Drug Policy 13, 85–94.

Rhodes, T., Davis, M., Judd, A., 2004. Hepatitis C and its risk management among drug injectors in London: renewing harm reduction in the context of uncertainty. Addiction 99, 621–633.

Rhodes, T., Singer, M., Bourgois, P., Friedman, S.R., Strathdee, S.A., 2005. The social structural production of HIV risk among injecting drug users. Social Science and Medicine 61, 1026–1044.

Rhodes, T., Treloar, C., 2008. The social production of hepatitis C risk among injecting drug users: a qualitative synthesis. Addiction 103, 1593–1603.

Rothman, K.J., Adami, H.O., Trichopoulos, D., 1998. Should the mission of epidemiology include the eradication of poverty? Lancet 352, 810–813.

Shenker, M., 1997. Biostatistics and Epidemiology. In: LaDou, J. (Ed.), Occupational and Environmental Medicine, Appleton Lange, California.

Shoveller, J.A., Johnson, J.L., 2006. Risky groups, risky behaviour, and risky persons: Dominating discourses on youth sexual health. Critical Public Health 16, 47–60.

Shy, C., 1997. The failure of academic epidemiology: witness for the prosecution. American Journal of Epidemiology 145, 479–484.

Southgate, E., Weatherall, A., Day, C., Dolan, K., 2005. What's in a virus? Folk understandings of hepatitis C infection and infectiousness among injecting drug users in Kings Cross, Sydney. International Journal for Equity in Health 4, 5.

Strathdee, S., Hallett, T., Bobrova, N., Rhodes, T., Booth, R., Abdool, R., Hankins, C., 2010. HIV and risk environment for injecting drug users: the past, present, and future. Lancet 376, 268–284.

Thomas, D.L., Astemborski, J., Rai, R.M., Anania, F.A., Schaeffer, M., Galai, N., Vlahov, D., 2000. The natural history of hepatitis C virus infection: host, viral, and environmental factors. Journal of the American Medical Association 284, 450–456.

Trostle, J.A., Sommerfeld, J., 1996. Medical anthropology and epidemiology. Annual Review of Anthropology 25, 253–274.

Wozniak, L., Prakash, M., Taylor, M., Wild, C., 2007. Everybody's got it, but situational and strategic participation in normalized HCV discourse among injection drug users in Edmonton, Canada. International Journal of Drug Policy 18, 388–396.

Chapter 9

Identity, Social Position, Well-Being, and Health: Insights from Australians Living with Hearing Loss

Anthony Hogan,[1] Katherine J. Reynolds,[2] and Don Byrne[2]

[1]*School of Sociology, The Australian National University, Canberra, Australia,* [2]*Department of Psychology, The Australian National University, Canberra, Australia*

THE SOCIAL EPIDEMIOLOGY OF HEARING LOSS

Hearing loss is a very common phenomenon in the Australian community, with 22% of the population having measurable hearing impairment (Wilson et al., 1992, 1999). This prevalence increases with age with 59% of people aged over 60 years having measurable hearing loss. Notably, hearing loss in itself is not a disease, even if at times the impairment itself may result from disease processes, or processes which for the convenience of the legal system (e.g., persistent exposure to long-term noise at work) are deemed to be disease processes (P. Niall, personal communication). Living with hearing loss has been associated with poorer physical and mental health outcomes (Hogan et al., 2001, 2009) and is ranked eighth in terms of burden of disease in Australia (Begg et al., 2008). Nonetheless, living with hearing loss has been identified as an underestimated public health problem (Wilson et al., 1992).

This chapter commences with a review of the literature on health outcomes for people living with hearing loss, addressing research on physical and mental health as well as health-related quality of life (HRQoL). It then applies insights from social psychology to interrogate why people living with hearing loss endure the ensuing health outcomes. To this end we consider the extent to which stressors arising from a contested communicative environment and social identity may contribute to the morbidity experienced by this cohort.

When Culture Impacts Health. http://dx.doi.org/10.1016/B978-0-12-415921-1.00009-9

HEARING LOSS AND PHYSICAL HEALTH

Men with uncorrected hearing loss have been reported to have a higher comparative mortality rate than the population (Apollonio et al., 1996), elevated risk rates for diabetes (Mitchell, 2002), high blood pressure (Wilson et al., 1992), a higher incidence of stroke (Mitchell, 2002), increased rates of heart attack (Hogan et al., 2001), and higher use of prescribed medications (Wilson et al., 1992). Those with moderate to severe hearing loss are three times more likely to see their doctor than members of the general population (Wilson et al., 1992), up to seven times more likely to require assistance in the home (Wilson et al., 1992), and fifteen times more likely to need assistance in activities of daily living (Wilson et al., 1992). It is not readily apparent from the literature why it is that microscopic damage to hair cells within the cochlea could be associated with such poor health outcomes. Preliminary consultations among general practitioners identified the possibility that concurrent disease processes (e.g., microvascular disease) may explain some of the comorbidities associated with hearing loss (B. Wu et al., unpublished observations). However, while such an outcome is mechanistically possible, a preliminary examination of available data suggests that this is not generally the case. Hogan et al. (2010) have demonstrated that the extent of cardiovascular disease (including diabetes, heart disease, heart attack, angina, and hypertension) associated with hearing loss only accounted for 10.1% of the primary health conditions reported by people with hearing loss. Moreover, disorders of the ear were identified as a primary condition reported by more than one-third of respondents, as were high levels of noise exposure. A more comprehensive explanation of the causal mechanisms, which underpin hearing and health outcomes, is therefore required.

HEARING LOSS AND MENTAL HEALTH

Studies consistently report that people with hearing loss experience varying degrees of psychological distress (Thomas, 1984; Rutman, 1989; Eriksson-Mangold and Carlsson, 1991; Hogan et al., 2009; Australian Senate, 2010). The literature notes that stress, anxiety, loss of security, depression, loneliness, low self-confidence, shame, and anger are commonly associated with living with hearing loss (Dye and Peak, 1983; Andersson et al., 1995; Hetu, 1996; Scherer and Frisina, 1998; Borg et al., 2002; Espmark et al., 2002; Kent, 2003; Tambs, 2004; Monzani et al., 2008; Lindley, 2009; Saunders and Griest, 2009). People with hearing loss notably report increased rates of affective mood disorders and poorer social relations (Mulrow et al., 1990; Ihara, 1993) and increased rates of psychiatric disorder, particularly those rating their hearing as poor (Hogan et al., 2001). Prima facie evidence then points to a possible connection between mental health, hearing, and more general health outcomes. However, such a position is also contested by studies that have critically reviewed the design and conclusions of such research (Rutman, 1989; Hogan et al., 2012). Methodologically,

Hogan et al. (2012) demonstrated that many papers associating hearing loss with mental illness are qualitative in nature. Second, they observed that most papers identifying adverse mental health outcomes are not based on an epidemiology of mental illness, but are based on generic measures of quality of life readily influenced by expectable problems associated with hearing loss, for example, fatigue from having to concentrate on conversation while under social pressure and relational conflict due to misunderstandings. As such, the work of Hogan et al. (2012) provided a substantiation of Rutman's (1989) early work in this field, where the relationship between hearing and relational conflict was first observed.

Notably across this literature, the fear and consequences of stigma are identified as central to the onset of these conditions (Hallberg and Carlsson, 1991; Hetu and Getty, 1991; Hogan, 2001; Gagné et al., 2009). Taking into account the psychosocial effects of stigma, Hogan et al. (2011) have argued that acquired hearing loss can disrupt existing interpersonal social relations and threaten social identity and status. Stigma and identity concerns can create psychological barriers that lead to denial and inhibit people from accepting the help that they need, even if not getting help poses disadvantages to their well-being.

Bringing this research together it becomes evident that a series of psychosocial factors are associated with living with hearing loss:

1. A highly stigmatized condition (Hogan, 1992; Hetu, 1996; St Claire and He, 2009; Hogan, 2012)
2. An associated fear of being stigmatized (Hetu and Getty, 1991)
3. Reluctance to acknowledge difficulties (Hetu and Getty, 1991)
4. Misperceiving the social effects of hearing loss as breakdowns in relationships (Hetu and Getty, 1991)
5. Misattributing reduced social contact due to hearing difficulties to changes in lifestyle preferences (Hetu and Getty, 1991)
6. A subsequent threat to social identity (Hogan et al., 2011).

HEARING LOSS AND HRQoL

Over the past 10 years two population studies have reported an association between hearing-related social participation difficulties and reduced HRQoL, using the SF 36 (Hogan et al., 2001, 2009). A threshold effect between HRQoL and communication difficulty (i.e., increasing communication disability as distinct from level of impaired hearing) has been observed. That is, up to a certain degree of communication difficulty, no health effect was found to be present, but after a certain degree of communication strain, health effects became evident (Hogan et al., 2001, 2009). Controlling for age, gender, and comorbidities, these studies reported a threshold effect associated with increasing communication difficulties and health, even when respondents were using hearing aids. The effect is presented in Figure 9.1. We observe that the pattern in the data is highly consistent with Cummins' (2010)

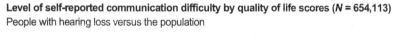

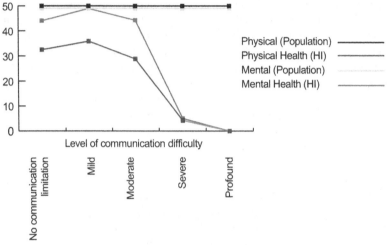

FIGURE 9.1 Level of self-reported communication difficulty by quality of life scores (*N* = 654,113) (Hogan et al., 2009).

threshold effect model of the effects of sustained stress on social well-being (see Figure 9.1).

The most adverse health effects of hearing-related communication difficulty are evident in the relatively small population of people with severe to profound hearing loss. However, the magnitude of the burden of disease associated with hearing loss is being generated by the very large numbers of aging people with mild to moderate hearing loss.

Bringing these respective insights together Hogan et al. (2009) argued that the stressors resulting from communicating with impaired hearing, in difficult communication environments, underpinned poorer health outcomes. Developing this insight we argue that when the social inclusion needs of people with hearing loss are not taken into account, contested social identity results, and this experience is associated with a psychologically reactive and physiologically damaging pathway:

1. As a result of problematic social encounters (such as those that may produce a fear of stigmatization or a sense of threatened identity), hearing loss becomes a salient psychological issue for the person concerned.
2. The individual spontaneously puts in place *ad hoc* and typically counterproductive coping strategies (reluctance to acknowledge hearing difficulties, avoiding problematic social encounters, bluffing, passing, minimizing, denial, etc.).

3. The psychosocially demanding situations become psychologically charged and are evidenced in undermanaged and unacknowledged stress, affective mood disorders, other psychiatric disorders, and poorer social relations.

4. In addition to relational distress, the individual's response to these psychologically charged situations results in the stimulation of the sympathetic nervous system.

5. The sympathetic nervous system is stimulated, for example, by fear responses associated with possible stigmatization, while anxiety responses to a sense of threatened identity activate the cortisol response.

6. This reaction cycle is repeated every time the individual faces the same or similarly psychologically charged social situations resulting in a chronic condition of overstimulation.

7. Chronic overstimulation results in additional morbidity.

This model aligns well with Cummins (2010, p. 1), who proposed a model of subjective well-being (SWB), which argues the following:

each person has a "set-point" for personal wellbeing that is internally maintained and defended (…). The provision of personal resources, such as money or relationships, cannot normally increase the set-point (but …) can strengthen defences against negative experience. Moreover, for someone who is facing homeostatic defeat, the provision of additional resources may allow them to regain control of wellbeing. In this case the provision of resources will cause personal wellbeing to rise until the set-point is achieved. Low levels of personal resources, such as occasioned by low income or absence of a partner, weakens homeostasis. If personal challenges such as stress or pain exceed resources, homeostasis is defeated, and subjective wellbeing decreases below its normal range.

Cummins (2010) argued that individuals can sustain their sense of SWB over time in the face of specific stressors. In the face of shorter term and even significant life stressors people can bounce back or be resilient. However, Cummins and colleagues argued that a threshold point exists with regards to the intensity and potential duration of persistent stressors, such that an individual's well-being breaks down. Their model is depicted in Figure 9.2.

Interestingly, further work on Cummins' model (O'Brien et al., 2012) shows that within the construct of SWB, strong connections with others are directly related to feelings of self-efficacy. Hogan et al. (2012) argued, however, that when faced with the threat of being stigmatized, to seemingly protect themselves individuals (to differing degrees) disconnect from their social supports, therein reducing their coping or adaptive capacity. The association between exposure to chronic stressors, such as stigma, social isolation, and subsequent social disconnection, results in poorer health outcomes. The key determinant of stress derives from the "fit" between the individual's characteristics and the perceived and objective demands of the environment. Stress is higher and

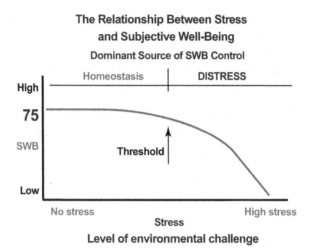

FIGURE 9.2   The relationship between stress and SWB (Cummins, 2010).

well-being lower where the fit between the person's coping capacity and environmental demands is poor.

ENHANCING THE WELL-BEING OF PEOPLE WITH HEARING LOSS

Hearing aids are inherently offered as the primary if not only intervention for people with hearing loss. The use of hearing aids has been shown to significantly improve HRQoL by as much as 50% (Hogan et al., 2001, 2009). However, significant international studies show that as many as 40% of people choose not to regularly use their devices (Smeeth et al., 2002) and 41% report dissatisfaction (Chisolm et al., 2007) with them. These problems occur for four basic reasons. First, hearing aids are essentially microphones with limited capacity to effectively manage the competing sound inputs that people with hearing loss require. Inherently, people with hearing loss simultaneously need assistance hearing high-frequency sounds (the sibilant sounds) while also hearing low-frequency sounds at normal levels. The most common problem people have is hearing conversational speech (containing lots of soft sounds that need amplification) in noisy settings. Background noises are typically low-frequency sounds. These *thicker*, low-frequency background noises easily drown out softer (*thinner*) high-frequency sounds, which make speech clear. Device manufacturers struggle with the design of devices that can both amplify the soft "voice" sounds people need to hear without also amplifying the less helpful background noises. While device manufacturers are making progress in addressing this problem, most device users will complain that they cannot hear in background noise, particularly when using devices.

Second, damage to the auditory pathway may mean that a person can no longer easily select out or focus on the sounds he or she wants to hear over other background sounds. Third, and most significantly, despite people with hearing loss constituting a significant social group, advocacy groups have enjoyed little success in securing a renegotiation of the social construction of communication. Notably though, early first signs of change are becoming evident as more and more baby boomers enter the critical age of having impaired hearing. Increasingly, acoustic treatments are being introduced to public spaces including hotels, restaurants, and airport lounges. Such treatments reduce reverberation and in turn reduce background noise. For the small number of people with hearing loss who use hearing devices, auditory access is becoming more possible at banks, cinemas, and government agencies through the increasing availability of hearing loop systems. Such systems cut out background noise by providing a signal from the speaker directly into a person's hearing aid—a closed circuit communication system if you will.

However, for social change to be truly effective, a shift is required in the way people interact so that people with hearing loss can socially participate without being stigmatized. Hogan et al. (2011) argued that social change needs to occur to group-based communicative norms, which underpin the way family and friends interact with each other on a daily basis. Such simple changes to social communication (e.g., reducing background noise, ensuring we face each other when speaking, etc.) within a person's immediate social network can provide the social support and practical solutions needed to minimize psychological distress. These efforts also can create a pool of people who are capable of mobilizing in the interests of broader destigmatization and social change.

METHODS USED IN THIS CHAPTER

A series of research methods underpins the material reported in this chapter. The preliminary insight that social factors were contributing to poor health outcomes arose from consultations with people with hearing loss in community settings. The second insight on this issue arose from a systematic review of the published literature, which in turn was extended through epidemiological analysis of population health data where outcomes for people with hearing loss were included in the study. Third, practical questioning was applied to the outcomes of the data, namely, questioning the extent to which current explanations of hearing and well-being logically fitted with the data as compared with the experiences of people living with hearing loss (see, for example, Australian Senate, 2010). Since existing interpretations were found wanting, it was necessary to return to the literature to examine how adverse health effects of living with other social stressors were understood. Notably, Mills' (1970) essential sociological question was brought to bear on the problem: Were these outcomes the unique problem of certain individuals or was there a more systemic social explanation available as to what was causing these problems? For full documentation of the research methods underpinning this chapter the reader is referred to Hogan (2012).

REFERENCES

Andersson, G., Melin, L., Lindberg, P., Scott, B., 1995. Dispositional optimism, dysphoria, health, and coping with hearing impairment in elderly adults. International Journal of Audiology 34 (2), 76–84.

Apollonio, I., Carabellese, C., Frattola, L., Trabucchi, M., 1996. Effects of sensory aids on the quality of life and mortality of elderly people - A multivariate analysis. Age and Ageing 25 (2), 89–96.

Australian Senate, 2010. Hear us! Inquiry into hearing and health in Australia. Parliament House, Canberra.

Begg, S.J., Vos, T., Barker, B., Stanley, L., Lopez, A.D., 2008. Burden of disease and injury in Australia in the new millennium: measuring health loss from diseases, injuries and risk factors. Medical Journal of Australia 188 (1), 36–40.

Borg, E., Danermark, B., Borg, B., 2002. Behavioural awareness, interaction and counselling education in audiological rehabilitation: development of methods and application in a pilot study. International Journal of Audiology 41, 308–322.

Chisolm, T.H., Johnson, C.E., Danhauer, J.L., Portz, L.J.P., Abrams, H.B., Lesner, S., McCarthy, P.A., Newman, C.W., 2007. A systematic review of health-related quality of life and hearing aids: final report of the American academy of audiology task force on the health-related quality of life benefits of amplification in adults. Journal of the American Academy of Audiology 18 (2), 151–183.

Cummins, R.A., 2010. Subjective wellbeing, homeostatically protected mood and depression: a synthesis. Journal of Happiness Studies 11, 1–17.

Dye, C., Peak, M.F., 1983. Influence of amplification on the psychosocial functioning of older adults with neurosensory hearing loss. Journal of the Academy of Rehabilitative Audiology 16, 210–220.

Eriksson-Mangold, M., Carlsson, S.G., 1991. Psychological and somatic distress in relation to perceived hearing disability, hearing handicap, and hearing measurements. Journal of Psychosomatic Research 35 (6), 729–740.

Espmark, A.K.K., Rosenhall, U., Erlandsson, S., Steen, B., 2002. The two faces of presbyacusis: hearing impairment and psychosocial consequences [Los dos rostros de la presbiacusia: impedimento auditivo y consecuencias psicosociales]. International Journal of Audiology 41 (2), 125–135.

Gagné, J.-P., Southall, K., Jennings, M.B., 2009. The psychological effects of social stigma: Applications to people with an acquired hearing loss. In: Montano, J., Spitzer, J. (Eds.), Adult Audiologic Rehabilitation, Plural, San Diego, CA, pp. 63–91.

Hallberg, L.R.M., Carlsson, A.G., 1991. A qualitative study of strategies for managing a hearing impairment. British Journal of Audiology 25, 201–211.

Hetu, R., 1996. The stigma attached to hearing impairment. Scandinavian Audiology 24 (43), 12–24.

Hetu, R., Getty, L., 1991. Development of a rehabilitation program for people affected with occupational hearing loss. 1. A new paradigm. Audiology 30, 305–316.

Hogan, A., 1992. Rehabilitation for workers with noise-induced hearing loss. University of Wollongong, New South Wales, Australia, Master's thesis.

Hogan, A., Taylor, A., Doyle, J., Osborn, R., Fitzmaurice, K., Kendig, H., 2001. The communication and health needs of older people with hearing loss: are hearing aids enough? Australian & New Zealand Journal of Audiology 23 (1), 11–18.

Hogan, A., O'Loughlin, K., Miller, P., Kendig, H., 2009. The health impact of a hearing disability on older people in Australia. Journal of Aging and Health 21, 1098–1111.

Hogan, A., Bryne, D., Reynolds, K., 2010. Beyond the gap: towards a more comprehensive structuring of hearing services. ENT & Audiology News 19 (2), 79–83.

Hogan, A., Reynolds, K.J., O'Brien, L., 2011. towards a social psychology of living with acquired hearing loss. Perspectives October 18 (1), 13–22.

Hogan, A., (Ed.), 2012. A Fairer Hearing. ANU E Press, Canberra.

Hogan, A., Reynolds, K.J., Latz, I., O'Brien, L., 2012. A social psychology of contested social identity. In: Hogan, A. (Ed.), A Fairer Hearing. ANU E Press, Canberra, 110–141.

Hogan, A., Scarr, E., Lockie, S., Chant, B., Alston, S., 2012. Ruptured identity of male farmers: subjective crisis and the risk of suicide. Journal of Rural Social Sciences, in press.

Ihara, K., 1993. Depressive states and their correlates in elderly people living in a rural community. Nippon Koshu Eisei Zasshi 40 (2), 85–94.

Kent, B.A., 2003. Identity issues for hard-of-hearing adolescents aged 11, 13, and 15 in mainstream setting. Journal of Deaf Studies and Deaf Education 8 (3), 315–324.

Lindley, P., 2009. The vicissitudes of life: Experiences of a consumer and significant other. Australian College of Audiology Newsletter. December issue: 6–13 Australia, Brisbane.

Mills, C.W., 1970. The Sociological Imagination. Penguin, Harmondsworth.

Mitchell, P., 2002. The prevalence, risk factors and impacts of hearing impairment in an older Australian community: The Blue Mountains Hearing Study. The 2002 Libby Harricks Memorial Oration. Delivered at the XXVI International Congress of Audiology. Deafness Forum, Melbourne, Australia March 21, 2002.

Monzani, D., Galeazzi, G.M., Genovese, E., Marrara, A., Martini, A., 2008. Psychological profile and social behaviour of working adults with mild or moderate hearing loss. Acta Otorhinolaryngologica Italica 28 (2), 61–66.

Mulrow, C.D., Aguilar, C., Endicott, J.E., Velez, R., 1990. Association between hearing impairment and the quality of life of elderly individuals. Journal of the American Geriatrics Society 38 (1), 45–50.

O'Brien, L., Berry, H.L., Hogan, A., 2012. The structure of overall life satisfaction: Insights from farmers and non-farmers in rural Australia during drought. Manuscript in preparation.

Rutman, D., 1989. The impact and experience of adventitious deafness. American Annals of the Deaf 4 (134), 305–310.

Saunders, G.H., Griest, S.E., 2009. Hearing loss in veterans and the need for hearing loss prevention programs. Noise and Health 11 (42), 14–21.

Scherer, M.J., Frisina, D.R., 1998. Characteristics associated with marginal hearing loss and subjective well-being among a sample of older adults. Development 35 (4), 420–426.

Smeeth, L., Fletcher, A.E., Ng, E.S., Stirling, S., Nunes, M., Breeze, E., Bulpitt, C.J., Jones, D., Tulloch, A., 2002. Reduced hearing, ownership and use of hearing aids in elderly people in the UK – the MRC trial of the assessment and management of older people in the community: a cross sectional survey. Lancet 359, 1466–1470.

St Claire, L., He, Y., 2009. How do I know if I need a hearing aid? Further support for the self-categorisation approach to symptom perception. Applied Psychology: An International Review 58, 24–41.

Tambs, K., 2004. Moderate effects of hearing loss on mental health and subjective well-being: results from the nord-trondelag hearing loss study. Psychosomatic Medicine 66 (5), 776–782.

Thomas, A.J., 1984. Acquired Hearing Loss: Psychological and Psychosocial Implications. Academic Press, London.

Wilson, D., Xibin, S., Read, P., Walsh, P., Esterman, A., 1992. Hearing loss - an underestimated public health problem. Australian Journal of Public Health 16, 282–286.

Wilson, D.H., Walsh, P.G., Sanchez, L., Davis, A.C., Taylor, A., Tucker, G., Meagher, I., 1999. Epidemiology of hearing impairment in an Australian adult population. International Journal of Epidemiology 28 (2), 247–252.

Chapter 10

Framing Debates about Risk for Skin Cancer and Vitamin D Deficiency in New Zealand: Ethnicity, Skin Color, and/or Cultural Practice?

Paul Callister and Judith Galtry

Victoria University, Wellington, New Zealand

INTRODUCTION

Every so often a miracle vitamin is identified. In 1964, a book titled *Vitamin E, Your Key to a Healthy Heart: The Suppressed Record of the Curative Value of This Remarkable Vitamin* was published (Baily, 1964).

Just six years later, Linus Pauling in *Vitamin C and the Common Cold* claimed that high daily doses of vitamin C would reduce the incidence of colds (Pauling, 1970). A 1979 review *Ascorbic Acid and Cancer* postulated that vitamin C might even protect against cancer (Cameron et al., 1979).

While the potential protective benefits of vitamin D (on colon cancer) had first been suggested many years earlier (Garland and Garland, 1980), now, in the early twenty-first century, it has been touted as the new "miracle" vitamin. In New Zealand, the journalist Ian Wishart (2008) has been an outspoken proponent of the purported "powers" of vitamin D, particularly that obtained through sun exposure. In a 2008 article titled *Cancer Society Wrong on Melanoma Risk—Sunlight: the Best Medicine?* Wishart announced:

Two new scientific studies out this month have added to the growing mountain of evidence that our obsession with reducing sun exposure and slathering ourselves in sunscreen could actually be killing us. At the heart of the debate is vitamin D—a crucial ingredient, it now turns out, in the battle against a whole range of modern illnesses.

When Culture Impacts Health. http://dx.doi.org/10.1016/B978-0-12-415921-1.00010-5

This article also cited a United States' newspaper report (Fauber, 2007), which asserted:

It seems too simple to be true: Expose most of your body to about 15 minutes of sunlight a day during the summer and take large doses of inexpensive vitamin D pills during the winter and maybe, just maybe, you will substantially reduce the risk of getting various cancers, the flu, diabetes, heart disease, autoimmune diseases and neurological disorders.

These promises are appealing when considering ways of improving overall population health. But in New Zealand, there is a particular emphasis on bettering health among Maori and Pacific groups. The higher incidence of cancer and other illnesses among these groups is regarded as a major contributor to ethnic health inequalities (New Zealand Ministry of Health, 2002).

In the early stages of the debates, the potential benefits of sun exposure seemed especially relevant to Maori and Pacific people based on evidence that people with dark skin are not only at lower risk of developing melanoma but also require more ultraviolet radiation (UVR) exposure to synthesize vitamin D.

But there were several methodological challenges inherent in the vitamin D and sun exposure debate. The first of these was determining what constitutes adequate serum vitamin D status. We begin by briefly discussing this and then highlight New Zealand research that has identified apparent vitamin D deficiency. This is followed by an examination of recent evidence showing increased melanoma incidence among Maori and, to a lesser extent, Pacific peoples. In doing so, we highlight some uncertainties around the definition and use of ethnicity in medical and wider social science literature. We also emphasize, in the absence of data, the danger of making a methodological leap from culturally defined measures of ethnicity to assumptions about skin color and, possibly, group behavior. Finally, drawing on international studies, we consider whether skin color, if measured, is sufficient for determining risk and targeting health advice. We conclude that while a complex set of individual variables needs to be considered when determining risk factors for both vitamin D deficiency and skin cancer, until better evidence is available some simple, universal behavioral messages about the risks and benefits of sun exposure may still be useful.

In endeavoring to understand the evolving history of debates about safe sun exposure in relation to both vitamin D and skin cancer we have drawn on a range of sources, including "participatory research." From 2003 to 2011, Judith Galtry was the Skin Cancer Advisor at the New Zealand Cancer Society and organized and participated in a range of research and policy forums on these issues. These forums led to the development of the Cancer Society's position statements on The Risks and Benefits of Sun Exposure in New Zealand 2008 and other relevant advice. In addition, we draw on peer-reviewed academic research and "gray" literature, as well as popular media.

RECENT CONCERNS ABOUT VITAMIN D

Key concerns relating to vitamin D have focused on what constitutes adequate blood levels, potential health outcomes, and the optimal way for the body to obtain it. Although it has long been known that vitamin D is important for bone and muscle health, medical debates have centered on wider potential health benefits. These include a possible inverse association between blood vitamin D levels and incidence and mortality from certain cancers (Scragg, 2007; Moan et al., 2008). This hypothesized association led various national cancer agencies to develop position statements on vitamin D and cancer risk, including a focus on the risks *and* benefits of sun exposure (e.g., Cancer Council Australia, 2007; Cancer Society of New Zealand, 2008; United States National Cancer Institute, 2009).

Some vitamin D can be obtained naturally from the diet (such as oily fish, eggs, and meat) or through supplements. However, traditionally the sun has been the primary source. But sun exposure has risks. Although amounts and patterns of sun exposure influence skin cancer risk, there is strong evidence that the three main types of skin cancer—cutaneous malignant melanoma, squamous cell carcinoma, and basal cell carcinoma—are caused by excess harmful sun exposure (Armstrong and Kricker, 2001). Due to a unique combination of factors, New Zealand and Australia lead the world in melanoma incidence (Parkin et al., 2007). In both countries, since the 1980s, there have been official campaigns to raise awareness about the need for sun protection during peak periods of UVR.

In contrast, the benefits of vitamin D have only recently been promoted, often via the media rather than through health promotion campaigns, with a focus on the possible health risks associated with low vitamin D status.

National and international attention on the purported health risks associated with poor vitamin D status led to increased demands on the health system, particularly among the "worried well," for blood tests to monitor vitamin D levels. Given that testing shows "deficiency" is quite common, vitamin D has also become a profitable new supplement. According to a 2010 article in *The New York Times*:

> ... *doctors are increasingly testing their patients' vitamin D levels and prescribing daily supplements to raise them. According to the lab company Quest Diagnostics, orders for vitamin D tests surged more than 50 percent in the fourth quarter of 2009, up from the same quarter a year earlier. And in 2008, consumers bought $235 million worth of vitamin D supplements, up from $40 million in 2001, according to Nutrition Business Journal.*

However, there has been difficulty in achieving scientific consensus on vitamin D sufficiency (United States National Cancer Institute, 2009), with recent agreement among several UK health agencies that 50 nmol/L is the benchmark for determining vitamin D adequacy (UK Consensus on Vitamin D, 2010).

Vitamin D Deficiency and Ethnicity in New Zealand

In recent years, there has been a plethora of research on vitamin D levels among various populations throughout the world. As an example, in New Zealand, based on the analysis of blood samples collected as part of the 2002 National Children's Nutrition Survey, Rockell et al. (2005) found that Maori and Pacific children have, on average, lower vitamin D levels than European children. However, the researchers acknowledged that a variety of other factors may have influenced levels, including obesity, diet, and exercise levels.

While supplementation is generally advised for individuals with vitamin D deficiency, in New Zealand it has also been suggested that Maori and Pacific peoples should increase their sun exposure (Scragg, 2007). Based on stereotypes about skin color, Maori and Pacific people have sometimes been assumed to not be at risk, or at low risk, of melanoma and therefore do not need to "cover up" in the same way as individuals with fair skin during the spring and summer months. Linked to this, there has been some suggestion that official "SunSmart" policies are inherently racist on the grounds that the recommended behaviors for the whole population (minimizing sun exposure through clothing, hats, and use of sunscreen) disadvantage particular ethnic groups. But the degree to which ethnicity is a predictor of risk depends on what it is being measured (Callister et al., 2011).

Increased Melanoma Incidence among Maori (and Pacific) Peoples

New Zealand has moved from measuring "race" to measuring "ethnicity" in statistical collections. Ethnicity is currently "culturally constructed" in New Zealand (Callister et al., 2007). In other words, individuals are free to "choose" their ethnicity. Given the often complex and intermarried backgrounds of people in settler societies, self-identification of ethnicity in response to official surveys is not always straightforward. In discussions of skin cancer risk, terminology often gets confused with regard to race, ethnicity, skin color, or perhaps some assumed group behavior.

Scientific evidence is reasonably clear that having fair skin increases the risk of skin cancer, including melanoma, especially when fair-skinned people migrate from low to high UVR environments and do not adapt their behaviors accordingly (Boyle et al., 2004). It has been estimated that, while potentially modifiable, as much as 90% of melanoma in Australasia is attributable to excess harmful sun exposure (Armstrong and Kricker, 1993). Boyle et al. (2004, p. 5) note:

The highest incidence rates of melanoma are reported from (essentially European migrant populations in) Australia and New Zealand (non-Maori population) where the annual incidence is more than double the highest rates recorded in Europe. Incidence rates have been increasing rapidly for several decades in all Caucasian populations although there is now an indication that in those areas where the incidence is highest, the mortality rate is beginning to stabilise or fall.

Caucasian is not an officially recognized ethnic group in New Zealand, but it is a term that has been used in skin cancer research to denote fair skin. For instance:

The main aetiological factor for melanoma is exposure of Caucasian skin to ultraviolet (UV) light, particularly intermittent exposure and particularly during childhood. The best avenue currently for melanoma prevention is believed to be by encouraging protection against sunburn, particularly in children, and in fair-haired and fair-skinned people.

Sneyd and Cox, 2006, p. 8

In the late 1980s, Shaw (1988) noted that malignant melanoma was rare among Maori. Twenty years later, in an editorial in the *New Zealand Medical Journal*, Shaw (2008, p. 6) continued to report that melanoma "is rare in non-Caucasians." In the New Zealand medical literature "European" is seen as equating to "Caucasian." Using Cancer Registry data, Sneyd and Cox (2009) examined trends in melanoma rates among Maori, Asian, and Pacific people in New Zealand. This showed a strong increase in incidence among Maori and, to a lesser extent, Pacific peoples, although from a relatively low base. Sneyd and Cox (2009) discussed the possible influence of changing (i.e., "lightening") skin color on melanoma incidence among Maori and Pacific groups, but acknowledged there is little research on this. Skin color is also not reported in statistical collections.

As a further confusing factor, medical researchers and policy makers sometimes use the term "Pakeha," although this is not a universally accepted term in New Zealand (e.g., Bedggood, 1997; Pearson and Sissons, 1997). Pakeha are also often defined in confusing ways, for example, as "New Zealanders of European descent" (Sibley and Liu, 2004). Although European is an ambiguous term in this context (denoting certain countries in the Northern Hemisphere), if this term is used, it can also be claimed that, due to a long history of intermarriage, almost all Maori are similarly "New Zealanders of European descent." Other New Zealand medical researchers simply divide the population into two groups: Maori and non-Maori, the latter not being an ethnic group but simply a residual group. Given that non-Maori are made up of a wide range of ethnic groups that differ in terms of skin color and cultural practices, any broad "group" characteristics have little relevance when considering the relative risks and benefits of sun exposure.

Despite skin color not being an explicit component of New Zealand's historical official statistics, it is sometimes directly discussed. For instance, there has been some discussion about the "browning of New Zealand" (e.g., Kiro, 2002), including in relation to national sports teams. Along with "ethnic or national origins" and "race," skin color is one of the 13 prohibited grounds for discrimination identified in the New Zealand Human Rights Act of 1993. However, one of the most common examples of use of skin color is likely to be by the police. For instance, it is not uncommon to hear a suspect described as Caucasian, meaning a fair-skinned person. Yet skin color, like many other physical characteristics, is increasingly unlikely to be a good predictor of ethnicity.

What Factors Should Sun-Related Messages Focus On?

What approach should public health strategies adopt in relation to the risks and benefits of sun exposure, both in terms of groups and individuals? As an example, in the *Medical Journal of Australia*, Lucas and Ponsonby (2002, pp. 597–598) make the following three recommendations:

1. If patients are likely to have low personal UVR exposure, doctors should encourage a diet high in vitamin D, monitor serum vitamin D levels, and, if low, consider vitamin D supplementation.
2. Excessive exposure to UVR should continue to be discouraged. However, we need to make sure this message is not taken to the opposite extreme of reducing beneficial UVR exposure, such as short exposures during winter.
3. Public health messages regarding sun exposure should be tailored to the population with regard to levels of pigmentation, behavioral practices, and regional and seasonal levels of ambient UVR.

These Australian recommendations refer to pigmentation rather than to ethnicity, and also to behavior. In some other articles, there is also an emphasis on culture. For example, skin color is an important variable in a review article considering risk factors for vitamin D in Denmark, but the challenges in determining risk based on a range of unclear variables, including ethnicity, are also noted (Mygind et al., 2011). Determining religious or cultural affiliation (such as whether a person is a Muslim) and immigrant status does not directly measure behavior but may be used to predict, possibly incorrectly, behaviors, such as the likelihood of sunbathing. Clothing, such as whether headscarves or long-sleeved shirts are worn, are better predictors of risk. But, ideally, these questions need to be asked alongside those concerning other risk factors, such as skin color. However, even when asked in a questionnaire, New Zealand research suggests that individuals often find it difficult to classify objectively their own skin color (Reeder et al., 2010).

Given that information on skin color, religion, and behavioral practices, including diet and exercise, is not collected in many studies, it is not surprising that ethnicity or race has been the variable emphasized for identifying risk and/or targeting health promotion messages for both skin cancer and vitamin D deficiency (e.g., Scragg, 2007; Shaw, 2008; Hu et al., 2009; Sneyd and Cox, 2009). Yet some of these studies already show that while race or ethnicity may have been a useful predictor of skin color and, possibly, sun-related behavior in the past, there is the potential for an increasingly imperfect fit between ethnicity and the risk of developing skin cancer. This weakening could be due to the effects of ethnic intermarriage or ethnic mobility, but it also might be exacerbated by a move toward culturally defined ethnicity.

Specific genetic risk factors for both low vitamin D status and melanoma are starting to be identified (Lin et al., 2008; Wang et al., 2010). It is also likely that a simple test to identify individuals with the highest genetic risk factors for vitamin

D deficiency will eventually be developed. In terms of UVR measurement, new technologies, such as clothing that provides real-time UVR readings, are also being developed. In the meantime, uncertain information has to be relied on.

Universal, Group, or Individual Sun-Related Messages?

At the height of publicity about the purported "miracles" of vitamin D, New Zealand SunSmart policy makers were asked to provide "ethnically targeted" messages (with a particular emphasis on Maori and Pacific people) about both the risks and benefits of sun exposure. Highlighting the challenges inherent in this, one body of research recommended that Maori and Pacific people should become more aware of potential melanoma risk; while elsewhere, based on less certain science, it was suggested these groups increase sun exposure in order to reduce potential risk for certain cancers. Advice was also seen to differ according to the particular season, location, and time of day.

So, as a practical example of this type of approach, in a classroom setting, a teacher would be faced with the dilemma of whether to insist that all or only some students, depending on race or skin color, "slop" on sunscreen and don sunhats before going outside in the peak of the New Zealand summer.

Clearly, policies like this would not only be impractical but, if adopted, would potentially emphasize "difference" and foster racism. But what about overall public health messages? In New Zealand, there used to be "universal" "burn time" messages (based on the time it took an individual with fair skin to sunburn) promoted through the media. For a variety of reasons, burn time advice was abandoned and replaced in 2003 by advice based on the Ultraviolet Index (UVI) (Bulliard and Reeder, 2001; Galtry, 2010). The UVI, which measures UVR, in many instances simply warns about predicted, not real-time, UVR. In both New Zealand and Australia there has been a universal recommendation to adopt SunSmart behaviors when the UVI is 3 or above (Cancer Council Australia, 2007; Cancer Society of New Zealand, 2008). This has also included advice for some unprotected sun exposure during winter and when UVR levels are low in summer, that is, early morning and late afternoon. Other ways of boosting vitamin D intake, such as through diet and supplementation (particularly for groups at risk of low vitamin D), are also recommended. In the face of imprecise science, individuals need to assess this advice based on their own known risk factors for both skin cancer and vitamin D deficiency.

CONCLUSION

Vitamin D has been touted as the latest "miracle vitamin." While some health benefits (for bone and muscle) have long been known, more evidence is still needed as to how much of a miracle it may really be with regard to health outcomes. While there is some consensus about the threshold for vitamin D adequacy, optimal levels are still unclear both for populations and for specific individuals. Also somewhat uncertain are specific risk factors for vitamin D deficiency. Skin color seems to be one, but there are also many other factors, including genetic factors, age, and a range of behaviors, such as diet and exercise. Often the full range of risk factors is not collected in studies in contrast to ethnicity or race data, which tend to be recorded.

The risk factors for skin cancer are better understood and include skin color. But behavior matters too. Ethnicity has been associated with risk in some studies, but it is becoming a less useful predictor over time.

So what about health policy? What should we do when we do not have all the necessary information on risk factors? It seems useful to fall back on some useful, universal messages, but with the expectation that individuals are provided with enough information about particular risk factors to make informed judgments about optimal behaviors. Hopefully advice will improve as studies provide a better understanding of the risks and benefits of sun exposure to specific individuals within increasingly diverse populations and environments.

EPILOGUE

This chapter was originally prepared for publication in 2011. However, the issue of protecting against both skin cancer and vitamin D deficiency continues to be an evolving and contested area of health policy. While a new consensus statement has recently emerged in New Zealand with revised recommendations, particularly with regard to identifying people at risk of vitamin D deficiency (New Zealand Ministry of Health and Cancer Society, 2012), contrary viewpoints continue to be strongly asserted (Wishart, 2012).

REFERENCES

Armstrong, B.K., Kricker, A., 2001. The epidemiology of UV induced skin cancer. Journal of photochemistry and photobiology B: Biology 63 (1–3), 8–18.

Baily, H., 1964. Vitamin E, Your Key to a Healthy Heart: The suppressed record of the curative value of this remarkable Vitamin. Chilton Books.

Bedggood, M., 1997. Pakeha ethnicity? Sites 35, 81–100.

Boyle, P., Jean-Francois Doré, J.-F., Autier, P., Ringborg, U., 2004. Cancer of the skin: a forgotten problem in Europe. Annals of Oncology 15, 5–6.

Bulliard, J.L., Reeder, A., 2001. Getting the message across: Sun protection information in media weather reports in New Zealand. New Zealand Medical Journal 23 (114(1126)), 67–70.

Callister, P., Didham, R., Potter, D., Blakely, T., 2007. Measuring ethnicity in New Zealand: developing tools for health outcomes analysis. Ethnicity & Health 12 (4), 1–22.

Callister, P., Galtry, J., Didham, R., 2011. The risks and benefits of sun exposure: should skin colour or ethnicity be the main variable for communicating health promotion messages in New Zealand? Ethnicity & Health 16 (1), 57–71.

Cameron, E., Pauling, l., Leibovitz, B., 1979. Ascorbic acid and cancer: a review. Cancer Research 39, 663–681.

Cancer Council of Australia, 2007. The risks and benefits of sun exposure in Australia. NSW: Cancer Council of Australia.

Cancer Society of New Zealand, 2008. The risks and benfits of sun exposure in New Zealand. Cancer Society of New Zealand, Wellington.

Fauber, J., 2007. Vitamin D—Cheap wonder drug? Milwaukee-Wisconsin Journal Sentinel. http://www.jsonline.com/features/29395959.html.

Galtry, J., 2010. The Ultraviolet Index: Health promotion tool or 'poisoned chalice'? Paper prepared for NIWA's Workshop on UV Radiation and its Effects: an update (2010). http://www.niwa.co.nz/sites/default/files/uv_index.pdf.

Garland, C., Garland, F., 1980. Do sunlight and vitamin D reduce the likelihood of colon cancer? International Journal of Epidemiology 9, 227–231.

Hu, S., Parmet, Y., Allen, G., Parker, D.F., Rouhani, P., Kirsner, R.S., 2009. Disparity in melanoma: a trend analysis of melanoma incidence and stage at diagnosis among whites, hispanics, and blacks in Florida. Archives of Dermatology 145, 1369–1374.

Kiro, C., 2002. When the invisible hand rocks the cradle: implications of the UNICEF report for public health in New Zealand. PHA News 5 (6), 1–3.

Lin, J., Hocker, T.L., Singh, M., Tsao, H., 2008. Genetics of melanoma predisposition. British Journal of Dermatology 159 (2), 286–289.

Lucas, R.M., Ponsonby, A.L., 2002. Ultraviolet radiation and health: friend and foe. Medical Journal of Australia 177 (11/12), 594–598.

New Zealand Ministry of Health, 2002. Reducing Inequalities. Ministry of Health, Wellington.

New Zealand Ministry of Health and the Cancer Society, 2012. Consensus Statement on Vitamin D and Sun Exposure in New Zealand Advice for use with the general population excluding pregnancy and infancy March 2012. Available from http://www.cancernz.org.nz/reducing-your-cancer-risk/sunsmart/vitamin-d/.

Moan, J., Porojnicu, A.C., Dahlback, A., Setlow, R.B., 2008. Addressing the health benefits and risks, involving vitamin D or skin cancer, of increased sun exposure. Proceedings of the National Academy of Sciences 105 (2), 668–673.

Mygind, A., Traulsen, J.M., Nørgaard, L.S., Bissell, P., 2011. The ambiguity of ethnicity as risk factor of vitamin D deficiency—a case study of danish vitamin D policy documents. Health Policy 102 (1), 56–63.

Parkin, D.M., Whelan, S.L., Ferlay, J., Teppo, L., Thomas, D.B., 2007. Cancer incidence in five continents. Vols. I to VIII International Agency for Research on Cancer, IARC CancerBase No. 7. Lyon, France. Available from http://www.iarc.fr/en/publications/pdfs-online/epi/index.php (accessed 9.09.2011.).

Pauling, L., 1970. Vitamin C and the Common Cold. Freeman, San Francisco, W. H.

Pearson, D., Sissons, J., 1997. Pakeha and never pakeha. Sites 35, 64–80.

Reeder, A.I., Hammond, V., Gray, A., 2010. Questionnaire items to assess skin color and erythemal sensitivity: reliability, validity, and the dark shift. Cancer Epidemiology Biomarkers & Prevention 19 (5), 1167–1173.

Rockell, J.E., Green, T.J., Skeaff, C.M., Whiting, S.J., Taylor, R.W., Williams, S.M., Parnell, W.R., Scragg, R., Wilson, N., Schaaf, D., Fitzgerald, E.D., Wohlers, M.W., 2005. Season and ethnicity are determinants of serum 25-hydroxyvitamin D concentrations in New Zealand children aged 5-14 y. Journal of Nutrition 135 (11), 2602–2608.

Scragg, R., 2007. Vitamin D, sun exposure and cancer: a review prepared for the Cancer Society of New Zealand by the School of Population Health. University of Auckland, Unpublished report. Available from http://www.cancernz.org.nz/assets/files/docs/National%20Office/Research_Reports/Vitamin%20D%20UV%20Cancer%20Review_03Sept07.pdf (accessed 18.11.09.).

Shaw, J.H., 1988. Malignant melanoma in Auckland, New Zealand. Surgery, Gynecology and Obstetrics 166 (5), 425–430.

Shaw, J.H., 2008. Melanoma in New Zealand: a problem that is not going away. New Zealand Medical Journal 121 (1279), 6–9, Available from http://www.nzma.org.nz/journal/121-1279/index.shtml (accessed 9.12.2009.).

Sibley, C.G., Liu, J.H., 2004. Attitudes towards biculturalism in New Zealand: social dominance and Pakeha attitudes towards the general principles and resource-specific aspects of bicultural policy. New Zealand Journal of Psychology 33, 88–99.

Sneyd, M.J., Cox, B., 2006. The control of melanoma in New Zealand. New Zealand Medical Journal 119 (1242), 1–11.

Sneyd, M.J., Cox, B., 2009. Melanoma in Māori, Asian, and Pacific peoples in New Zealand. Cancer Epidemiology Biomarkers and Prevention 18 (6), 1706–1713.

UK Consensus Vitamin D Position Statement, 2010. UK: British Association of Dermatologists, Cancer Research UK, Diabetes UK, the Multiple Sclerosis Society, the National Heart Forum, the National Osteoporosis Society and the Primary Care Dermatology Society. Available from http://www.sunsmart.org.uk/prod_consump/groups/cr_common/@nre/@sun/documents/generalcontent/cr_052628.pdf.

United States National Cancer Institute, 2009. Vitamin D and cancer prevention: strengths and limits of the evidence [online]. Factsheet. United States National Cancer Institute, Bethesda, MD. Available from http://www.cancer.gov/cancertopics/factsheet/prevention/vitamin-D (accessed 12.06.2009.).

Wang, T.J., et al., 2010. Common genetic determinants of vitamin D insufficiency: a genome-wide association study. Lancet 376 (9736), 180–188.

Wishart, I., 2008. Cancer Society wrong on melanoma risk—Sunlight: the best medicine? http://www.thebriefingroom.com/archives/2008/08/cancer_society.html.

Wishart, I., 2012. Vitamin D: Is this the miracle vitamin? Howling at the Moon Publishing, Auckland.

Chapter 11

Analyzing Smoking Using Te Whare Tapa Wha

Marewa Glover

University of Auckland, New Zealand

Tobacco smoking is the biggest killer of Maori people, killing about 440 annually based on 1989–1993 Maori deaths (Laugesen and Clements, 1998). Maori have the highest death rates from coronary heart disease in the group of countries under the Organisation for Economic Co-operation and Development, and Maori women have the highest rate of lung cancer in the world and suffer cervical cancer at more than twice the national rate (22.4 vs. 10.4 per 100,000 annual average from 1993 to 1995) (Ministry of Health, 1998). High rates of smoking among Maori women during pregnancy (two-thirds of Maori women smoked during peak child rearing age; Glover and Kira, 2011) contribute to higher rates of miscarriage, preterm births, low birth weight babies, and other difficulties during childbirth (Pomare et al., 1995). In 1996, the Maori sudden infant death syndrome rate was approximately five times higher than that of non-Maori (4.6 vs. 0.9 deaths per 1,000 live births) (Ministry of Health, 1998). From birth, Maori have proportionately higher rates of hospital admission for asthma and glue ear (Pomare et al., 1995). Through adulthood Maori suffer disproportionately higher hospitalization rates for smoking-related chronic obstructive respiratory disease, hypertensive disease, and other forms of heart disease and cancers. In addition to the impact of illness and death from tobacco, "tobacco use has dramatically affected Maori cultural, social and economic development" (Reid and Pouwhare, 1991, p. 59). "Smoking desecrates the mana of our marae" (Ellis, 1995, p. 1) and it brings about the early death of kaumātua, which represents a vital loss (Te Puni Kokiri, 1998) as "they are the storehouses of our culture" (Fisher, cited in Health Research Council, 1996). Maori economic development is also undermined by tobacco use with the tax take per annum from Maori smokers approximating $260 million (Apaarangi Tautoko Auahi Kore, 2003).

In 1976, nearly 60% of Maori smoked. This rate dropped to 50% by 1991 and 49% in 2001, which was double the non-Maori non-Pacific rate (Ministry of Health, 2003). Higher smoking rates are concentrated in younger people. Nearly 60% of Maori women between 15 and 44 were smokers (Ministry of Health, 1999). The highest smoking rate (46%) among Maori men was for those between 25 and 39 (Statistics New Zealand, 1997). Among women aged 15 and

When Culture Impacts Health. http://dx.doi.org/10.1016/B978-0-12-415921-1.00011-7

over, Maori had the highest smoking rates (48%) compared with Pakeha (22%), Pacific (19%), and other women (5%) (Ministry of Health, 1999).

The goal of this chapter is to understand how to reduce Maori smoking, while employing a kaupapa Maori methodology, which preferences Maori theories.

TE WHARE TAPA WHA

A number of Maori models of health have been developed (reviewed in Durie, 1994). Te Whare Tapa Wha (Figure 11.1), however, has achieved status as a paradigm. According to Kuhn's (1962) definition, a paradigm is an accepted model that has attracted an enduring group of adherents away from competing modes of scientific activity and is sufficiently open-ended, leaving problems to be resolved. Te Whare Tapa Wha is applied to a variety of situations to reveal a Maori perspective. It became widely accepted as the preferred Maori defini- tion of health during the 1980s (Durie, 1994) and has since achieved wide and common usage as a Maori model of health. Objective 1.2 of the Ministry of Health's (2002) Maori Health Strategy policy, He Korowai Oranga, specifically encouraged the use of Te Whare Tapa Wha. Te Whare Tapa Wha gives rise to predictions about Maori scientific activity, such as this chapter seeks to explore. It is attractive for its simplicity, metaphorical resonance for Maori, and basis in a Maori worldview, which can facilitate comprehension of scientific findings beyond academia.

Using the analogy of a wharenui (meeting house), all aspects of well-being are represented while reflecting fundamental tenets of Maori epistemology and remaining consistent with contemporary Maori thinking, as illustrated in Figure 11.1. The four sides of the whare represent the immediate effects on an individual; te taha wairua, the spiritual realm; te taha hinengaro, the psychological realm; te taha tinana, the physical body; and te taha whānau, the family and wider community. The whare as a whole illustrates the

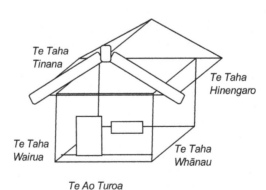

FIGURE 11.1   Te Whare Tapa Wha.

holistic interdependent relationship between all aspects. Balance is required to enjoy stability, and poor health is regarded as a manifestation of a breakdown in harmony within the individual and between the individual and the wider environment. Originally intended to refer to environmental health (Whaia Te Hauora, 1994), an additional aspect, te ao turoa, is used in this study to provide a category for the contextual, political, and environmental influences effecting health.

METHOD

One hundred thirty smokers who self-identified as Maori and who were intending to quit smoking were interviewed. Participants ranged in age from 16 to 62 (the average age was 35). Seventy-eight percent were women. Participants lived in the northern half of the North Island. A mix of closed and open-ended questions about participants' thoughts and behavior, family and social relationships, and environmental influences on smoking were asked. Where possible, questionnaire responses were quantified. Thematic analysis was done manually on some open-ended questions resulting in a coding set. Using SPSS for Windows, Release 6.1.3, standard frequency analysis for each variable was calculated for descriptive information. Logistic regression was performed to detect predictors of outcome variables, such as not smoking at follow-up. The significance level (the p value) was rounded up to three decimal places. The taped interviews were transcribed, formatted, and entered into QSR NUD*IST Release V.4.0. Data were coded according to Te Whare Tapa Wha. Analysis across both the quantitative and qualitative data was then conducted using a general inductive approach (Thomas, 2006). Analysis was more deductive than inductive in that Te Whare Tapa Wha was used as the analytic framework, rather than using a model or theory developed from the data.

The University of Auckland Human Participants Ethics Committee provided ethical approval.

RESULTS

The data distributed across the categories provided by Te Whare Tapa Wha are presented here. The biological and physical aspects of smoking were categorized under te taha tinana. Te taha hinengaro includes the information on participants' beliefs about the reasons for smoking and quitting. How familial and social influences contribute to smoking were classified under te taha whānau. Finally, the effects on and role of te taha wairua, the spiritual aspect, are presented.

Te Taha Tinana

Smoking is a physical behavior; thus, the data on how long participants had smoked, previous quit attempts and times off smoking, current type, and brand and number of cigarettes smoked per day were included under te taha tinana. On average, participants estimated that they had smoked for 18 of their years. Most (88%) had tried to quit an average of 2.5 times. Average consumption at first interview was 16 cigarettes per day. Half the participants smoked factory-made cigarettes and half smoked roll-your-owns (rollies) or both factory-mades and rollies.

Six questions from the Fagerstrom Test for Nicotine Dependency (FTND) and an exhaled carbon monoxide (CO) reading were included in the realm of te taha tinana, because the CO reading is a physical measure and the FTND purports to measure the strength of the physical addiction to nicotine. For example, the FTND asks: How soon after waking is the first cigarette smoked? Fifty-eight participants smoked their first cigarette within 30 minutes of waking up, indicating a medium to strong dependency on nicotine.

What participants did to prepare their body for quitting, for example, reducing the body's dependency on nicotine by cutting down smoking or using nicotine patches, was included under te taha tinana, as were other methods used to quit, such as going cold turkey. What physically happened when participants stopped smoking—the withdrawal symptoms such as increased appetite, agitation, anger, disrupted sleeping patterns, and increased coughing—were categorized under te taha tinana, as were any lasting changes relating to quitters' physical well-being, such as improved fitness reported by participants who were smoke free at follow-up. Participants who had relapsed to smoking by the follow-up interview experienced additional withdrawal symptoms, such as cravings. For some participants the strength of the symptoms caused them to relapse. Analysis of time to relapse showed that over half (54%) of the unaided quitters relapsed within the first week.

Severity of nicotine dependency, indicated by number of cigarettes smoked per day and CO reading, were predictive of success at quitting (Table 11.1). That is, the less that participants said they smoked and the lower their CO reading, the more likely they were to stop smoking.

Te Taha Hinengaro

While chemical and other changes may be occurring in the body/the realm of te taha tinana, the subjective experience, the interpretation occurs in te taha hinengaro. Participants' beliefs about their smoking behavior, such as their reasons for smoking and motivation for quitting, were categorized under te taha hinengaro. Participants were assessed in terms of their Stage of Change, that is, whether they were in precontemplation, contemplation, or action, which was based on when they intended to quit (within the next 6 months or within the next 30 days). Participants' explanation for choice of quitting method, self-efficacy (belief that they could quit), and their understanding of why they relapsed were considered under ta taha hinengaro.

TABLE 11.1 Potential Predictors for Quitting (N = 85)

	Stopped smoking		Still/Back smoking		Combined	
Average actual no. smoked per day**	9.1	SD = 8.47	17.3	SD = 14.7	16.1	SD = 13.1
Average CO reading**	11.2	SD = 9.43	17.5	SD = 9.15	16.7	
Self-efficacy**	5.8	SD = 1.5	4.7	SD = 1.5	4.8	
Difficulty score**						
Average	3.3	SD = 2.1	5.5	SD = 1.7	5.2	
Mode	1		7		7	

**Indicates a statistically significant difference (p < 0.05). SD, standard deviation.

Reasons for Smoking

Participants could list as many reasons for smoking as they wished (Table 11.2).

The most cited reason for smoking was habit. Participants spoke about the automatic, routine nature of their smoking.

It's like getting up in the morning and washing your face. I mean it's just become something that's part of my day. It's normal.

TABLE 11.2 Reasons for Smoking

	N = 130	%
Habit	95	73
Stress	63	48
Addiction	51	39
Social	44	34
Boredom	38	29
Enjoyment	33	25
Emotions	30	23
Time Out	22	17
Its Normal	15	11.5
Weight Control	6	5
Stimulant	6	5
Availability	5	4
Other	3	2
Don't Know	5	4

Some (11.5%) participants smoked because it was normal, which was distinguished from habit by statements about smoking being the norm, for instance, "because everyone else smokes."

Nearly half (48%) of the participants used smoking to cope with stress specifically, and 23% said they smoked to deal with emotions in general. They smoked to relieve anxiety, to release anger, to quell worries, to calm down, and to relax.

I find that I smoke more when I've got problems ... and I find it relaxes me quite a lot after an argument or if I'm having a confrontation with one of my whānau.... If I sit there and I puff away it helps to release the anger and stress.

Thirty-nine percent said they were addicted. As one person explained:

When you're spending $9 on a packet and smoking it in 2 days and ya know you can't really afford to spend money on something else, but you're racking your brain looking for a few extra dollars for a packet of cigarettes, yeah, well that's an addiction.

Smoking when socializing or drinking was the next most frequently cited reason for smoking. For some participants companionship and socializing with whānau and friends who smoke triggered them to smoke, and for others their smoking increased particularly when they were drinking alcohol.

When I'm with friends that are smokers, then I'll smoke.
I'm a proper little chain smoker when I'm drinking alcohol.

Twenty-nine percent of participants smoked when they were bored or had "nothing else to do." Some participants had no job, no friends because they were new to the area, lived in a rural area geographically isolated from others, or could not do things because of physical ailments.

A quarter of participants said they smoked because they enjoyed it.

The truth is I actually enjoy smoking. I don't know whether it's actual smoke I enjoy, it's the whole feeling. I enjoy the feeling.
I like the taste. I love the smell.

Seventeen percent of participants used smoking as a way of taking time out and rewarding themselves.

It sort of helps me to get through the day. It's like maybe a reward sort of thing. After you've mowed the lawns or something, you've done some chores and stuff, you sit down and have a smoke.

Motivation to Quit

Participants cited multiple reasons for quitting (Table 11.3). Most (85%) participants wanted to stop smoking for health reasons. About half of these participants were concerned about their declining physical health. Their complaints

TABLE 11.3 Reasons for Quitting

N = 130		%
Health	111	85
Cost	69	53
Children	67	51.5
Walk the Talk	33	25
Sick of It	28	21.5
Fitness/Sports	25	19
Others Don't Like It	14	11
Death of Others	4	3
Pregnancy	4	4
Other	41	31.5
Don't Know	1	1

ranged from poor "stamina" and "shortness of breath" to "stroke," "diabetes," and "emphysema." One-quarter had decided "it's time" because of how long they had been smoking and how old they were. A typical comment was:

I'm getting older … somewhere along the line I'm going to have to stop doing all these things to my body and start looking after it.

About one-quarter spoke of their hope for a long, good quality life. They wanted to be around "to enjoy life with my children and hopefully when they're my age I'll be able to do things with them" and "not to be dependent on other people or on any medication." Some of them were sure "it's going to end up killing me." Most of the participants (73%) reported having physical illnesses.

Cost was a motivating reason to quit for just over half (53%) of participants mainly because they could see how the money could be put to better use.

I would rather that money goes somewhere where I can see the benefits coming back to me than going up in a puff of smoke … between us we can be saving $100–120 a month, which is about $1000–1200 a year. That's a lot of money.

About half (51.5%) of the participants wanted to stop smoking for the sake of children. Some wanted to be smoke free role models for their own or other people's children and others believed that their children would learn from their example and follow them into smoking.

I don't want my boys to smoke. When you see something all your life it's something that's easy to get into. It's not okay and I don't want them to think it is.

One-quarter of participants wanted to stop smoking so they could be a better role model and or be more consistent with their own image of themselves, for example, because they were a nurse, teacher, drug and alcohol counselor, or youth worker. They spoke of feeling "hypocritical" and needing to "walk the talk."

Some participants (21.5%) said they were sick of smoking and some (19%) wanted to stop to improve their fitness or performance in sports. A few (11%) were stopping because other people did not like their smoking. Other reasons included stopping for religious or spiritual reasons and trying to start a whole new beginning, such as giving up alcohol or marijuana. Only four participants cited a current or planned pregnancy as a reason for stopping smoking.

Stage of Change

As recruitment focused on finding smokers who were intending to quit, most (83%) of the participants were in the action stage of change. The other 17% were in the contemplation or precontemplation stage of change.

Proposed Method of Quitting

Proposed method of quitting was categorized under te taha hinengaro as it reflects participants' beliefs about quitting methods and their intention. Twenty-six of the participants were undertaking a noho marae stop smoking program. The remaining participants were enlisted as a control group of unaided quitters. At the time of the study there were no government-funded or subsidized smoking cessation programs.

The unaided quitters were planning to stop smoking using a range of methods. Thirty percent were going to stop "cold turkey" using "probably sheer will-power." Many participants said they had previously tried to stop cold turkey but found it too hard so they would need to try a different method this time. A similar number of participants (28.5%) were going to slowly wean off smoking. Various ways of cutting down included lengthening the time between cigarettes or trying to go without a cigarette for as long as possible. A few of the unaided quitters were planning to attend a smoking cessation program, for example, a Seventh Day Adventist program. Several more said they would attend a program if one was available. Several participants were planning to use nicotine replacement products and a few were thinking about trying herbal cigarettes, homeopathic remedies, Nicobrevin, or Chinese medicine. Six percent did not know how they were going to stop.

Self-efficacy

Most of the participants were reasonably confident that they would succeed at quitting this time. On a scale from 1 to 7, the average score was 4.8. Self-efficacy was predictive of success at quitting (Table 11.1). Self-efficacy was also correlated with length of abstinence: the more confident were more likely to stop and they stayed stopped for longer. Participants that were smoke free at follow-up said quitting was easier than those who relapsed. Participants who relapsed tended to attribute blame to themselves and express poorer self-esteem.

Te Taha Whānau

Participants recalled starting to experiment with smoking on average at 12 years of age. The average age for starting to smoke regularly was 16 years. They reported that smoking initiation predominantly occurred either with whānau or in the whānau environment or with school peers or in the school environment (Table 11.4). Thinking back to childhood, about 70% of the participants said their parents smoked.

Few participants lived alone and as many as 65% lived with others who smoked. Of those participants who had a partner, 63% had a partner who smoked, although some of them were also intending to stop smoking. Whānau and friends were more likely to be smokers. Even though it was not as easy to smoke at work, about half still worked with and smoked with work colleagues.

Living with smokers was a predictor of relapse. More of the participants who stopped smoking were able to make their house smoke free. They also seemed to have whānau supportive of quitting, who had either quit themselves or were trying to quit. Some whānau were not supportive of quitting and encouraged relapse to smoking by offering cigarettes to the recent ex-smoker and deliberately trying to trigger cravings, for example, by blowing smoke in the face of the recent ex-smoker. Indirect acts included not respecting and supporting the provision of smoke-free environments, or withholding support. Some participants received no support or help with their quit attempt.

While 77% of participants recalled being advised by a health professional to quit, only 28% said the advice had influenced their decision to quit. Pressure from children to quit was perceived to be as influential as advice from a health professional.

Te Taha Wairua

The noho marae stop smoking program included activities for preparing spiritually for quitting. Tikanga (traditional protocols) were observed, including starting with a powhiri (opening ceremony) and ending with a poroporoake (closing ceremony). Karakia (prayer), waiata (song), mirimiri (massage), and visiting wahi tapu (sacred places) were some of the activities recognizing and tending

TABLE 11.4 Socialization to Smoke

Why started smoking	N = 130	%
Whānau	74	57
Peers school	73	56
Peers work	35	27
Everyone smoked	34	26
It was cool	26	20
Others smoked	25	19

to te taha wairua. Few of the unaided participants spoke of preparing spiritually for quitting. At the follow-up interview participants were more likely to speak of the changes in their wairua and the damage that smoking had done. Experientially participants reported effects on their taha wairua during withdrawal from nicotine, including experiencing an imbalance, vivid dreams, and visions. Some participants who stopped smoking confirmed a positive effect on their wairua. They experienced a "clarity" along with improved "sensibility." In retrospect, they could see how smoking had clouded or "blocked" their wairua like a fog.

Implications for Smoking Cessation

Smoking is sustained by a synergy of physiological, psychological, and social factors. In addition, there are spiritual and cultural factors unique to Maori that encourage and support Maori smoking. To be more effective at supporting smoking cessation among Maori, it is proposed that interventions need to acknowledge and address the effects of smoking in each of the realms provided for by Te Whare Tapa Wha.

Quitting was more likely the less people smoked per day, that is, the less severe their dependency on nicotine. Consistent with this, relapse was largely due to inability to survive nicotine withdrawal. Nicotine dependency and nicotine withdrawal syndrome, which are mostly experienced in te taha tinana, can be treated with interventions that focus on changes at a biochemical level, such as nicotine replacement products or cessation medications (McRobbie et al., 2008). Physical activity that brings about physical and biochemical changes, such as walking, playing sport, meditation, and extra sleep, can support smoking cessation. Making dietary changes could either support or hinder smoking cessation. For example, some participants underwent a detox diet, which assisted cessation. Others found they ate more and/or they ate more high-fat foods, which for some participants eventually led to weight gain, a commonly cited reason for relapse.

After the first fortnight, it was socializing and others' smoking that were the main triggers for participants' relapse. Once they had stopped smoking, participants had to learn other ways of coping with what may have been pre-existing depression or relationship difficulties. Lack of alternative coping skills, especially how to cope with overwhelming stress, may undermine attempts to stay smoke free. Participants who relapsed reported what can be termed a negative "aftermath" (Boustead, 1996). That is, they tended to blame themselves and shared negative self-judgments. They took returning to smoking as evidence of a weak personality. Thus, it was bad for their self-esteem, which could contribute to reduced self-efficacy for subsequent quit attempts. Unhelpful reactions from others, such as put-downs, tended to worsen negative aftermath. Participants who experienced negative aftermath were more likely to share lay beliefs about smoking, that is, they minimized the addictiveness of nicotine and believed quitting was dependent on "sheer determination." Some participants had unrealistic expectations about their level of dependency. Thus, an overemphasis on a psychosocial explanation of smoking behavior can inadvertently reinforce the stigma of weakness that attaches to ex-smokers who relapse. Self-efficacy, which was predictive of quitting success, should be able to be improved through the provision of cognitive behavioral therapy and support. Cessation services should encourage the use of effective smoking cessation methods, provide accurate information about the quitting process, and try to prevent relapse through skill building. Negative aftermath could be reduced if smokers were helped to understand how addictive nicotine is.

Individual smoking occurs within a whānau and social context. Biochemical drives to smoke are moderated by cultural and social norms, their expression shaped by the rules and fashions of the time. The whānau and immediate social group are where the rules and rebellions are played out, negotiated, conveyed to others, and passed intergenerationally. If smoking is the norm within the whānau environment, as it has been for well over half of Maori for over a century now, then children's adoption of adult practices like smoking is, as participants suggested, unremarkable. Maori children experiment with smoking to demonstrate and ensure their membership in the family and in their peer group. There is nothing rebellious about adopting a "normal" behavior everyone else is engaged in. Rather, in this context, smoking is an act of seeking to be similar to adults and significant others, that is, smoking uptake is an approval-seeking behavior. When both the whānau and social group smoke as a norm, smoking uptake is more likely. The child-rearing Maori population have the highest smoking prevalence rates in the country (around 60%). Smoking cessation for parents should be a priority for intervention. As this study showed, Maori home and social environments were largely permissive of smoking. To be effective, smoking-cessation interventions should assess the home and whānau environment and facilitate changes, such as making the house smoke free and offering cessation support to other smokers in the home, whānau, and social network of the intended quitter.

Nicotine is a psychoactive drug. Introduced to the body, it alters natural functioning, including consciousness. The smokers change: their thinking is altered, their priorities are changed, and their behavior changes. These changes are largely chemically induced. Whether the drug is heroin, cannabis, alcohol, nicotine, or caffeine, the *natural* person is temporarily lost. Unfortunately, regular use incurs more permanent changes, whether it be from neuroadaptation (e.g., an increased number of brain nicotine receptors) or cell damage, in which case the natural person is forever lost. This concept is expressed in the Maori slogan "Tobacco attacks our potential" (Department of Health, 1991). Smoking is a fundamental breach of tapu (sacredness) in a number of ways and can lead to breaches in tikanga. First, the origin and treatment of the plant itself could have ramifications for users. The plant has been removed from the guardianship of a particular Native American tribe and commercialized for individual profit. Native American tradition that dictated the occasional, highly ritualized use of tobacco was not appropriated along with the plant. The integral mana (power and status) of the tobacco plant has been abused as have the Native Americans from whom the plant was taken. The process of production of cigarettes incurs damaging costs to both the people employed in its growth and production, but also environmentally, for example, tobacco plantations have displaced food crops and forests. The integral mana of the consumer is similarly exploited, as they are conned into purchase of a product that, if used as intended, will kill half of its users (Doll et al., 1994).

It has been argued that tobacco was used to manipulate and control early Maori. There are recorded incidents of tobacco being used as a koha (reciprocal gift), a bribe, and an item of trade, for instance, in the purchase of land. Tobacco was also exchanged as part of the Treaty of Waitangi signing process (Broughton, 1996). It may be that tobacco's role in the colonization of Maori has negative ramifications for today's Maori and Pakeha tobacco users. Smokers trample upon their own mana when they smoke, as the smoke is consumed through the breath, which is tapu, but if classified as food, is noa (of common status). The psychoactive substances in tobacco "intoxicate" the user, inhibiting their wairua, damaging their tinana, reorienting their thinking, and changing their behavior toward others. Nicotine dependency causes people to prioritize their individual tobacco use and in the process they sideline fundamental Maori values, such as manaakitanga (caring), aroha (love), and whakapapa (geneology). For example, children do sometimes go without, as what little money there is in some families is spent on tobacco. Babies and children are frequently made ill through passive smoking and sometimes they die from smoking-related or exacerbated illnesses. Other whānau also sometimes die from smoking-related illnesses from passive smoking. At the extreme, nicotine dependency drives people to steal from others; for example, cash and tobacco are increasingly the target of aggravated robberies of shops and gas stations. Thus, smoking can lead people to breach tikanga. Interventions wanting to acknowledge te taha wairua may want to discuss the effects of smoking on te taha wairua with smokers. Interventions should at least operate in accordance with tikanga, using karakia where appropriate and if necessary referring clients to tohunga (experts) of rongoa (healing methods) or mate kite (seers) to assist with the care of te taha wairua.

Individual and familial behavior change can be encouraged and supported by public health programs and policies, classified here under te ao turoa. This research suggests that increasing smoke free environments and diminishing smoking prevalence in one's immediate whānau, social, and work environments creates pressure to quit. This supports the need to extend smoking bans and intensify campaigns that promote smoke free homes and discourage smoking around others.

Seventy-three percent of participants in this research reported having current illnesses, presumably requiring contact with primary health care providers. Screening for smoking should be an integral part of primary and secondary health care, and smoking cessation should be a treatment goal for all clients pre-senting with smoking-related illnesses and illnesses exacerbated by smoking. Other health professionals, such as dentists, physiotherapists, and psychologists could be mobilized to support the promotion of smoking cessation. Drug and alcohol services, experienced as they are in treating drug dependency, could also assist with nicotine dependency.

CONCLUSION

Compartmentalizing aspects of smoking into the four categories provided by Te Whare Tapa Wha may be artificial and the designation of some factors as physical and some as mental could be debated. The application of Te Whare Tapa Wha, however, to a problematic behavior such as smoking, can facilitate comprehension and assist the design of interventions aiming to deliver holisti-cally. That is, a more effective intervention to reduce Maori smoking preva-lence would include components that address smoking damage to the physical, mental, and spiritual health of the person and their whānau. Smoking-cessation treatment would treat the physical dependency on nicotine, include a cognitive behavioral component, and be delivered in a culturally appropriate way to the whole whānau. Effectiveness could be further improved by increasing the inten-sity of public health policies, campaigns, and programs.

ACKNOWLEDGMENTS

This research was funded by the Health Research Council of New Zealand.

REFERENCES

Apaarangi Tautoko Auahi Kore. National Mäori Tobacco Control Strategy 2003 to 2007. Welling-ton: Apaarangi Tautoko Auahi Kore.

Broughton, J., 1996. Puffing up a storm, Volume 1: "Kapai te torori." University of Otago, Te Ropu Rangahau Hauora Maori o Ngai Tahu, Dunedin.

Boustead, C., 1996. Grounded theory: Smoking cessation in the long term. Unpublished master's thesis, Newcastle University, United Kingdom.

Department of Health, 1991. Tobacco attacks our potential. [Poster Code 4330.] Department of Health, Wellington.

Doll, R., Peto, R., Wheatley, K., Gray, R., Sutherland, I., 1994. Mortality in relation to smoking: 40 years' observations on male British doctors. BMJ 309, 901–911.

Durie, M.H., 1994. Whaiora: Maori health development. Oxford University Press, Auckland.

Ellis, R., 1995. Ko tenei te whare auahi kore mo te oranga o nga tamariki! This is a smokefree whare for the health of our kids! A Health Research Council student summership report.

Glover, M., Kira, A., 2011. Why Maori women continue to smoke while pregnant. N. Z. Med. J. 124 (1339), 22–31.

Health Research Council of New Zealand, 1996, December. Iwi identifies kaumatua health needs. Health Research Council of New Zealand Newsletter 19.

Kuhn, T.S., 1962. The structure of scientific revolutions. The University of Chicago Press, Chicago.

Laugesen, M., Clements, M., 1998. Cigarette smoking mortality among Maori, 1954–2028. Te Puni Kokiri, Wellington.

McRobbie, H., Bullen, C., Glover, M., Whittaker, R., Wallace-Bell, M., Fraser, T., 20 June 2008. New Zealand smoking cessation guidelines. New Zealand Medical Journal 121 (1276), 57–70.

Ministry of Health, 1998. Progress on health outcome targets. Te haere whakamua ki nga whainga hua mo te hauora: The state of the public health in New Zealand. Ministry of Health, Wellington.

Ministry of Health, 1999. Taking the pulse: The 1996/97 New Zealand Health Survey. Ministry of Health, Wellington.

Ministry of Health, 2002. He Korowai Oranga: Maori health strategy. Ministry of Health, Wellington.

Ministry of Health, 2003. Tobacco facts 2003. Ministry of Health, Wellington.

Pomare, E., Keefe-Ormsby, V., Ormsby, C., Pearce, N., Reid, P., Robson, B., Watene-Haydon, N., 1995. Hauora: Maori standards of health III. Wellington School of Medicine, Wellington Te Ropu Rangahau Hauora a Eru Pomare.

Reid, P., Pouwhare, R., 1991. Te-Taonga-mai-Tawhiti: The gift from a distant place. Niho Taniwha, Auckland.

Statistics New Zealand, 1997. Highlights: Maori 1996 Census of Population and Dwellings. Statistics New Zealand, Wellington.

Te Puni Kokiri, 1998. Maori towards 2000. Whakapakari: Tatauranga Taupori, 1. Te Puni Kokiri, Wellington.

Thomas, D.R., 2006. A general inductive approach for qualitative data analysis. American Journal of Evaluation 27, 237–246. http://dx.doi.org/10.1177/1098214005283748.

Whaia, Te Hauora, 1994. Philosophy and Planning Document: 1994/95. Northland Health, Health Promotion Unit, Whangarei.

Chapter 12

Thirty Years of New Zealand Smoking Advances a Case for Cultural Epidemiology and Cultural Geography

John D. Glover,[1] Jane Dixon,[2] Cathy Banwell,[2] Sarah Tennant,[1] and Matthew Freeman[1]

[1]University of Adelaide, Australia, [2]The Australian National University, Canberra, Australia

INTRODUCTION

Despite 40 years of public health activity, approximately one in five males continue to smoke in most European countries and non-European countries of the Organization for Economic Co-operation and Development (Giskes et al., 2005). Current data undermine earlier predictions that the twentieth century smoking epidemic in affluent countries would pass as the generation of older smokers died (those born between the 1930s and 1950) (Lopez et al., 1994). What is now clear is that their ranks are replenished by successive waves of young smokers and by larger proportions of female regular smokers (Graham et al., 2006; White et al., 2006; Pampel, 2007). The uptake by young people of a behavior that contributes most to the burden of disease in many countries has been identified by the Nuffield Centre on Bioethics (2007) as a major issue for government attention.

Until recently, there has been consensus that population levels of smoking can be explained by a general theory of diffusion whereby the socially margin-alized follow the socially advantaged in adopting and then repudiating smoking (Lopez et al., 1994; Mackenbach, 2006; Chapman, 2007). This sociocultural process creates a lagged effect and health inequalities follow in the short term; however, it was assumed that as the current cohort of socially marginalized groups quit, the smoking epidemic would disappear over the longer term.

This chapter uses data on 30 years of smoking in New Zealand, and applies a mix of theories regarding social diffusion, the influence of social networks on behaviors, and cultural normalization and distinction to try to illustrate what would be needed to explain the variety of smoking patterns across the life course of different ethnic groups. We propose that attention must begin to be paid to

When Culture Impacts Health. http://dx.doi.org/10.1016/B978-0-12-415921-1.00012-9

the sociocultural processes that underpin the smoking patterns evident from the social epidemiology. What is required is twofold: the development of more sensitive individual-level sociocultural variables alongside sustained ethnographic research among subpopulations to elicit information on interpretations of, and responses to, the social context which smokers inhabit.

THIRTY YEARS OF SMOKING IN NEW ZEALAND: WHAT WE KNOW

Since 1976, the New Zealand Census has had a prescient eye to population inequalities. Compared to many countries, it has 30 years of data on an unparalleled range of socioeconomic, ethnic, and other factors useful for describing and monitoring deprivation. As a result, that country's social epidemiologists and medical geographers have vigorously pursued a social determinant of health research agenda, with a singular focus on smoking behavior and health-related outcomes (Barnett et al., 2004, 2005, 2009, p. 881; Salmond et al., 2011). The analyses consistently find entrenched and growing inequalities between socioeconomic, ethnic, and gender groups over 30 years, despite concerted government smoking-prevention strategies (Glover and Cowie, 2010; Salmond et al., 2011), and despite decreasing gaps in employment, educational, and income achievement between Maori and non-Maori since the 1980s (Blakely et al., 2006; Barnett et al., 2009). In explaining recent temporal, spatial, and subpopulation trends, the neo-liberal policy of economic deregulation that was a feature of New Zealand society in the 1980s has been invoked. The policy is reasoned to have harmed some groups directly through extending the reach of absolute deprivation and indirectly by deepening relative inequality (see Barnett et al., 2005; Anderson et al., 2006).

We are concerned about a lower level of sociocultural dynamic, which operates at the national level: the sociocultural processes that take place in subpopulation communities. Why have successive marginalized cohorts not followed more advantaged socioeconomic status (SES) groups in both abstaining from smoking altogether or relinquishing smoking after the teenage years? Thus our interest is in the uptake of smoking among recent cohorts and the non-quitting behaviors among young people as they progress into adulthood.

Specifically, we obtained New Zealand census data for smoking status (current smoking, ex-smoker, and never smoked), age (from 15 years of age, in 5-year age groups, to 85 years and over), gender, labor force status (employed, unemployed, and not in the labor force), place of residence (main urban area, secondary urban area, minor urban area, rural center, and rural and other areas), and ethnicity (European, Maori, Pacific people, Asian) for the years 1976, 1981, 1996, and 2006. These data provide information about subpopulation movements between the censuses. We have used age group data to ascertain life course patterning by gendered ethnic groups and gendered labor force status.

Broadly, this cohort analysis shows that the adult smoking population almost halved between 1976 and 2006, with most of the decline taking place in the earlier years: the overall annual decline from 1996 to 2006 (1.2%) was almost half that of the previous 20 years (2.0%). As Barnett et al. (2004, 2005) have noted, any population-wide decline masks gross ethnic, gender, and labor force status inequalities, which "cannot be simply accounted for by ethnic differences in socioeconomic status" (Barnett et al., 2009, p. 881).

While levels of ethnic disparity across the whole population declined in five of seven social indicators (exceptions being Maori higher education and social housing tenancy), between 1996 and 2006 there has been no significant impact on Maori–European differentials in smoking cessation rates. More than one in two Maori adults smoked in 2006 compared with one in five for the European population, and the gap in rates between Maori and European has widened substantially for both men and women over this 30-year period. Pacific people and Asians (albeit with much lower smoking rates) show the greatest persistence of smoking into older age. Groups who are marginalized on the basis of SES have also not improved their smoking risk to the extent of the whole population: smoking rates among the unemployed are almost 60% above those of the employed, a substantially larger gap than existed in 1976, when the differential was 25.8%.

Trends in the Age Groups of Successive Cohorts

Using the census data, prevalence rates were calculated for current smoking for each age group between 15 and 64 years, by gender. Our focus was on age of beginning smoking by different groups and on prevalence trends within subpopulations over time to see whether smoking prevalence in more recent cohorts simply constitutes a rite of passage to be dropped early in people's twenties or whether it persists despite the obvious health risks.

Age Trends across the Whole Population

Smoking rates have declined in all age groups over the 30 years to 2006, other than for 20- to 24-year-old females, for whom the rate in 1981 is above the rate in 1976. Around half as many people are smoking at 15–64 years in 2006 as were smoking at those ages in 1976, with fewer than half of 60- to 64-year-olds smoking in 2006 as did 30 years earlier. But the decline appears to have stalled in the later years, other than in the 20–34-year age groups, as illustrated by the relatively smaller gap between the 1996 and 2006 lines in Figure 12.1.

As noted by Barnett et al. (2005), ethnic differences in smoking prevalence have been growing over the last 25 years. For Maori, smoking rates are substantially above those for Europeans in each age group (Figure 12.2), with the largest differentials at the three latest time points (Table 12.1). Pacific people have rates at similar levels to Europeans in the earlier years (1976 and 1981), but do

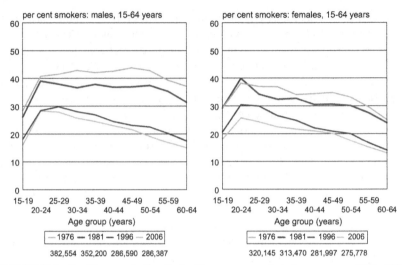

FIGURE 12.1   Smoking rates in New Zealand by age group, selected census years, 1976– 2006, males and females.

not exhibit a decline in 1996 and 2006 in those under 40 years of age. Rates for Asians are the lowest of the ethnic groups examined, and follow the pattern of decline seen earlier, other than at ages 15–18 and 20–24 years.

However, there are notable differences in smoking rates among males and females within these ethnic groups. For both European and Maori, it is largely related to differences in rates (higher for European males and for Maori females), and a slower rate of decline in the later years for females than is the case for males. For Pacific people, while rates for males are similar to those for Europeans, the pattern is very different for females, with rates for those under 40 years of age highest in the latest years.

For both males and females, smoking rates increase from the major urban areas, through secondary and minor urban areas, to the highest rates in the rural centers; the lowest rates are reported in the "other" rural areas (Figure 12.3). These (the most rural of areas) areas have experienced population growth over this period, in particular from the main urban areas (http://www.stats.govt.nz/ Publications/PopulationStatistics/internal-migration/urban-rural-migration .aspx). The greatest rate of decline in smoking rates is found in the main urban areas, and the pattern shown previously is repeated in each of the urban/rural classes, with the largest decline occurring before 1996, and a much smaller change taking place from 1996 to 2006.

Key Findings

In the section that follows, we expand on sociocultural explanations for the major findings.

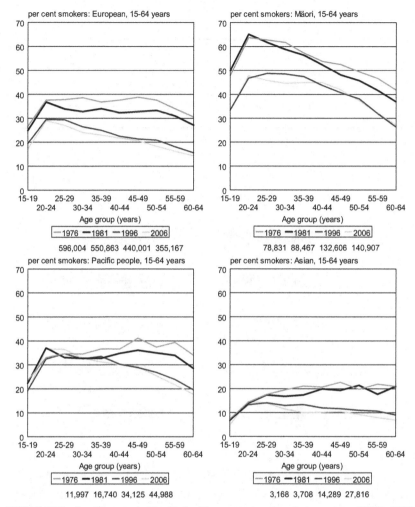

FIGURE 12.2   Smoking rates in New Zealand by age group, selected census years, 1976 to 2006, ethnicity.

The Residual Nature of Smoking among Successive Waves of Socially Disadvantaged Smokers

Despite the fact that rates and intercensual changes for Maori and Pacific people smoking is dramatically different from the European population, smoking is a residual activity among successive cohorts of low SES groups within each of the three ethnic groups. There are numerous possible competing explanations:

• A materialist explanation regarding the structures of disadvantage that shape health behaviors over the life course (Graham et al., 2006). Debates regarding the causal factors of smoking variations generally oscillate between

TABLE 12.1 Maori–Euro % and Rate Ratio				
Ethnicity	1976	1981	1996	2006
Maori	55.6%	55.0%	42.6%	41.2%
European	33.3%	29.8%	23.5%	21.9%
Rate ratio[a]	1.67	1.85	1.81	1.88

[a]Rate ratio is the ratio of the smoking rate for Maori to that for Europeans.

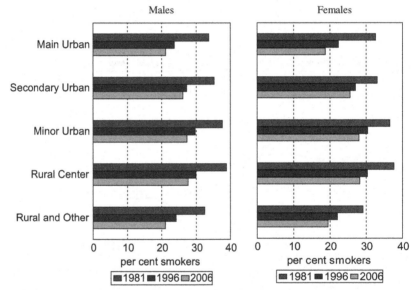

FIGURE 12.3   Smoking rates in New Zealand, by sex, selected census years, 1976 to 2006, by urban/rural location.

relative and absolute inequality at the population level versus income or income inequality at the individual level (see O'Dea and Howden-Chapman, 2000; Barnett et al., 2004, 2009; Blakeley et al., 2006). Smoking could be difficult to stop among all low SES groups because it is widely entrenched among the parents' generation. In the case of Maori and Pacific people, smoke-free environments are not a feature of daily life and the cost of quitting can be a barrier (Abel et al., 2001; Lanumata and Thomson, 2009; Glover and Cowie, 2010).

- A hybrid materialist–social network explanation. Health sociologists have been attempting to sharpen the rather opaque theory of diffusion by identifying the role of social networks in the transmission of smoking (Pampel, 2005; Christakis and Fowler, 2008). Social networks are described as vectors for the transmission of risky emotions and practices, offering a plausible explanation for the embodiment of contextual factors. Social networks are not hierarchical unlike social status groups, and in the case of smoking are comprised of people who are related familially or through friendship. Christakis and Fowler (2008) found that the SES of friends is relevant to quitting.

- A psychosocial explanation, which proposes that smoking is an easily accessible and affordable way to manage stress for economically disadvantaged Maori (Barnett et al., 2005), although the stress argument is disputed beyond the individual level (Pampel, 2005).
- A behavioral economics perspective about the pertinence of expectations of leading a healthy life and smoking (Lawlor et al., 2003, p. 267). If this is low among low SES groups then they may be predisposed to view smoking as culturally acceptable.

Applying a range of social science theories, including social network theories, to 100 years of data from the U.S. General Social Surveys, Pampel (2005) demonstrated that current SES differences in smoking are best explained by accounting for the cohort-specific social conditions, or period, through which adolescents pass. However, the mechanisms for the differential embodiment of population-wide policies and commercial campaigns remain a mystery.

Less attention has been paid to Pacific peoples' patterns of smoking (see Lanumata and Thomson, 2009), but cultural histories show that the Pacific Island groups (Samoan, Tongan, Cook Islanders, and Nuiean) have not experienced colonization and alienation from land and culture in the same way that Maori have. Many Pacific people migrated to New Zealand, particularly in the 1960s, looking for a higher standard of living and as a result of demand for labor. They have been exposed to Pakeha (i.e., New Zealanders of European descent) urban life for a shorter period, and in all four cultures, strong family and church networks are important but are dissipating among younger generations born in New Zealand (Abel et al., 2001). Church-based affiliations are also likely to discourage smoking particularly among older Pacific Island women. Thus the upward trends in Pacific peoples' smoking lends support to the thesis of acculturation: the longer the Pacific people are exposed to the effects of social marginalization, the more likely they are to behave in ways common to other marginalized peoples.

Spatial Patterning

From our analysis it appears that smoking cessation by men and women in secondary urban, minor urban, and rural centers has slowed down. Medical geographers are advancing the case for a cultural geography of health, where the focus lies with the intersecting characteristics of place and population cultural attributes (Gesler and Kearns, 2002). The clear and stable urban to rural center gradients evident over the past quarter century of smoking in New Zealand mask the socioeconomic and ethnic differences shown by other studies and surveys. For instance, the 2003 New Zealand Health Survey revealed that the prevalence of current smoking increased significantly with deprivation for both males and females in urban areas, but not rural areas (Ministry of Health, 2007). Moreover from the work of Barnett and colleagues, the differential impact of urban and rural inequality on men's and women's smoking in New Zealand is notable. Maori women in particular appear to be more prone to smoke in situations of urban inequality than Maori men. To explain the interactions between behaviors and environments requires not only knowing about the qualitative meanings subpopulations provide for their actions and their environments (Frohlich et al., 2002, p. 1413), but also an understanding of the impact of demographic shifts, such as the large proportions of single Maori women moving to cities away from their communities during the 1950s (Goldman, 1957; Metge and Cambell, 1958). Did this movement contribute to today's relative levels of urban and rural inequality and provide unintended exposure to a dangerous commodity?

Life Course and Gender Patterning

There are consistent age-period peaks and declines for Europeans and Maori, respectively, at each time period, and consistent patterns for Pacific people and Asians in 1996 and 2006. However, it does not appear that smoking is merely a rite of passage among the young, only to be left behind by their mid-twenties, in recent Maori or Pacific Island cohorts. With approximately 45% of Maori and 30% of Pacific people smoking into their early forties in 2006, the situation is worse than in 1996. These data show that later quitting occurs less frequently, possibly in part due to contemporary tobacco's high addictiveness. While before Maori quit smoking over the life course, their overall rates are much higher than other groups, and almost twice as many of them continue to smoke into their fifties and sixties compared to the European population.

While the gender differences in smoking have reduced, there is pronounced variability among men and women in different ethnic groups across the different life stages. Since 1976, and contrary to the general argument about the foreseeable end to the epidemic, New Zealand women have not followed men in their smoking "careers" by shunning smoking at the same rate. Figure 12.2 clearly indicates that women have adopted smoking at higher rates from the 15-to 19-year-old group for 30 years or more.

In terms of period effects on smoking, earlier generations, and males in particular, were exposed to the celebration of smoking, whereas from the 1970s women were a major target of cigarette advertising. This commercial "intervention" could be interrogated in concert with cultural histories that reveal a tradition of strong outspoken Maori women and how the combined commercial cultural influences may encourage the consumption of a high-risk commodity, like cigarettes. Whether this sociocultural explanation is stronger than the socioeconomic argument of Maori women responding to area-level inequality by smoking is yet to be tested. What is unclear in contemporary contexts is why being a young female, especially a disadvantaged one, raises the risk of smoking.

CONCLUSION

The urgency to halt the decline in smoking cessation among current cohorts is highlighted by the argument that future generations of smokers are likely to be increasingly disadvantaged and nicotine dependent (Graham et al., 2006, p. ii9). Social network researchers suggest that interventions that target the behaviors of peer groups, social networks, and family groups could be more effective than mass education campaigns. Certainly they are more politically palatable than targeting a major determinant of smoking: namely, income inequalities. However, this analysis suggests that greater understanding of the subpopulation cultural transmission of risk, pleasure, and social solidarity and identity across space and periods is required before we can sensibly conclude that a more targeted diffusion of expert knowledge and healthy role modeling by network members is the best way forward.

The Need for a Multimethod, Multisite, and Team-Based Approach

The availability of high-quality census data covering three decades provides a unique opportunity to track changes in population-wide smoking rates for different age and ethnic groups and compare across two generations. However, tracking this change does not explain what processes are generating health behavior patterns.

The different life course smoking careers exhibited by social–gender and ethnic–gender groups in different localities supports the current interest in social networks as vectors for risky emotions and practices and supports conjecture that cultural factors—such as learned behaviors, peer group influence, and the sociocultural status of men and women within society at large and within their ethnic groups—play an important role in perpetuating smoking behaviors (Dixon and Banwell, 2009). The differential "hold" by social networks over individuals and ethnic groups in urban and rural areas is not known, and qualitative studies are required to augment the census data and the social indicator trends referred to earlier. In this regard, the application of cultural geographic methods, which combine area mapping of services and opportunities with sociocultural assessments of the area, are pertinent (see Gesler and Kearns, 2002, chap. 3; Ellaway and Macintyre, 2009). In relation to youth smoking, Frohlich et al. (2002) have cautioned against a predictable patterning between behaviors and area characteristics and urged focus groups and interviews to explain the spatial epidemiology.

In other words, it is not sufficient to simply add new and improved cultural variables into large surveys. An integrated multimethod design incorporating age–period–cohort quantitative analyses plus qualitative analyses of rationales for behavioral routines and perceptions of areas could be built in at the outset to test alternative theories of risk behavior transmission. One approach involves nested ethnographic studies located across the country on identified SES, ethnic, and geographic differences from census data. An example is the highly innovative "Place of Alcohol in the Lives of New Zealand Women" study conducted in the mid-1980s, which included six locations and nine targeted studies with groups such as Cook Islanders, Maori, young people, and career women. A shared methodology was employed in all studies, based on in-depth interviews, focus groups, and diaries to collect alcohol consumption data (Park, 2001).

New Zealand researchers continue to provide leadership in relation to qualitative approaches to studying smoking. For example, Lanumata's (2009) explication of qualitative research among Pacific people's communities and Marewa Glover's (2005) adoption of a Maori perspective on health, Te Whare Tapa Wha (see Chapter 11), to guide an interview protocol with smokers. This perspective incorporates four aspects that are assumed to be inter-related: the spiritual, physical, psychological, and family and community realms. Glover (2005) considered these realms within the environmental and political contexts of interviewees. Put together, she provides a culturally attuned description of smoking behavior triggers, leading to more nuanced intervention options than typically follow from research designs that omit the sociocultural aspect.

REFERENCES

Abel, S., Park, J., Tipene-Leach, D., Finau, S., Lennan, M., 2001. Infant care practices in New Zealand: a cross-cultural qualitative study. Social Science & Medicine 53, 1135–1148.

Anderson, I., Crengle, S., Kamaka, M., Chen, T.-H., Palafox, P., Jackson-Pulver, L., 2006. Indigenous health in Australia, New Zealand and the Pacific. Lancet 367.

Barnett, R., Moon, G., Kearns, R., 2004. Social inequality and ethnic differences in smoking in New Zealand. Social Science & Medicine 59, 129–143.

Barnett, R., Pearce, J., Moon, G., 2005. Does social inequality matter? changing ethnic socioeconomic disparities and Maori smoking in New Zealand. Social Science & Medicine 60, 1515–1526.

Barnett, R., Pearce, J., Moon, G., 2009. Community inequality and smoking cessation in New Zealand, 1981-2006. Social Science & Medicine 68, 876–884.

Blakely, T., Fawcett, J., Hunt, D., Wilson, N., 2006. What is the contribution of smoking and socioeconomic position to ethnic inequalities in mortality in New Zealand? Lancet 368, 44–52.

Chapman, S., 2007. Health advocacy and tobacco control. Making smoking history. Blackwell Publishing, Oxford.

Christakis, N., Fowler, J., 2008. The collective dynamics of smoking in large social network. New England Journal of Medicine 358, 2249–2258.

Dixon, J., Banwell, C., 2009. Theoretically-driven research for explaining health risk transitions: the case of smoking. Social Science & Medicine 68, 2206–2214.

Ellaway, A., Macintyre, S., 2009. Are perceived neighbourhood problems associated with the likelihood of smoking? Journal of Epidemiology and Community Health 63, 78–80.

Frohlich, K., Potvin, L., Chabot, P., Corin, E., 2002. A theoretical and empirical analysis of context: neighbourhoods, smoking and youth. Social Science & Medicine 54, 1401–1417.

Gesler, W., Kearns, R., 2002. Culture/place/health. Routledge, London.

Giskes, K., Kunst, A., Benach, J., Borrell, C., Costa, G., Dahl, E. et al (2005) Trends in smoking behaviour between 1985 and 2000 in nine European countries by education. Journal of Epi and Community Health 59(5), 395–401.

Glover, M., 2005. Analysing smoking using Te Whare Tapa Wha. New Zealand Journal of Psychology 34, 13–19.

Glover, M., Cowie, N., 2010. Increasing delivery of smoking cessation treatments to Maori and Pacific smokers. New Zealand Medical Journal 123, 6–8.

Goldman, I., 1957. Variations in Polynesian social organization. Journal of Political Science 66, 146–155.

Graham, H., Inskip, H.M., Francis, B., Harman, J., 2006. Pathways of disadvantage and smoking careers: evidence and policy implications. Journal of Epidemiology and Community Health 60, ii7–ii12.

Lanumata, T., Thomson, G., 2009. Unequal risks, unmet needs: the tobacco burden for Pacific peoples in New Zealand. New Zealand Medical Journal 122, 39–53.

Lawlor, D., Frankel, S., Shaw, M., Ebrahim, S., Davey Smith, G., 2003. Smoking and ill-health: does lay epidemiology explain failure of smoking cessation programs among deprived populations? American Journal of Public Health 93, 266–270.

Lopez, A., Collishaw, N., Piha, T., 1994. A descriptive model of the cigarette epidemic in developed countries. Tobacco Control 3, 242–247.

Mackenbach, J., 2006. Health inequalities: Europe in profile. Erasmus MC University Medical Center, Rotterdam.

Metge, M., Cambell, D., 1958. The Rakau Maori studies: a review article. Journal of the Polynesian Society 67, 352–358.

Ministry of Health, 2007. Urban-rural health comparisons: key results of the 2002/03 New Zealand Health Survey. Public Health Intelligence Occasional Bulletin. Ministry of Health, Wellington.

Nuffield Council on Bioethics, 2007. Public health: ethical issues, Cambridge.

O'Dea, D., Howden-Chapman, P., 2000. Income and income inequality in health. In: Howden-Chapman, P., Tobias, M. (Eds.), Social inequalities and health: New Zealand, Ministry of Health, Wellington.

Pampel, F., 2005. Diffusion, cohort change, and social patterns of smoking. Social Science Research 34, 117–139.

Pampel, F., 2007. Persistence of education differences in smoking, United States 1976–2005. Institute of Behavioural Science. University of Colorado, Boulder.

Park, J., 1991. Ladies bring a plate: Change and continuity in the lives of New Zealand women. Auckland University Press, Auckland.

Salmond, C., Crampton, P., Atkinson, J., Edwards, R., 2011. A decade of tobacco control efforts in New Zealand (1996–2006): impacts on inequalities in census-derived smoking prevalence. Nicotine & Tobacco Research. 14, 664–673.

White, V., Hayman, J., 2006. Smoking behaviours of Australian secondary students in 2005. Australian Government Department of Health and Ageing. Drug Strategy Branch, Canberra.

Chapter 13

On Slimming Pills, Growth Hormones, and Plastic Surgery: The Socioeconomic Value of the Body in South Korea

Daniel Schwekendiek,[1] Minhee Yeo,[2] and Stanley Ulijaszek[2]

[1]Sungkyunkwan University, Jongno-gu, Seoul, Republic of Korea and [2]Institute of Social and Cultural Anthropology, University of Oxford, UK

INTRODUCTION

Obsession with one's appearance, specifically height, slimness, and body shape, is a modern social phenomenon in South Korea that has now reached unparalleled proportions. The result is now widespread hormonal growth treatment, demand for slimming pills, and rampant plastic surgery. This chapter discusses the socioeconomic value of the (ideal) body in South Korea, and it also provides a model that contextualizes these phenomena from macrohistorical and multivariate perspectives.

Interestingly, from a historical and cultural point of view, the body has never been an object of obsession let alone something that should be modified in Korean society. On the contrary, under Confucianism, which became the state ideology in Korea during the Joseon dynasty (1392–1910), the body was considered as an object that was naturally inherited from one's ancestors and therefore a part of the collective family (Kim, 2009). Hence, for about 500 years, manipulation of the body and any part of it was considered inappropriate, as it would have violated the Confucian dogma of filial piety and was seen as a rejection of one's natural inheritance. Regarding physical idealization, the corporeal ideal for males was to maintain the family body through ancestor worship, thus making male physical attractiveness per se secondary. Women's corresponding corporeal ideal was bearing a son in order to continue the family line, thus maintaining the family body in the material world. Beauty and physical attractiveness were less important compared to child-bearing or labor abilities (Kim, 2003).

In transitioning South Korea, the body became a political object and part of the social body of the nation. From the mid-1950s to mid-1980s, South Korea was mostly ruled by autocratic if not totalitarian leaders. For political reasons,

When Culture Impacts Health. http://dx.doi.org/10.1016/B978-0-12-415921-1.00013-0

141

individuality was frowned upon, and the ideals of beauty and physical appearance were dictated by the state. For instance, short hair was ordered to be worn by boys at all schools, thus making it the epitome of maleness, whereas long hair was condemned as rebellious. Yet, distinct from Joseon dynasty, women became a part of the work force in industrializing South Korea, as their labor was needed to expand the industrial sector. Whereas Confucianism limited Korean women to a domestic setting through social and legal regulations (Deuchler, 1992), postcolonial Korean women became a part of public life while also constituting a more powerful income group (Kim, 2003).

In the 1990s, with the election of the first democratic South Korean presidents, who in turn also introduced market and media liberalization, and with South Korea emerging as a global player and a fully postindustrialized nation, consumer markets and the media began to influence society's conception of the ideal body. As a result, male and female Korean stars began to modify their bodies in order to obtain more individual conceptions of maleness or femininity, and the masses largely responded to these new ideals. Koreans obsessively started to exercise and diet, with females, especially, often resorting to plastic surgery to obtain an edge in the emerging and highly competitive media star market (Kim, 2009). Not only did Korean media stars start to promote an idealized and manipulated body type, beauty companies also started fiercely competing against each other by actively advertising in order to sell their products and jump on the emerging consumer market bandwagon. In the 1990s, the number of advertisements in Korean magazines about the body drastically increased from a single to double digit number under autocratic rule to 220 in 2001 under democratic leadership (Ham, 2006). Moreover, dieting and slimness were emphasized in the media from the mid-to late 1990s: in the 1980s, three to nine advertisements appeared, whereas in 1999, 65 pieces, more than in the entire 1980s, were published (Ham, 2006). Moreover, males started to dye their hair and began wearing earrings or long hair (Kim, 2009), a corporeal manipulation that was previously stigmatized by the authoritarian government. More important, similar to the slimness craze that was in part enhanced by Korean media stars, the plastic surgery industry started to advertise aggressively: while only approximately 5 of these advertisements surfaced per year in the 1980s, between 10 and 30 were published in the 1990s, and about 70 in the 2000s (Ham, 2006). In summation, during the 1990s, with political democratization and a booming domestic consumer market, modification of the body was no longer taboo. On the contrary, it had become a uniform phenomenon in modern Korean society.

In the late 2000s, besides growing interest in dieting and cosmetic surgery, obsession with height, especially for males, became a burgeoning trend in Korean society (*New York Times*, 2009; *Korea Times*, November 30, 2009), often resulting in hormonal treatment and the expansion of growth clinics. Another major change in the late 2000s was the idealization of (Western) sexy body shapes by a rather conservative Korean society. For females, the ideal of an "S-line" (a Korean–English neologism referring to an hour-glass shape with emphasis on the hips and breasts), and for males, the ideal of an "M-line" (emphasis on the abdominals), emerged in commercials and the media (*Korea Times*, May 8, 2009). Besides dieting and exercise, (sexy) fashion became an important vehicle to achieve such an idealized body shape, resulting in micro miniskirts, extremely tall high heels, and demand for wonder bras or bra padding. For instance, in 2009, miniskirts as short as 23 cm and high heels as tall as 14 cm were sold in major Korean department stores, both new national records (*Joongang Ilbo*, 2009). This was an extreme development for Korean society, which had traditionally been conservative. For instance, women were only a few years earlier expected to wear shirts over their swimsuits (*Korea Times*, January 4, 2009). Of note, the previous de-sexualization of fashion in Korea was likely a remnant of Confucian gender discrimination that forbade a woman from showing any part of her body to unauthorized eyes in order to keep them in the household (Deuchler, 1992).

This article draws on a vast array of sources. Most important, from a methodological point of view, statistical figures employed in this article were taken from secondary literature, most of which comprise articles that recently appeared in major Korean newspapers such as the *Korea Times*, *Choson Ilbo*, or *Joongang Ilbo*. This research also considered further widely read Korean newspapers such as *Hankoreh*, *Korea Herald*, or the *Donga Ilbo*; however, articles appearing in these newspapers were not relevant enough for this project. Today, Korean newspapers oftentimes report on contemporary or emerging trends in Korean society by resorting to comprehensive social surveys carried out by the government or private researchers. Most of the primary data cannot be accessed due to data protection issues. Hence, we are limited to re-citing the survey figures reported in the newspapers. As a consequence, we only provide a contextualized descriptive analysis, rather than testing for statistical significances. Multivariate, advanced statistical analysis is needed in the future.

EMERGENCE OF A WESTERN CORPOREAL IDEAL IN KOREA

The new ideal body type shaped by the media in Korea is primarily a Western body. Corporeal ideals have clearly moved away from the traditional Mongolian body that has been the natural norm on the peninsula for millennia. The idealization of the Western body probably started somewhere in the 1990s due to expanding domestic consumer markets, higher purchasing power of the masses due to economic growth, and, last but not least, selection of the media as a "strategic" industry and engine of growth by the government (Shim, 2005). This not only resulted in drastic liberalization of the media and consumer industry per se, but also major changes in advertisement and marketing laws. For instance, a major revision of the national law in 1994 allowed Korean advertising companies to make use of foreign celebrities and models, which resulted in Korean women's magazines advertising Western looks to their readers (Kim, 2003).

Needless to say, these changes were instrumental, if not causal, in effectively transplanting Western corporeal ideals into traditional Korean society. Although more Asian models seem to appear in Korean commercials today, all of these models have strikingly Western facial features that give them a clear Eurasian look. Korean models are thus cementing Western beauty norms in consumer markets. For instance, the round Korean face, which used to be the standard in Korean society, is now looked down on by the masses, and Koreans today are offended and ashamed if they are told to have a classic "moon face."

Beyond this, Kim (2008) notes that these new (Western) ideals are a result of America's political, military, and media dominance in Asia (especially in postcolonial Korea) in the new world order after World War II. In almost all Southeast and Northeast Asian societies, where America maintains its military bases and political presence, the phenomenon of double eyelid surgeries is common in Asian women who desire to look more Western. In this light, another factor that has increased the idealization of Western looks in South Korea is America's military and economic superiority (and presence) in Asia, resulting in a new form of (cultural) imperialism in the postcolonial era and indirectly dictating American beauty norms to the masses. As correctly pointed out by Kim (2003): "Many of the articles and beauty tips in these [Korean] magazines function on the assumption that the Korean body is flawed while the white body is the standard norm."

In summation, America's economic, political, and media imperialism might have led to the biocultural idealization of Westerners, which, in turn, was picked up and exaggerated by the postcolonial Korean media, thereby creating unrealistic Western corporeal standards in contemporary Korean society.

Socioeconomic Value of the Body

The idealized body is an asset in highly competitive markets in Korea. In the job market, according to a poll by Unilever that was conducted among women in Asia, only 33% of the respondents in South Korea, and thus the lowest rate among all countries in the region, were satisfied with their looks. It was concluded that Koreans were the most insecure about their physical appearance in Asia (*Chosun Ilbo*, September 26, 2009). Similarly, research among 15- to 59-year-old Koreans found that 63% of those who went on a diet in 2008 actually were of normal weight (below a BMI of 25; *Chosun Ilbo*, March 27, 2010). This finding likewise indicates that Koreans seem to be dissatisfied with their bodies even though they are actually healthy by international and national standards. As an explanation, a survey among 243 South Korean job recruiters found that 67% of the employers admitted that the appearance of an applicant does affect their decisions, and a survey among 609 South Korean job hunters found that 25% seemed to have been discriminated against by the job recruiter because of their appearance (*Chosun Ilbo*, November 20, 2009). In other terms, physical appearance is a major criterion in the South Korean job market, as admitted openly by both job hunters and job recruiters. This differs from other (Western) developed countries, where employers have to hire on an equal opportunity job basis. Thus, due to cultural and formal reasons, appearance instead of ability is more often, but certainly not always, a major criterion to landing a job in South Korea (Figure 13.1).

Regarding the marriage markets, the aforementioned poll by Unilever found that 98% of South Korean women indicated that men value the looks of women above everything else. According to a South Korean matchmaking agency surveying 494 single females, 53% of the women indicated that they already had or would like to have plastic surgery to meet a potential husband (*Korea Times*, January 20, 2010). A study among 975 singles aged 20–39 by a South Korean matchmaking agency found that besides financial assets, education, and job security, height is a crucial criterion for the ideal husband, as women expect the prospective husband to stand at 175–180 cm (*Chosun Ilbo*, December 24, 2009). Interestingly, the average height of males in the relevant age group is around 172 cm (Table 13.2), which makes the desired average of 175–180 cm correspond to the top 10% of the South Korean population, further reinforcing the strong desire for an idealized (Western) body. A similar survey among 2,550 Korean adults found that 74% of the female respondents said that height is the main criterion for their dating partners, with an expected height of 180 cm (*Korea Times*, November 30, 2009). According to a much cited quote in a popular TV talk show: "Height is a measure of competitiveness. I think a man who is short is a loser" (*Korea Times*, November 30, 2009). This is an interesting finding, as shortness has historically been idealized, as reflected in two common Korean proverbs: "Little peppers are spicier" and "Tallness is tasteless." In

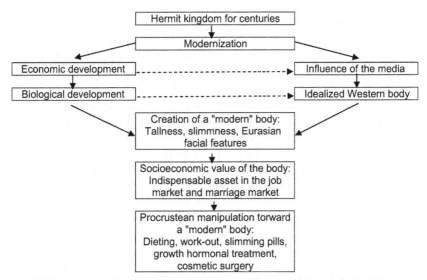

FIGURE 13.1   A model explaining the development of the value of the body in South Korea.

a similar vein, blind dates arranged by friends ("sogaetting") are a common way of dating in Korean society, and Koreans are now primarily interested in knowing the anthropometric measurements of their potential dating partner. In comparison, just a decade earlier, Koreans were primarily interested only in whether or not their prospective dating partner was good looking. Not only are idealized anthropometric measurements important criteria for spouses, now even South Korean parents have high expectations regarding the growth of their offspring. A survey among 400 parents found that the ideal height for sons is 181 cm and for daughters 167 cm. Interestingly, again, these desired heights are far from reality as they correspond to the top 10% of the tallest males and females in South Korea (Table 13.2). However, they almost perfectly correspond to the average heights of South Korean superstars in the media (Table 13.1), who are slightly above the averages of Americans (Table 13.2), again suggesting that media and Western ideals have largely shaped these expectations. All of these findings indicate that there seems to be a recent and extreme shift in the idealized Korean body and its socioeconomic value. Not surprisingly, what can also be seen in Table 13.2 is that both female and male Korean media stars not only correspond to the tallest 10% of the Korean population, but also to the very slimmest 10% of the Korean (and American) population.

Procrustean Manipulation Toward a "Modern" Body

Manipulation toward a normative body is rampant in contemporary South Korean society, ranging from dieting and exercise, facial surgery, growth hormone treatment, and consumption of appetite suppressants. These are elaborated upon in the following section.

The rate of plastic surgery in South Korea is known to be the highest in the world with 17% having gone under the knife and an additional 53% indicating that they have considered it (*Chosun Ilbo*, September 26, 2009). Limiting factors for those who have not undergone surgery but are willing are usually financial constraints. Thus, an incredible rate of 7 in 10 persons seems to demand plastic surgery in Korea. Beyond this, South Korea has now become a major hub for plastic surgery tourism in Asia, with 1,242 plastic surgeons as of 2009 (*Chosun Ilbo*, September 8, 2009). An almost linear increase in plastic surgery clinics has occurred since the 1990s in Korea (Ham, 2006).

Biochemical manipulation for achieving an ideal body has recently become another widespread phenomenon in Korean society. Out of 1,000 respondents surveyed by Consumer Korea in 2008, 13% said they took slimming pills (*Chosun Ilbo*, March 27, 2009). Not only are some of these pills, including appetite suppressants that are arguably narcotics, banned in many countries such as the European Union, many South Koreans of normal weight seem to demand them and corrupt doctors often supply them. The market for slimming pills has grown fourfold from 2003 to 2008 in Korea, and the country is now even ranked second and third in the world in consumption of the appetite suppressants

TABLE 13.1 Anthropometry of Top 10 Stars in South Korea in 2009

Income rank 2009	Western name (leader of band)	Gender	Job	Birth year	Height	Weight	BMI
1	TVXQ (Jung Yun Ho)	Male	Singer, dancer, model	1986	1.84	66	19.49
2	Rain	Male	Actor, singer	1982	1.84	75	22.15
3	Big Bang (Kwon Ji-Yong)	Male	Rapper, singer, producer	1988	1.77	58	18.51
4	Super Junior (Park Jung-Soo)	Male	Singer, dancer, actor	1983	1.78	59	18.62
5	Kim Hyun Joong	Male	Actor, singer	1986	1.80	68	20.99
6	Ko Hyun Jung	Female	Actress, model, singer	1971	1.72	54	18.25
7	Girls' Generation (Kim Tae-yeon)	Female	Singer	1989	1.62	44	16.77
8	Lee Byung Hun	Male	Actor, singer	1970	1.78	68	21.46
9	Yoo Jae Suk	Male	Comedian	1972	n/a	n/a	n/a
10	Kang Ho Dong	Male	Comedian, wrestler	1970	n/a	n/a	n/a

Source: All K-Pop, "VXQ are top earners in Korea for 2009," under: http://www.allkpop.com/2009/12/tvxq_top_earnings_in_korea_for_2009 (accessed online 12 July 2010); various star profiles from http://wiki.d-addicts.com (accessed online 12 July 2010).

TABLE 13.2 Height and BMI of Korean Top Stars, Average Koreans, and Average Americans

Anthropometry	Mean	Centiles				
		10th	25th	50th	75th	90th
Height Korean males (25–29 years)	172.5 cm	165.5 cm	169.2 cm	172.5 cm	176.5 cm	179.5 cm
Height U.S.–American males (20–29 years)	177.6 cm	167.1 cm	172.3 cm	177.8 cm	183.0 cm	186.8 cm
Height Korean male top stars	180.2 cm					
Height Korean females (25–29 years)	159.3 cm	152.7 cm	155.7 cm	159.0 cm	163.0 cm	166.0 cm
Height U.S.–American females (20–29 years)	163.2 cm	154.8 cm	158.7 cm	163.0 cm	167.9 cm	171.4 cm
Height Korean female top stars	167.0 cm					
BMI Korean males	23.0*	20.0	21.0	23.0	25.0	27.0
BMI U.S.–American males (20–29 years)	27.0	20.7	23.1	25.8	30.1	34.2
BMI Korean male top stars	20.2					
BMI Korean females	22.0*	19.0	20.0	22.0	24.0	26.0
BMI U.S.–American females (20–29 years)	26.5	19.4	21.4	24.4	30.0	35.9
BMI Korean female top stars	19.1					

*Indicates median because means were were not reported.
Source: McDowell et al. (2008), The Korean Society of the Study of Obesity, "Report of Obesity in Korea," under: http://www.iotf.org/oonet/korea2.htm (accessed online 12 July 2010); Korean Agency for Technology and Standards (2004); Data for Korean media top stars from Table 13.1.

phendimetrazine and phentermine, despite the finding that Korea already has one of the lowest obesity rates in the developed world. Previous research has found that Koreans are much more influenced by diet pill advertisements (rather than active exercising) compared to Western consumers (Kim and Lennon, 2006).

A similar expansion has started to occur in the growth hormone treatment market. An increasing number of South Koreans now resort to hormone treatment to improve their stature, an extreme and questionable manipulation of the body such that even the *New York Times* (*Korea Times*, November 30, 2009) recently featured a full-length article. Many South Korean parents from the middle class, being worried about their offspring's anthropometric development, today even give vitamins and concoctions (that are advertised to stimulate growth) to their children. Upper-class parents spend as much as $2,500 to send their children to clinics where they receive hormone shots to boost their stature. Although most of these medical and pseudomedical treatments have not even been proven to raise stature, this clearly reflects a new body craze that is perhaps unparalleled in modern history; to our knowledge, no other society in the world values stature as much as South Korea apparently does.

A Model Explaining the Biosocial Value of the Body

Our model attempts to contextualize the aforementioned findings in a multivariate, more casual way (see Figure 13.1). After centuries of self-imposed isolation from the West, (forced) socioeconomic modernization suddenly began in the early twentieth century with Japanese colonization and was continued under American occupancy after liberation and American political assistance during the Cold War.

We suggest that two major developments took place. First, the South Korean economy rose dramatically within just a few decades, which led to better biological living standards for the Korean people and anthropometry levels approaching those of developed (thus Western) nations (Schwekendiek and Jun, 2010). It is important to realize that these biosocial secular improvements in body size occurred naturally and in a steady but accelerating process over a few decades. Second, another major change occurred in the media in postindustrialized Korea, which underwent sudden political and economic liberalization resulting in emerging domestic consumer markets as well as revision of the marketing law contributing to the rise of the advertising industry. The media , targeted as a "cultural technology" by the new Korean government (Shim, 2005), developed from a minor and regulated infant industry under military dictatorship to a key industry under democratic leadership. As a manifestation of the growing power of the media, a survey among South Korean schoolchildren found that in the early 1980s, thus before expansion of the media industry, the majority wanted to become scientists (23%), followed by teachers (14%), judges (12%), and doctors (11%). However, these days, some 42% want to be singers, followed by actors (9%), whereas the proportion of South Korean schoolchildren desiring to become scientists has fallen to below 1% (*Chosun Ilbo*, March 3, 2010). This clearly shows that the power of the media has risen dramatically in the postindustrialized era. More important, as laid out in great depth above, the media, for example, its stars and models, largely started to represent Western beauty and corporeal ideals, which in turn began influencing the masses toward an idealized "modern" body while stigmatizing the classical and natural Korean (i.e., Mongolian) phenotype.

Two side developments are worth pointing out. First, economic development of (postindustrialized) South Korea has largely occurred via new (visual) media, comprising the Internet, mobile phones, and computers, where beauty and design play important roles. As an illustration of this, it should be taken into consideration that South Korea is the largest producer of flat screens, second and third largest producer of mobile phones, and represents the sixth largest nation in both broadband and e-commerce in the world (Foster-Carter, 2009). Engines of economic growth have largely shifted away from traditional sectors such as the textile industry or heavy industry to (visual) consumer electronics, which has resulted in expansion of Korea's visual media sector (not to mention that the movie and music industry per se was targeted by the government in the 1990s).

A second side development has resulted from (naturally) improving anthropometry due to economic growth. South Koreans underwent dramatic increases in growth and are now the tallest in East Asia and probably among the entire Mongolian race; moreover, they are rapidly catching up to Western anthropometric levels (Schwekendiek and Jun, 2010). This finding might have led to new body awareness, which could have been partially utilized by the media and marketing industry to transplant the Western body into Korean society. Interestingly, Korea's media idol, Hollywood, does not seem to promote extraordinarily tall or extremely slim ideals, as many male and female Hollywood stars are rather short and not necessarily extremely underweight. On the contrary, according to a former applicant in Hollywood, the media industry seems to prefer smaller actors because they look better from most camera angles (Schwekendiek, 2010). In a similar vein, Hollywood does not promote plastic surgery among its actors and actresses at all; American actors are primarily selected for their acting and natural looks, whereas candidates who have received plastic surgery are even disadvantaged (*Chosun Ilbo*, July 23, 2010). A major difference is that Korean superstars are recruited early in their careers by professional entertainment agencies, whereupon they receive all-around training in various disciplines, as can also be seen in Table 13.1 where many Korean stars are singers, actors, dancers, and models at the same time. Many of these roles require a rather tall stature, a perfect body weight, and extreme beauty, which might largely explain why South Korean superstars are more often selected for their extraordinary physical appearance than ability alone compared to movie and music stars in the West. Further, Korean entertainment agencies expect media stars to be quite present and socially interacting, for example, on TV shows or live events, such that not only beauty but also anthropometry becomes a *conditio sine qua non* to become a media star.

The combination of (natural) secular improvements in the anthropometry of Koreans due to economic development and the increasing power of the media and consumer markets worshipping a westernized body has led to the creation of a new body awareness in postindustrialized Korea. Tallness, slimness, and Eurasian facial features constitute this modern body, which has quickly become the "state of the art" of the masses. The problem now is that this new (overidealized) body also has become the norm in the highly competitive job and marriage markets, where women and men who do not correspond to these new beauty standards are marginalized and discriminated against, even when they have better abilities. Hence, the perfect body per se becomes an indispensable asset for these perhaps two most important spheres of life, landing a job and finding a partner.

Finally, because only very few fulfill these idealized norms, the masses rampantly start manipulating their bodies toward the desired (Western) media ideal by dieting, exercising, or taking slimming pills to achieve a perfect body weight, or by resorting to medical (or pseudomedical) treatment to improve their stature. Last, the masses are rampantly undergoing surgery, often starting in middle school and at the latest before going on a marriage date or to a job interview.

Implications

Let's discuss some implications of this article. On the positive side, South Korea seems to be a place that has high body awareness, leading to healthy lifestyles such as fitness and balanced nutrition. South Korea has one of the lowest obesity rates in the developed world and has avoided the obesity problems that have plagued almost all Western nations in the late twentieth century. Our model suggests that Koreans opt for healthy living because anthropometry represents embodied capital in Korea's highly competitive job and marriage markets and because Koreans are largely influenced by the media. It has been suggested that the extraordinary low rate of obesity in postindustrialized Korea can be explained by active government intervention that has banned fast-food restaurants close to schools or fast-food commercials on TV. Previous research also suggested that the retention of traditional healthy food elements in the Korean diet as well as the continuation of Korean cooking practices have contributed to a relatively low-fat diet in Korea (Kim et al., 2001; Lee et al., 2002). We suggest that nutritional asceticism, that is, intrinsic motivation not to overeat as an investment into the future job and marriage markets, represents a major determinant of body weight in Korea. Hence, according to our model, the low prevalence of obesity in Korean society can be explained by *food demand* factors rather than (governmental or traditional) *food supply* factors alone.

On the other hand, a number of health risks have resulted from rampant body manipulation in Korean society. Although the nation has seemingly avoided the negative effects of obesity-related diseases such as diabetes and heart disease and stroke, there is tentative evidence for anorexia resulting from Korea's obsession with slimness as well as completely new health risks emerging from rampant use of appetite suppressants and growth hormone injections (whose side effects are unknown). In a similar vein, it seems that there are a number of unlicensed plastic surgeons operating due to high demand, even though such double-eyelid surgeries and nose jobs represent a certain health risk while having no medical advantage.

Perhaps the most dangerous development in Korea is that ethic discussion of corporeal ideals does not take place or is completely ignored by the masses. The recent development toward growth hormone treatment and consumption of appetite suppressants is dangerous as it is the beginning of a new form of biosocial engineering. The question then becomes: What is next on the biosocial agenda? Is it blue eyes? Is it genetic manipulation? This raises a historical discussion on eugenics and biological Darwinism, a questionable ideal that is resurfacing in Korea now.

In addition, our article found that social stress seems to have increased dramatically over the last decade. Koreans, from middle school age onward, are already concerned, if not obsessed, with their bodies. Adults in the job and marriage markets as well as those pursuing a professional career are indirectly pressured to go under the knife if they do not correspond to the corporeal ideal. As suggested, this is a matter of economic survival and of avoiding social stigmatization. As a result, it is creating a new form of biosocial stress, the extent of which does not exist anywhere else in the world.

Finally, this article supports active policy interventions in Korea to relieve social stress from the masses and break the vicious circle of biosocial manipulation. We have argued that liberalization of the media in Korea has resulted in enormous economic success and expansion of an industry that now seems to influence the masses more than anything else. Korean policy makers would be advised to encourage advertising companies, the media industry, and entertainment agencies to return to a more realistic image of media stars that reflects the Korean population rather than an exaggerated (Western) media ideal.

From a methodological point of view, this article is limited to secondary sources because of data inaccessibility issues. As a result, we have only provided a descriptive analysis of major reported survey findings, which we contextualized and explained. Future research will have to apply advanced data analysis to test for statistical significances and differences among respondents. As social survey data from governments oftentimes cannot be accessed due to privacy protection of individuals or formal issues, researchers will have to implement their own social surveys. This can be easily done by conducting random telephone interviews. This is a common and reliable sampling method in the United States when there is no underlying population data from the government or other institutions. Such a generated dataset will also allow multivariate testing of hypotheses.

ACKNOWLEDGMENTS

Daniel Schwekendiek was supported by the National Research Foundation of Korea by the Korean Government (MEST) (NRF-2007-361-AL0014).

REFERENCES

Chosun Ilbo, 8 September 2009, "Plastic Surgery All the Rage Among College Students."
Chosun Ilbo, 26 September 2009, "Korean Women Among Region's Most Insecure: Poll."
Chosun Ilbo, 20 November 2009, "More Koreans Pin Job Hopes on Plastic Surgery."
Chosun Ilbo, 24 December 2009, "What Makes the Perfect Potential Spouse?"
Chosun Ilbo, 3 March 2010, "Young Koreans' Obsession with Stardom Is a Deep Concern."
Chosun Ilbo, 27 March 2010, "Koreans Overdose on Diet Pills."
Chosun Ilbo, 23 July 2010, "Hollywood Leans Toward More Natural Looks."
Deuchler, M., 1992. The Confucian Transformation: A Study of Society and Ideology. Harvard University Asia Center, Cambridge.
Foster-Carter, A., 2009. North & South Korea: Two Crises—One Future? www.menas.co.uk/newsroom/Korea.pdf.
Ham, I., 2006. Korean Culture of Daily Life and Body. Ewha Womans University Press, Seoul.
Joongang Ilbo, 15 December 2009, "Miniskirts Tell Tale of Rough Economy."
Kim, E.-S., 2009. The Politics of the Body in Contemporary Korea. Korea Journal. Autumn, 5–14.
Kim, M., Lennon, S.J., 2006. Content analysis of diet advertisements: a cross-national comparison of Korean and U.S. women's magazines. Clothing and Textiles Research Journal 24, 345–362.
Kim, N., 2008. Imperial Citizens: Koreans and Race from Seoul to LA. Stanford University Press, Stanford.
Kim, S., Moon, S., Popkin, B., 2001. Nutrition transition in the Republic of Korea. Asia Pacific Journal of Clinical Nutrition 10, 848–856.
Kim, T., 2003. Neo-confucian body techniques: women's bodies in korea's consumer Society. Body & Society 9, 97–113.
Korea Times, 4 January 2009, "Ads Mirroring Social Changes."
Korea Times, 8 May 2009, "Korean Women Are Not Alphabets."
Korea Times, 30 November 2009, "'Tall Man' Industry Thriving."
Korea Times, 20 January 2010, "Women Willing to Undergo Surgery for Marriage."
Lee, M.-J., Popkin, B., Kim, S., 2002. The unique aspects of the nutrition transition in South Korea: the retention of healthful elements in their traditional diet. Public Health Nutrition 5, 197–203.
McDowell, M.A., Fryar, C.D., Ogden, C.L., Flegal, K.M., 2008. Anthropometric Reference Data for Children and Adults: United States, 2003-2006. National Health Statistics Report Number 10.
New York Times, 23 December 2009, "South Korea Stretches Standards for Success."
Schwekendiek, D., 3 March 2010. "Korea: Indications and Implications, " Unit for Biocultural Variation and Obesity Seminar. University of Oxford, Online under http://media.podcasts.ox.ac.uk/socanth/ubvo/Schwekendiek03Mar10.mp3.
Schwekendiek, D., Jun, S.-H., 2010. From the poorest to the tallest in East-Asia: the secular trend in height of South Koreans. Korea Journal 50, 151–175.
Shim, D., 2005. Globalization and Cinema Regionalization in East Asia. Korean Journal. Fall, 233–260.

Economically Transitioning Societies

Tacking between Disciplines: Approaches to Tuberculosis in New Zealand, the Cook Islands, and Tuvalu

Julie Park and Judith Littleton

Department of Anthropology, The University of Auckland, New Zealand

We are frequently being urged to broaden our perspectives to adopt more holistic frameworks whether they are cultural epidemiology, social epidemiology, or political ecology (Baer, 1996; Kreiger, 2001; Trostle, 2004). Rather than simply adding more levels to an analysis or attempting an "add and stir" approach to multidisciplinarity, we are arguing in this chapter for an approach that tacks between disciplines, recognizing the different logics that underlie approaches and seeing the gaps between as areas for exploration. We further argue that anthropological theory (in its entirety, which extends well beyond culture theory) and approaches to public health can be usefully married with (but not absorbed into) an epidemiological approach. A more generic social science approach is clearly useful in some respects, but we suggest that maintaining tension between different approaches to public health issues is more creative.

In our research we are building a picture of tuberculosis (TB), which includes problematic categories such as "migrant TB," that acknowledges historical arrangements and seeks linkages between biological entities and socioeconomic arrangements in the context of lived experience. Within the "Transnational Pacific Health through the Lens of TB" project, we and our students have tended not to give primacy to one method or one discipline but tacked between. The result is a complex web of causation and lived experience. In this chapter we analyze aspects of historical and contemporary tuberculosis in Polynesia (including New Zealand) to demonstrate how multiple, separate disciplines contribute to a deeper understanding.

When Culture Impacts Health. http://dx.doi.org/10.1016/B978-0-12-415921-1.00014-2

QUESTIONING EPIDEMIOLOGY: TB AND MIGRANTS

In 1972, A.R. Kerr, Secretary of the Thoracic Society, wrote to the editor of the *New Zealand Medical Journal* about the Society's concern with the high incidence of active TB among recently arrived Pacific Island immigrants. He included in his letter a long extract from Dr. Ryan, the tuberculosis officer for the Auckland Hospital Board. Ryan claimed that more than one-third (37%) of the TB cases in Auckland were recent Pacific migrants who had brought TB with them. Ryan was of course concerned about the spread of the disease, but he also emphasized the financial cost these new settlers placed on the New Zealand tax payer: "The arrival of active cases of tuberculosis from overseas constitutes a public health hazard and represents a financial burden to the New Zealand tax-payer" (Ryan, quoted in Kerr 1972, p. 295). This emphasis suggests that Pacific people in New Zealand were not tax payers, and perhaps not New Zealanders, despite the special status as citizens of many of these migrants and the other arrangements in place for permanent residency and acquiring citizenship.[1] The debate played out in the pages of the *New Zealand Medical Journal*. In reply Mackay, a doctor in Wellington, acknowledged the high TB rates among Maori and Pacific peoples in New Zealand, but presented the epidemiological information for both his and Ryan's patients. This showed that because many of them were born in New Zealand and others had been here for years, it was impossible for most of them to have brought in TB (Dunsford et al., 2011, p. 68). As he stated: "During 1970 and 1971, 28 immigrants to New Zealand were discovered to have tuberculosis within one year of arrival, but only six of these were immigrants from the Pacific Islands" (Mackay, 1972, p. 449). An analysis of ethnicity and TB data by Swinburn (1973) indicated a much lower proportion (15.5%) of admissions from Pacific people than that suggested by Ryan.

This debate could perhaps be seen as simply a case of good versus bad epidemiology: the "immigrant TB" trope laid to rest once and for all by properly analyzed, reliable data. But such an explanation is unsatisfactory because the trope persists into the twenty-first century, despite evidence to the contrary (Das et al., 2006; Littleton et al., 2010). Admittedly, the category of migrant now includes a much wider range of groups than only those from the Pacific. This association of tuberculosis with certain (often highly visible) migrant groups (Lawrence et al., 2008) and the tacit exclusion of members of those groups from full citizenship takes concrete form in debates about the legitimacy of access of migrants with TB to New Zealand's public health services. Exclusionary views are not confined to certain fringe groups but can be heard in the national Parliament in an effort to appeal to voters (Park and Littleton, 2007). Epidemiology

---

1. Cook Islanders, Niueans, and Tokelauans are New Zealand citizens, and a variety of special arrangements were in place for Samoans, some of whom were citizens, and later for Tongans and Tuvaluans.

cannot explain this persistence or the attraction of the idea of immigrant TB, but anthropology and history can, using the social theories that have been developed in these and related social science disciplines.

One useful theory is that of "Anglo decline." This theory addresses the sense of decline in power and influence experienced by sectors of society that were the unquestioned "national managers," to use Ghassan Hage's term (Hage, 1998). The multicultural realities created through population mobility and multinational movement of capital mean that formerly dominant sectors of society have to yield space to newer groups, and newer interest groups and experience a loss of their formerly unquestioned right to enjoy life in the ways to which they had become accustomed. As a result, they blame newly arrived groups for these losses and unpleasant experiences of no longer being in control. Such targeting finds expression in parliamentary debates, newspaper commentaries, and general discourse around particular groups of immigrants and disease (Park and Littleton, 2007; Lawrence et al., 2008).

Agamben's (1998) distinction between *zoe* and *bios* or full life and bare life is also useful here. Migrants may be welcomed as laboring bodies, for example, but most are unwelcome as full citizens and political subjects. The ideological categorization of workers as a "labor resource" or "input factor" separate from the worker-person enables the host society to ignore migrants' rights apart from a right to bare life. This distinction is clearly made above in Ryan's comments, which focus upon the category of temporary work permit holders and contrasts that with New Zealand citizens who are tax payers. (Temporary work permit holders of course were also tax payers, but this seems to have escaped notice.)

Both epidemiology and these social sciences are needed together to counteract the prejudicial beliefs that load the blame for TB in New Zealand onto new migrants, or to address the social and physical conditions that allow TB and other infectious diseases to flourish in some communities (Park and Littleton, 2007). Migrants are frequently targeted as a source of TB infection and they do experience higher rates of TB than many host populations (Das et al., 2006; Littleton et al., 2008), but this epidemiological fact is not a "natural fact." It masks the complexity around the categorization of peoples and the identification of particular groups as problems, and draws attention away from social inequalities, which can be explored and explained through social theory. But further than this, we have found that to understand the current rates of TB among Pacific Islanders requires attention to history as well as contemporary circumstances.

THE MATTERS OF HISTORY: WHY HISTORICAL POLITICAL ECOLOGY IS NECESSARY

In New Zealand, one recently arrived group of Pacific migrants is from Tuvalu. It was only in the 1990s that their numbers exceeded 1,000 and at the time of writing it is estimated that this community may number 3,500–4,000.[2] Approximately 11,000 Tuvaluans reside in their home islands where they confront many challenges, especially related to the effects of climate change and other forms of globalization. Although the TB rates in Tuvalu have begun to tumble since the 1990s, they are still very high according to World Health Organization standards. In Auckland, Tuvaluans are estimated to have roughly ten times the TB rates of other Pacific peoples. These high TB rates can be explained in a number of ways such as crowded living conditions, much interhousehold movement, a sometimes inadequate diet, and syndemic interactions between these socioeconomic conditions, other diseases, such as diabetes, and a large amount of latent TB in this community (Littleton and Park, 2009). However, this framework is inadequate without a basis in historical political economy, since it fails to explain why this particular community is affected in such a manner.

In a recent paper (Park et al., 2011) we have argued that the high TB rates among Tuvaluans at the turn of the twenty-first century cannot be completely understood without knowing the historical background of colonization of Tuvalu by Britain. From the London center of this empire, Tuvalu (then the Ellice Islands and part of the Gilbert and Ellice Islands Protectorate) was at the end of a very tenuous line. Even with the Western Pacific High Commission, of which it was part, based in relatively nearby Suva, Fiji, contemporary reports during the colonial era demonstrate that the Ellice Islands were too far away, and granted too few resources, for the type of health care that would help combat rampant TB. The situation was exacerbated because Ellice Islanders along with Gilbertise were involved in contract labor for the British Phosphate Company, especially in the nearby phosphate islands where conditions were often harsh and conducive to the development and spread of TB. By the 1970s when the Ellice Islands separated from the Gilberts and became independent, TB was still an important health problem, 20 years after effective detection, treatment, and prevention were available (Resture, 2010). It took newly independent Tuvalu another 20 years before those TB rates showed improvement. Hence the current TB situation in New Zealand and in Tuvalu is hopefully the tail end of a TB epidemic introduced with colonial contact and maintained through colonial practices as well as current socioeconomic conditions.

At the other end of the spectrum is the situation of the Cook Islands where TB rates are so low they are almost indiscernible; one case might pop up every two or three years. Yet in Auckland, there are several cases each year with Cook Islands people. Again a historical approach is needed (Futter Puati, 2010). Unlike Tuvalu, the Cook Islands were much closer to the center of its colonial power, New Zealand. The parallels drawn by both Cook Islands and New Zealand doctors between Cook Islanders and Maori and persistent work to implement prevention and treatment that was acceptable to the local people led to successful

---

2. The 2006 census enumerated 2,625 (Statistics New Zealand, 2008).

control of tuberculosis. By the 1970s TB was no longer a serious health problem for the Cook Islands. Leading biomedically trained Cook Islands doctors recognized and respected the cultural knowledge of local people and local expert healers in relation to health risks and healing. They worked with them rather than against them. At the same time, the historical records suggest that what might be interpreted as an authoritarian regime of surveillance, isolation, and treatment was very largely accepted by the people as care, necessary to rid them of TB. Indeed, our recent research (2010 and 2011) on the island of Atiu in the southern Cook Islands suggests this interpretation of care is still very current. Whether it is the quarterly inspections of all houses and yards to check that living conditions are health giving and there are no breeding grounds for mosquitoes, or the full turnout of everyone eligible (and quite a few who were over the target age) for human papillomavirus vaccinations, the accepting, and indeed welcoming, of this kind of intensive attention for the good of the community is very striking. Detailed historical and ethnographic research provides a community-based perspective to try to tease out the principles and relationships that made the Cook Islands' efforts to reduce and prevent TB so successful. Yet if that is the case then why does TB occur among Cook Islanders resident in Auckland, albeit at lower rates than among the Tuvaluan community?

CONTEMPORARY TB: NEW THEORETICAL FRAMEWORKS

Setting the frame more broadly, TB among Pacific peoples in New Zealand has a different epidemiological distribution to other ethnic groups. Rates among Pacific people in total are higher than among Maori or Pakeha but lower than among a large category called Asian. However, as alluded to above, dividing the category "Pacific" into island groupings shows great degrees of variation that partially reflect historic experiences as described above. What is also different about the epidemiology of TB among Pacific people in New Zealand is that, contrary to most other ethnic categories, high rates of TB among the elderly are accompanied by active transmission among children.

A powerful explanation is that compared to other groups in New Zealand, Pacific people live in poorer socioeconomic circumstances, one factor of which is household crowding. That relationship between household crowding and infectious disease was clearly demonstrated in an analysis of an epidemic of meningococcal disease and tuberculosis (Baker et al., 2008). However, we would argue that the situation is more complex than a social determinants of health framework might suggest and that a syndemic perspective might be usefully applied. *Syndemic* is a term coined by Merrill Singer and colleagues to refer to "two or more afflictions, interacting synergistically, contributing to excess burden of disease in a population" (Syndemics Prevention Network, 2005). Alternative terms include disease clusters and coexisting epidemics, but such terms suggest a simultaneous occurrence whereas the seeds for a syndemic may be sown over time. We have suggested that such is the case for Pacific peoples in New Zealand (Littleton and Park, 2009). Contemporary tuberculosis among these groups is a historical legacy of high rates of infection among children and adults during the 1950s to 1970s (and later for Tuvalu). However, that legacy of TB infection that can reactivate to active disease is experienced within a community now facing a major epidemic of obesity and diabetes. TB and diabetes interact: pre-existing diabetes is associated with a higher rate of reactivation of TB infection to disease, and it makes for a more difficult diagnosis of tuberculosis and a more difficult and prolonged treatment regimen. It is suspected that TB disease also contributes to the development of diabetes. Furthermore, noxious social conditions such as household crowding, poor nutrition, and exposure to smoke contribute to both conditions. In the case of Pacific people in New Zealand, these interactions occur in the context of crowded households, households where grandparents and other elders who are susceptible to both TB and diabetes are providing childcare to young children, and where household composition fluctuates in response to transnational movement. Movement to New Zealand is movement into a context where housing and food is dependent upon cash in contrast to the islands where many people pay no rent and where much of their food can be raised or caught. We have argued, based on our ethnographic research as well as analysis of demographic and epidemiological data, that this syndemic interaction explains why the epidemiological pattern of tuberculosis for Pacific peoples is different than for other ethnicities in New Zealand.

Adopting a syndemic orientation therefore ensures that we focus on the connections between health-related problems rather than focus upon a particular disease. Those connections include social conditions and addressing them involves social change and social policy (Syndemics Prevention Network, 2005). The syndemic perspective drawn earlier, however, leaves out one important aspect of social policy, namely immigration status. Cook Islanders in New Zealand are New Zealand citizens with free access to hospital and public health services. Rates of TB are higher among Cook Islanders living in Auckland than in the Cook Islands for a range of reasons. Living conditions are difficult and the health consequences of household crowding are more acute in New Zealand, thus TB transmission is more likely. Activation of latent TB infection into TB disease as a consequence of comorbidity is also likely. Furthermore, some Cook Islanders come to New Zealand because of complex health problems, such as treatment for cancer and diabetes. What distinguishes a Cook Islanders experience of TB in New Zealand from a Tuvaluan one is that immigration status does not have to be considered, much less worried about, in diagnosis or treatment of the disease, as Cook Islanders are New Zealand citizens. For Tuvaluans, however, uncertain migration status is a major problem. Historical factors mean that there is not a single "tuberculosis" for Pacific people.

An outbreak of TB among Tuvaluan families in Auckland in 2002–2003 highlighted these issues. Voss et al. (2006) described the course of the disease through the children while ethnographic interviews by Ng Shiu (2006) and Hay (2009) showed the difficulties faced by Pacific households touched by the disease and the health workers working with them, given uncertain immigration status and frequent transnational movement combined with a lack of resources. As Hay (2009, p. 63) wrote of one of her participants:

Ioane lives rurally and took time from work to transport his father, translate for him and keep him company in a foreign country. Each trip to the nearest hospital was an hour's drive. Once Betero was back at his son's place, the PHN or Public Health Assistant had to make the journey to his house every day to give daily DOT. The landline was disconnected and usually Ioane's mobile phone was not answered so that it was impossible for the PHN to know whether Betero and any others she needed to visit were actually at home. Ioane had to be at home for testing of other family members because he was the only English speaker and there were no interpreters available for their language. Ioane and others in the households with TB or LTBI had to take time off work and drive to a laboratory for blood tests. The laboratory nearest to them was some kilometres away and had limited opening hours...Ioane is still paying for his father's hospital stay because his doctors did not apply to the MoH for a Section 10 letter....

Gaining a sense of this lived experience through ethnographic fieldwork, which in this case has involved life history interviews, participant observation at clinic appointments, and other community events, has brought to the fore two separate matters of policy: the role of immigration policy in constructing health and public health risks, and the need for an effective public health service provision.

As detailed previously New Zealand does not have a "special" relationship with Tuvalu. Tuvaluans may apply for immigration to New Zealand and 75 places are available each year for families with offers of employment. These places are rarely filled given the stringent requirements (Malua, 2011). An additional avenue of temporary immigration is the Recognized Seasonal Employment Scheme, which allows for groups of up to 50 people to come for a period of nine months to work in seasonal employment such as fruit picking. Such schemes are closely monitored to ensure that those workers return to their home countries at the end of the period of employment. At the same time, however, Tuvaluans are increasingly concerned about the impact of climate change on Tuvalu and the long-term chances of their children and wishing to establish transnational networks so that they may have options should Tuvalu become uninhabitable. New Zealand is, because of historical links and geographic proximity, an obvious option. As a result there is a growing Tuvaluan community with undocumented migration status. The TB research demonstrates how this contributes to health issues and work by Malua (2011) has shown the strain the current immigration policy places upon families and the community. We, along with Bedford and Bedford (2010), have argued that given the inevitability of climate-forced migration, changes to immigration policy now are desirable (Park and Littleton, 2011).

The other side of the equation is the need for effective health services that can work with such communities. In Auckland, the public health services are organized on a regional basis with contact tracing and delivery of TB medication (whether as directly observed therapy or self-administered) undertaken by a team of public health nurses and workers. As studies of TB outbreaks have demonstrated, such work can be extremely challenging in the context of a stigmatized condition like TB and the fear of immigration authorities. Ethnographic research including participant observation with patients and occasionally with nurses, and especially interviews and casual conversations, has shown that the role of the public health nurse (PHN) was much more than that of a dispenser and observer of therapy. She (nearly all were women) was someone who "walked with" the patient through the difficult and onerous treatment program. She was there to sound off to; to intervene with government departments so that entitlements to housing and income support were received; to provide comfort, encouragement, and friendship; to celebrate the milestones of treatment; and to provide, especially from the resources of the Lung Health Association, taxi chits and sometimes food vouchers, to allow appointments to be met and food on the table. Some patients used phrases such as "I love my PHN." "I owe my life to her." Although patients realized that the PHNs were monitoring their treatment, they too, like the Cook Islanders, felt this as care. In an early publication from our project we used the phrase "alliance and compliance" (Searle et al., 2007), but this sense of being cared for went well beyond the Pakeha (European) population on which that paper was based and included Maori (Oh, 2005), a variety of Asian groups (Anderson, 2008), and an African refugee population (Lawrence, 2008), as well as several Pacific groups (Ng Shiu, 2008). Yet changes in health service delivery mean that such services can be at risk as was so clearly demonstrated in New York in the early 1990s (Wallace and Wallace, 1998). It is the ethnographic work that shows the important content of the work of PHNs in walking alongside their patients.

CONCLUSION

We adopted TB as a focus for our work initially because of fears that it was a growing problem in New Zealand. Over the course of our research the rates of TB have stopped growing yet it has remained a useful focus for research. TB is a condition that places people into prolonged contact with the health care system and as such it has highlighted for us the cracks and inequalities within our societies. Equally important, it has forced us to focus and adopt a range of disciplinary perspectives from epidemiology, anthropology, history, health promotion, political studies, development studies, and geography. Through the work of all of the different investigators involved in the project, different questions, conundrums, and perspectives have been highlighted and explored. The result is (as is clear in this chapter) not just a single narrative, and we have moved over the course of our work from the importance and historical construction of stigma to a much broader sense of the role of transnationalism in constructing contemporary health experiences. This is not a straight disciplinary path but a tacking between.

REFERENCES

Agamben, G., 1998. Homo sacer: Sovereign power and bare life. Stanford University Press, Stanford.

Anderson, A., 2008. Mark of shame: Social stigma, tuberculosis and Asian immigrants to New Zealand. In: Farmer, T., Herring, J., Littleton, J., Park, J. (Eds.), Multiplying and Dividing: Tuberculosis in Canada and Aotearoa New Zealand, RAL-e 2, Auckland, pp. 196–204.

Baer, H., 1996. Bringing political ecology into critical medical anthropology: a challenge to biomedial approaches. Medical Anthropology 17, 129–141.

Baker, M., Das, D., Vengopal, K., Howden-Chapman, P., 2008. Tuberculosis associated with household crowding in a developed country. Journal of Epidemiological and Community Health 62, 715–721.

Bedford, R., Bedford, C., 2010. International Migration and Climate Change: A post-Copenhagen perspective on options for Kiribati and Tuvalu. In: Burson, B. (Ed.), Climate Change and Migration: A South Pacific Perspective, Institute of Policy Studies, Wellington, pp. 89–134.

Das, D., Baker, M., Venugopal, K., McAllister, S., 2006. Why the tuberculosis incidence rate is not falling in New Zealand. New Zealand Medical Journal 119, U2248.

Dunsford, D., Park, J., Littleton, J., Friesen, W., Herda, P., Neuwelt, P., Hand, J., Blackmore, P., Malua, S., Grant, J., Kearns, R.A., Bryder, L., Underhill-Sem, Y., 2011. Better Lives: The Struggle for Health of Transnational Pacific Peoples in New Zealand, 1950-2000. RAL 9, University of Auckland, Auckland.

Futter-Puati, D., 2010. Maki Maro - Tuberculosis in the Cook Islands, A social history 1896–1975 Unpublished Master's Thesis in History. University of Auckland, Auckland.

Hage, G., 1998. White nation: Fantasies of White Supremacy in a Multicultural Society. Pluto Press, Annandale, NSW.

Hay, D., 2009. The experience of having tuberculosis (TB) treatment in Auckland, School of Population Health, Unpublished Master's Dissertation in Public Health. University of Auckland, Auckland.

Kerr, A.R., 1972. TB and Polynesians, Letter. New Zealand Medical Journal 76, 295.

Krieger, N., 2001. Theories for social epidemiology in the 21st century: an ecosocial perspective. International Journal of Epidemiology 30, 668–677.

Lawrence, J., 2008. Health, wellbeing and diaspora: The lived experience(s) of TB in a refugee community in Auckland, New Zealand. In: Farmer, T., Herring, J., Littleton, J., Park, J. (Eds.), Multiplying and Dividing: Tuberculosis in Canada and Aotearoa New Zealand, RAL-e 2, Auckland, pp. 205–217.

Lawrence, J., Kearns, R.A., Park, J., Bryder, L., Worth, H., 2008. Discourses of disease: representations of tuberculosis within New Zealand newspapers 2002–2004. Social Science & Medicine 66, 727–739.

Littleton, J., Park, J., 2009. Tuberculosis and syndemics: implications for pacific health in New Zealand. Social Science & Medicine 69, 1674–1680.

Littleton, J., Park, J., Bryder, L., 2010. End of the plague? Tuberculosis in New Zealand. In: Herring, D.A., Swedlund, A.C. (Eds.), Plagues and Epidemics: Infected Spaces Past and Present, Berg, Oxford, pp. 119–136.

Littleton, J., Park, J., Thornley, C., Anderson, A., Lawrence, J., 2008. Migrants and tuberculosis: analysing epidemiological data with ethnography. Australian and New Zealand Journal of Public Health 32, 142–149.

Mackay, J.B., 1972. Tuberculosis in polynesians (Letter to the Editor). New Zealand Medical Journal 76, 449.

Malua, S., 2011. The effects of immigration policy changes on Pacific migrants: A case study of migrants in Auckland, New Zealand. Unpublished Dissertation for Post Graduate Diploma of Arts in Anthropology. The University of Auckland, Auckland.

Ng Shiu, R., 2006. The place of tuberculosis: The lived experience of Pacific peoples in Auckland and Samoa, Unpublished Master's Thesis in Geography. University of Auckland, Auckland.

Oh, M., 2005. He Korowai Oranga—Maori health strategy: An effectivie partnership? A Critique from the Perspective of TB Care, Unpublished Master's thesis in Political Studies. University of Auckland, Auckland.

Park, J., Littleton, J., 2007. Beyond ethnography in the political ecology of TB. SITES: A Journal of Social Anthropology and Cultural Studies 4, 3–24.

Park, J., Littleton, J., Chambers, A., Chambers, K., 2011. Whakapapa in anthropological research on tuberculosis in the Pacific. SITES: A Journal of Social Anthropology and Cultural Studies 8, 6–31.

Resture, S.A., 2010. Te Maama Pala: Continuity and change in coping with tuberculosis in Tuvalu, Unpublished Master's Thesis in History. University of Auckland, Auckland.

Searle, A., Park, J., Littleton, J., 2007. Alliance and compliance in tuberculosis of older pakeha people in Auckland, New Zealand. International Journal of Tuberculosis & Lung Disease 11, 72–76.

Statistics New Zealand, 2008. Tuvaluan People in New Zealand: 2006. Statistics New Zealand, Wellington.

Swinburn, P., 1973. Tuberculosis in Auckland. New Zealand Medical Journal 78, 520–525.

Syndemics Prevention Network, 2005. Syndemics Overview, Centres for Disease Control. http://www.cdc.gov/syndemics/overview-principles.htm.

Trostle, J.A., 2004. Epidemiology and Culture. Cambridge University Press, Cambridge & New York.

Voss, L., Campbell, M., Tildesley, C., Hay, D., Vaughan, A., Thornley, C., 2006. Paediatric tuberculosis in a Pacific Islands community in New Zealand. Journal of Paediatrics & Child Health 42, 118–122.

Wallace, D., Wallace, R., 1998. A Plague on Your Houses. Verso, New York.

Chapter 15

Cultural Epidemiology: The Example of Pari Village, Papua

Ian Maddocks

Flinders University of South Australia, Bedford Park, Australia

"Culture," a common term for the rich tapestry of human practice and meanings in which any human group is embedded, is constructed by the group's values, beliefs, and social norms. Culture changes with time and the pace of that change has nowhere been more rapid than in Papua New Guinea, characterized as "One Thousand Years in a Lifetime," by Papuan leader Albert Maori Kiki (Kiki, 1968).

In any community, simple epidemiological techniques using numerator and denominator data can be used in assessments of its "health," and may be tracked over time, allowing a monitoring of changes in the distribution of disease.

Culture has its own numerators and denominators, but these are not easily "counted," making its effect on disease patterns less definite. In situations of rapid change, however, the relationship may be persuasive.

CULTURE AND DISEASE IN TRADITIONAL TIMES

Papua New Guinea has offered some intriguing examples of diseases in which traditional customary practice was a major determinant of a particular disease.

- **Kuru.** This is the best known. The custom among the Fore people of opening a dead body, handling, and even ingesting its parts, led to an epidemic of infection of the central nervous system by prion particles, with inevitable progressive disability and death.
- **Pig-Bel.** The ingestion of an unusually large meal of pig meat on feasting occasions encouraged intestinal growth of *Clostridia* organisms and bowel gangrene.
- **Donovanosis.** As described by Dutch observers, the custom of initiating adolescents by anal intercourse in men's houses encouraged this unsightly ulcerating venereal infection.

The first European visitors found, among Papuans, diseases that they regarded as indicative of a primitive culture. They were repelled, associating obvious

When Culture Impacts Health. http://dx.doi.org/10.1016/B978-0-12-415921-1.00015-4

167

skin diseases with a lack of both cleanliness and godliness. Many were infections associated with exposure to the insects and organisms of a tropical environment (malaria), to close skin contact transmitting disease from one to another (yaws, leprosy, tinea), or to infection after trauma (tropical ulcer). Infection with bowel parasites was encouraged by rudimentary hygiene and sanitation.

That exposure, determined largely by their environmental situation, was a major influence on both culture and health of the people. Almost any tropical community lacking metal, having no fiber suitable for making cloth, and needing to live close together in small houses, might incur the same diseases.

CASE STUDY METHODOLOGY

The initial methodology, which underlies the descriptions that follow and the specific case studies, might be termed "study by immersion." By taking up residence in the community, and providing a primary health care service, which was accepted quite enthusiastically, we "health intruders" were confronted daily with circumstances that needed explanation or interpretation. Friendships with village identities allowed us to hear, from willing informants, legends, songs, and stories that reflected earlier times.

By keeping careful records of all illness from trivial to major, we were able to chart the high prevalence of particular minor illnesses, for example, roundworm infestations or cuts to the feet, for which village daily activity provided context and causation. By undertaking targeted surveys in this largely receptive and compliant population we were able to add quantitative data that strengthened daily impressions.

Background of the Community Case Study: Pari Village

Pari is a community of the Motu people, set about 5 km from the center of Port Moresby. It has been the subject of personal study for more than 40 years, including a period of 6 years of family residence, 1968–1974 (Maddocks, 1978).

In the 1960s the arrangement of village houses was little changed from what is shown in a photograph taken about 40 years previously (see Plate 1).

Traditional Economy

The traditional economy was subsistence: food and the equipment for everyday life were obtained from the sea and the gardens and the bush using direct human effort and local materials; digging sticks, stone axes, and adzes obtained by trade with inland tribe; trees for canoes and houses through trade with coastal neighbors; nets fashioned from local fibers for fishing or trapping wallabies; pottery dishes and urns for cooking and storage and trade (Plate 2).

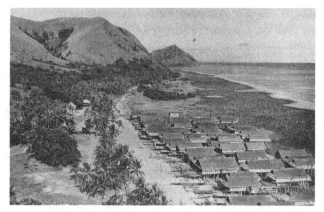

PLATE 1   Pari 1924. *(From Annual Report for Papua, 1925.)*

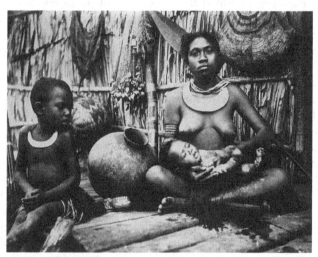

PLATE 2   Motu mother and child, 1880s. Every item depicted in this nineteenth century photo-graph was made on site or obtained through exchange (except the Pears soap). *(From New Guinea Collection, University of Papua New Guinea.)*

Communal Activities

In traditional life, Pari celebrated particular seasons with special activities that required much cooperative effort, and each was attended by careful rituals of song and action.

- **Dubu.** The death of a clan leader called for the accumulation of garden pro-duce over months, leading up to their display on a tall platform. The occa-sion was attended by song and dance with the distribution of the foodstuffs to honor the dead and bring status to the organizer of the feast.

- **Kidukidu.** A major Pari myth explained the seasonal arrival of schools of southern blue fin tuna to the waters of nearby Bootless Inlet (in Motu, *Daugolata*). Generations earlier, the story tells that a named Pari woman, Uguta Vani, gave birth to five tuna fish, but kept it secret. Her husband caught one and cooked it, so she sent the others to the deep sea, warning them to come to be caught only if men who had not slept with their wives made a net. The rituals associated with the netting of tuna were strictly followed; the successful leader of the enterprise, the *varo tauna* (net man), stood to gain high repute.
- **Hiri.** Dangerous trading voyages were mounted annually to the Gulf of Papua to exchange pots for canoe logs, and especially sago, which would provide food for the village through the hungry wet season. Again there were rituals of song and sexual abstinence. There was status to be won for those who completed the enterprise, and their daughters sported special tattoos.

It was important to respect the set and known rituals decreed by custom for every major seasonal activity because adherence to those rituals determined success. Everyone knew what was required, and there was always an explanation when an enterprise failed: someone had not adhered to the necessary taboos and rituals.

Similarly, in crisis situations, such as illness or accident, there were established mechanisms for investigating why this had occurred and ways of seeking to redress the situation. Causes commonly implicated were a breakdown in relationships, expressions of anger or hostility, and a failure to share.

Pari families knew that the ancestor spirits of former generations stayed close by the hearth in the center of the house (the *irutahuna*) and observed behavior. They intruded in daily life, rewarding good behavior or punishing faults and bringing well-being or sickness or success or failure. Serious illness occurred when sorcerers or *"Vada"* men (malevolent ghosts) worked powerful magic. This could be invoked by rivals or enemies, and significant illness needed the services of a *Babalau* (Diviner) to find the persons responsible (Plate 3).

Confronted with misfortune or sickness, the families knew what to do. By confession and restitution of wrongs, healing might be won; by the employment of a *Babalau*, the sorcerer could be identified and negotiation commenced to restore well-being. This gave the people of Pari a sense of "control." Control is a basic component of health, which is strongly influenced by cultural understandings and practices.

Colonial Change and the Health Transition

In the latter nineteenth and early twentieth century, missionaries, colonial powers, and traders brought new diseases to Papua: tuberculosis, gonorrhea, epidemics of dysentery, measles, whooping cough, and influenza. Some had a mortality estimated at up to 10%. The tendency to seek a cooling stream for reducing fever was thought to contribute to influenza mortality, but again, these

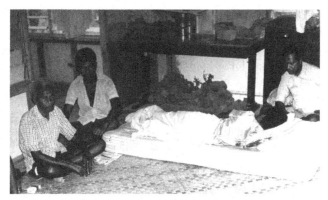

PLATE 3 A *Babalau* working with a Pari patient. The *Babalau* (left) is sitting in with the patient and the family, hearing the story of the illness, and working toward identifying who might have caused the sorcery. *(Photography by Ian Maddocks, 1974.)*

infections are to a large extent "culture independent"—their severity related primarily to new organisms affecting nonimmune populations.

Demographic Shifts

From 1880 to1940 the village comprised a population of approximately 350 persons, and successive census counts indicated a high fertility and high infant mortality allowing little increase in that number. There were approximately five persons per house. The houses were all of bush materials, sited along the beach, and extended into the sea on high posts. Only a small stone church and a house for the pastor were sited inland from the beach. Photographs through that time showed many outrigger canoes standing along the beach; fishing with nets from these canoe platforms was a daily occupation for groups of men, and fish was a major part of the village diet.

During the Pacific War the village was compulsorily re-sited away from proximity to Port Moresby to a "safer" location approximately 100 km east along the coast. Following return to the old site, re-construction conformed to the earlier pattern of clan groups but utilized sawed timber and corrugated iron acquired from abandoned army camps. Some houses began to be sited on the land rather than over the sea. Fishing remained an important activity, and many canoes went out each week.

In 1974 the village numbered 1,200 persons in 100 houses (12 persons per house) and houses were beginning to be built away from the sea.

By 2010, the village had over 5,000 people, accommodated now 20 persons to a house, and a majority of the houses were inland rather than over the sea. The most impressive structure in the village was a large church. No canoes could be seen; net fishing by groups of men had been abandoned. Individual line fishing was now the preferred technique, using a small number of dinghies with out-board motors able to travel beyond the over-fished closer reefs.

Infant Mortality

The rapid increase in population over 40 years was due largely to a decrease in infant mortality for which the increased use of clinic and hospital services for antenatal, delivery, and infant care may be partly responsible. From the 1960s there was a simultaneous increase in maternal fertility through loss of older sanctions about periods of abstinence from intercourse. Table 15.1 shows the birth records of two families in Pari. In one, births occurred up to 1950 and of 11 pregnancies to two mothers only three children survived; in the other there were 13 births to one mother subsequent to 1945 and all survived (Table 15.1).[1]

Environmental Changes

Environmental changes have accompanied Pari's rapid population increase. In 1960, houses were in orderly clan lines, that of the "chief" of each clan closest to the beach. The trees shading the edge of the beach were predominantly coconut trees, and the women drew their water from a shallow village well. A rough gravel road of 2 km permitted access from the closest town suburb.

TABLE 15.1 Birth Records of Two Pari Families

GAUDI HETAU m Boio GUBA		DONISI OALA m Roda TOM
1. Hetau GAUDI1922	Died	1. Asi DONISI 1945
2. Hare GAUDI 1925	Died	2. TOI DONISI 1948
3. GAUDI GAUDI 1928	Died	3. ENOKA DONISI 1949
4. GUBA GAUDI 1930		4. Godidi DONISI 1950
5. MAVARA GAUDI 1932	Died	5. Udu DONISI 1951
6. ISI GAUDI 1934	Died	6. Dika DONISI 1954
[At this time Boio GUBA died, GAUDI HETAU then m Igo ARIA]		
7. Maodi GAUDI 1943		7. Nou DONISI 1956
8. IGO GAUDI 1945	Died	8. OALA DONISI 1958
9. Nauna GAUDI 1947	Died	9. DAROA DONISI 1960
10. Hetau GAUDI 1948		10. TOM DONISI 1963
11. ISI GAUDI 1950	Died	11. Segana DONISI 1964
		12. KAROHO DONISI 1968

1. From family records collected by Ian Maddocks 1968–1974.

In the five years leading up to national independence in 1975, increasing numbers of houses were being built on land. Sites were determined by negotiation between families and followed no plan. Around the same time the village was connected to town services: water (piped to communal stand-pipes), electricity (to street lights along the beach), and several telephones had been connected (e.g., to the Pastor's house).

By 2010 shady trees had taken advantage of more generous availability of water and surrounded the majority of houses extending up the nearby slopes; the houses continued to be haphazardly placed with no planned road access, drainage, or sanitation. Electricity made television accessible and was connected to many houses, but being individually metered was often unavailable. Services had not matched growth; there was no plan in place for street layout, drainage, or sewage, and no there was no garbage collection.

The connection of piped water, of electric light, or telephones might be counted as developments consistent with improvement in Community Health. In Pari, however, the water supply has been intermittent and inadequate for the increased population; payments for water and power falter, making them inaccessible; and pipes and power lines are tapped illegally. Telephone lines have been sabotaged for their copper wire, and mobile phones are more reliable but expensive. After the 2 km road from the closest town suburb was tarred, it quickly became dangerously pot-holed.

The town of Port Moresby began to grow rapidly after 1950, and brought opportunities for employment. The availability of cash allowed the purchase of new food items (rice, tinned fish, and alcohol) and clothing, tools, and transport. In the 1960s Pari men were in demand as carpenters, and were employed by firms profiting from a buoyant housing industry. Other enterprises were tried, and some exploited traditional skills such as dancing for overseas tourists or fabricating shell bangles and necklaces to sell in the town.

The Cultural Epidemiology of Three Health Conditions

Helminth Infestation

Large numbers of small children, playing and defecating in the beach sand, create concentrations of maturing helminth ova, and there was almost universal child infection with ascaris and trichuris worms. The greater concentration of small children playing on the beach had an increased the risk of transmission (Plate 4).

Method

In 1973, a house-to-house visitation by a Pari assistant distributed small containers with an explanation of the microscopy to be undertaken for stool parasites and a request that stool samples be collected. In spite of traditional concerns about the potential for using feces for sorcery, most were returned the next day and specimens from an approximately 50% sample of the child population were obtained for examination (Table 15.2).

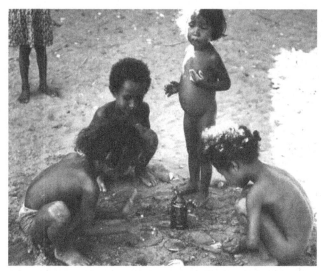

PLATE 4   Pari children playing in beach sand. *(Photographed by Ian Maddocks, 1972.)*

TABLE 15.2 Prevalence of Helminth Ova in Stool of Young Pari Populations

Age groups	Number tested	Ascaris	%	Trichuris	%
Male					
0–5	27	17	62	23	85
5–10	51	44	86	51	100
10–15	29	24	83	29	100
15–20	2	1	50	1	50
Female					
0–5	34	24	70	26	76
5–10	45	39	86	43	96
10–15	39	31	79	36	92
15–20	13	6	46	10	76

Near 100% prevalence of worm infestation was demonstrated; egg numbers were also estimated, and demonstrated that many carried very heavy helminth loads.

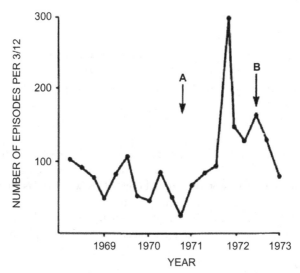

A = Non-returnable bottles introduced

B = Non-returnable bottles prohibited

FIGURE 15.1   Three-month record of episodes of cut feet presenting to the village clinic together with approximate dates of changes in legislation relating to returnable bottles.

Comment

Only by matching clinical data with a targeted survey can a fuller epidemiological picture be obtained; however, this needs a cultural understanding to achieve a complete picture, such as watching our own toddler playing with peers in the beach sand.

Cut Feet

Method

Clinic records were readily analyzed month by month. They showed a rapid increase in the incidence of cuts to the feet (mainly in school-age children) in late 1972, a few months after the 5 cent returnable bottle fee was stopped by Parliament. Only after lobbying (in which these results played a part) and repeal of the legislation did the epidemic decline (Figure 15.1).

Comment

People went barefoot and children played in the beach sand or explored in shallow waters where beer bottles were increasingly discarded and often deliberately smashed. Employed men found pleasure in spending some of their weekly wage on beer; once emptied, the only remaining satisfaction left was to hurl the bottle and watch it smash. When an empty bottle became worth something again, it was preserved. Political action is sometimes the only effective path to health improvement.

Change in Body Weight
Method

House-to-house visits on repeated occasions allowed records of body weight over a period of 10 years (Maddocks and Maddocks, 1977). Cohorts of single decade age groups showed consistent increases in body weight from 1964 to 1974 (Figure 15.2).

Comment

The well-muscled men of the past were disappearing. Obesity began to coexist with hunger, as the busy round of subsistence living was replaced with sedentary employment and store-purchased diets. This was the first indication of predictable increases in the prevalence of hypertension, diabetes, stroke, and myocardial infarction among Pari adults, virtually unknown in the 1960s, but now common causes of hospital admission and sudden death in the village.

DISCUSSION

Changes in "Control"

Until 1960, Port Moresby was a place of the Motu. Numbering about 3,000 they were the dominant language group of the area, along with some hundreds of white families (largely Australians). By 2010, Port Moresby had become a multiethnic metropolis of some 400,000 persons; the Motu were now a small minority, swamped by Highland immigrants and displaced from influence and employment.

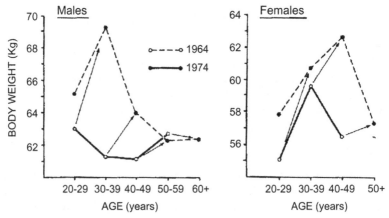

FIGURE 15.2 Changes in body weight of cohorts of Pari adults through one decade. Measurements by Ian Maddocks, 1964 and 1974.

Through its proximity to the seat of government and the many services available in the city, Pari would seem to have been well placed to capitalize on the advantages of development and achieve higher standards of health than were previously available.

This has not occurred, and to some extent it has been the holding on to old cultural norms that has prevented this population from making effective use of the opportunities the town presents.

In cosmopolitan Port Moresby the old rituals outlined by Groves in another Motu Village 50 years ago (Groves, 1957) have no power; it is now largely through nepotism, corruption, and bribery that influence and position are obtained, and they are used for the narrow benefit of one of the hundreds of tribal groups that have thronged into the town. Papuans and New Guineans have faced a huge change from old rituals to modern ways of gaining control, as was suggested by several papers at the 2010 Wagani Seminar in Port Moresby (Wai, 2010; Henao, 2010).

Compared with Highlanders, the Motu are seen as passive, avoiding confrontation, anger, and conflict. This may be seen as "cultural," but others see it as a consequence of long subservience to white dominance for 100 years, compared with the relatively recent introduction of the outside world to the large Highland populations.

In the 1960s, Pari men were in demand as carpenters within the colonial rule when bosses were mainly Australians and Papuan salaries were very small. The traditional resources of garden and sea were still exploited by the local villagers, and employment income was an "extra."

In the 2000s widespread unemployment was more the norm in the Motu villages near Port Moresby. Corrupt politicians and bureaucrats in league with individual entrepreneurs have ensured wealth for a few, but in Pari there is real poverty and fear of gang violence in the town. Pari attempts to build an income have been tentative and often unsuccessful. A handful of fishermen sell at the local market, but the local reefs are being fished out, and the illegal distillation of alcohol (known as "steam") from cane sugar is more profitable.

We Don't Know What to Do about These Changes

In 2007, a consultation with the Pari church members explored how they assessed current village life and well-being. This list points to the major concerns they expressed:

- "No caring and sharing"; decay of old obligations
- Violence and drug abuse, brewing alcohol, youth indiscipline
- Town water and power supply irregular and costly
- Intrusion of foreigners stealing from gardens, "crashing" parties and feasts
- Dynamiting destroying the reefs
- Corrupt leadership; ineffective local government

- Expense of school fees, "drop-outs" unable to complete schooling
- Absence of employment opportunities
- Danger on the road from foreign "rascals"
- Hunger—children sent to school without breakfast or lunch

The common element in this liturgy of complaints is the loss of control—"We don't know what to do about these changes."

In the past, observing the proper rules, singing the necessary songs, keeping the powerful taboos, and maintaining good relationships with neighbors kept the ancestors content and the *Vadas* away (Groves, 1957). Even under the major constraints of subsistence living and tropical disease, these observances were held to ensure a good outcome for the individual, the family, and the village, and was the path to health.

In modern times, however, there are no known rituals that will ensure passing an examination, and no songs that will help get a job. The former rules no longer seem to apply, the songs have no force, the taboos are widely ignored, and one no longer knows what to do or how to succeed. The sacred hearth where the help of the ancestral spirits was invoked is replaced by the kerosene or electric stove in the back kitchen. The hospital is a frightening place where dangerous spirits thrive and doctors are strangers and were the path to health.

CONCLUSION

To preserve individual and community health, a population needs to understand the likely causes of sickness or disaster and ownership of the resources needed to confront and manage those difficulties. Pari had its own understanding and own resources in traditional times, but multiple outside pressures have eroded that control and diminished community health, in spite of the availability of effective medical treatments and improved survival.

Despite its clinic, its low infant mortality, its outboards, and mobile phones, Pari village is, in many ways, less "healthy" now than in the nineteenth century when the cohort who survived childhood had repulsive diseases, but understood agreed ways to confront and manage them.

Pari—A Local Tale of Global Consequence?

What is happening to this small Papuan community is occurring throughout the world, often on a much larger scale. In the face of global problems, any of us may experience a pervasive sense of powerlessness: the scale is too large, what we confront is outside our past experience, and what worked for us formerly seems inadequate. Old cultural norms of kindness, frugality, and group solidarity have eroded.

Citizens of the new age, moving increasingly into urban environments, are called to find new ways to control their lives through cooperation across new, poorly understood boundaries. In spite of amazing potential for connecting via social electronic communication, only a few seem to have exploited the new opportunities with any sense of confidence or control. The consequences for health, in its broadest sense, of the global urbanization movement are attracting increasing concern (Moore et al., 2003). The lack of caring and sharing is widespread, with a focus on whatever brings short-term advantage to individuals, sectional groups, dominant communities, or nations. The result is, as Deputy Prime Minister Puka Temu noted in 2010 when commenting on Papua New Guinea's development record, "Our nation is not peaceful and harmonious, and our people are not prosperous and are disempowered" (Temu, 2010).

REFERENCES

Groves, Murray, 1957. Sacred Past and Profane Present. Quadrant 1(Winter), 38–47.

Heano, Loani, 2010. Church, Election and Corruption. In: Maddocks, I., Wolfers, E.P. (Eds.), Living History and Evolving Democracy, University of Papua New Guinea Press, Port Moresby, pp. 191–194.

Kiki Albert Maori, 1968. Kiki: Ten Thousand Years in a Lifetime: A New Guinea Autobiography. Cheshire, Melbourne.

Maddocks, D.L., Maddocks, I., 1977. The Health of Young Adults in Pari Village. Papua New Guinea Medical Journal 20 (3), 110–116.

Maddocks, I., 1978. Pari Village. In: Hetzel, B.S. (Ed.), Basic Health Care in Developing Countries. An Epidemiological Perspective, Oxford University Press, pp. 403–415.

Moore, M., Gould, P., Keary, B.S., 2003. Global urbanisation and impact on health. International Journal of Hygiene and Environmental Health 206, 269–278.

Temu, P., 2010. Long Term Development Strategy and Wealth Creation: A Paradigm Shift Platform. In: Maddocks, I., Wolfers, E.P. (Eds.), Living History and Evolving Democracy, University of Papua New Guinea Press, Port Moresby, pp. 108–113.

Wai, Simeon, 2010. Democracy versis Bigmanship. In: Maddocks, I., Wolfers, E.P. (Eds.), Living History and Evolving Democracy, University of Papua New Guinea Press, Port Moresby, pp. 176–190.

Chapter 16

Life and Well-Being under Historical Ecological Variation: The Epidemiology of Disease and of Representations

Robert Attenborough[1] and Don Gardner[1,2]

[1]*The Australian National University, Canberra, Australia,* [2]*Universitaet Luzern/University of Lucerne, Switzerland*

INTRODUCTION

In this chapter we report on aspects of research undertaken among a small population (the Mian) living on the northern fringes of New Guinea's mountainous backbone. The ethnographic setting is empirically unusual in important respects, and while our research demonstrates that cultural factors are integral to the epidemiological and broader social history of the population, it raises questions about the methodological shape of cultural epidemiology.

CULTURAL EPIDEMIOLOGY OF THE MIAN

Most of the field research we discuss in this chapter was conducted in 1986, the year *Writing Culture*, by Clifford and Marcus, was published. This volume did much to publicize the doubts some cultural anthropologists had about the concept that had long been taken to be at the heart of their discipline. Responding to the realities of a decolonizing world and critiques from neighboring disciplines, these anthropologists expressed their concern at the way anthropological conceptions of culture tended to essentialize other ways of life and to ignore political and historical processes as well as individual agency (see Chapter 2).

In this context, a relevant theoretical intervention in the debates about culture is that of the cognitive anthropologist, Dan Sperber, and his colleagues. Although the vigorously formulated arguments of this European wing of the "evolutionary psychology" movement have not proved popular with cultural anthropologists, we mention them here precisely because—as any Internet search engine will demonstrate—the term "cultural epidemiology" is sometimes applied to

When Culture Impacts Health. http://dx.doi.org/10.1016/B978-0-12-415921-1.00016-6
181

Sperber's view that the distribution of (mental and public) representations within a population of interacting individuals (an "epidemiology of representations") is precisely what constitutes a local culture (Sperber, 1996; Heintz, 2010). According to this perspective, the distribution of representations (and institutions) in a population depends upon the general psychological or cognitive capacities of humans, the properties of representations themselves, and the ecological context (which is sociological no less than biological) in which they subsist.

Although we will *not* use the term cultural epidemiology to refer to Sperber's approach, our research is precisely concerned with the distribution of practices (and the concepts, beliefs, preferences, and values—"representations"—they implicate) among a historically and linguistically defined population that is distributed across a biologically significant altitudinal cline. Our research is predicated on the view that people's understandings, values, and preferences are no less part of the etiology of patterns of sickness and well-being than such environmental factors as climate or mosquito-biting densities. Yet while cultural representations/meanings make a difference to Mian historical trajectories, their heterogeneity and contingency on other aspects of social existence give their analysis an irreducibly idiographic form. Our emphasis, consequently, also contrasts with the pioneers of the epidemiology of representations, because it is more focused on the socioecology of representation (as process *and* product) than on its cognitive basis. Gardner's Ph.D. thesis (1981) at least made it clear that data on the ecological setting, horticultural productivity, and morbidity and mortality of Mian communities could not be omitted from a convincing account of the historical development of the marked cultural variation within the Mian population.

The research discussed in this chapter was part of the effort to develop a better model of those historical processes. We believe our case demonstrates that, even in the face of overwhelming biomedical threats, populations like the Mian interpret and respond to events in ways essential to their historical fate.[1] The relevance of this case to a volume on culture-in-health (or cultural epidemiology) depends upon seeing the *necessity* of the specification of responses to events—and,

---

1. Although our epidemiological research sought to make clearer some of the dynamics underlying the precolonial distribution of Mian speakers, practices, and representations, we do not wish to suggest that these can simply be read off from the situation that ensued after the advent of Australian colonial control. On the contrary, precisely because the interactions between all dimensions of social life continued, the *Pax Australiana*, through government directives and Christian missions (which dispensed medical treatments and advice along with new practices relevant to the organization of bodies, souls, and relations between persons and groups), changed the historical trajectory of the Mian way of life quite dramatically. Nevertheless, it did so through processes at work prior to colonization. While we can only speak to the general dynamics of the postcontact history of Mian communities in passing, given the aims of this chapter, we nevertheless acknowledge that the vicissitudes of state control, mineral exploration in the area, and the interpretive synthesis of Christian and earlier understandings of how life might be lived (Robbins, 2004) have significantly impacted the cultural epidemiology of the region.

hence, the dispositions that generate them—to historical outcomes. As Sahlins has argued (since 1976), the overdetermination of local cultural conditions by "externalities" like natural disasters, colonial intrusion, or—more to our point—variation in the prevalence of malaria, merely goes to the fact of cultural response, not the character of the response, which is a necessary condition of downstream events. In short, our case depends upon sheer ethnographic specificity no less than do those of cultural epidemiologists, even if we characterize cultural meanings in terms some among them would wish to challenge.

Mian Social Life

The Mian are the most northerly of the 15 populations of the Mountain Ok language family: south of them live another, larger Mountain Ok group, the Telefolmin; to their north dwell lowlands and riverine peoples speaking languages of different phyla; their western neighbors are another Mountain Ok group, the Atbalmin, while to the east live several small Ok and Ok-like groups. Although long-term settlements are rare above 1,100 m, the land in the southern portion of the Mian area contains peaks of 3,000 m, while the plains in northern and western parts are only about 200 m above sea level. Yet even higher altitude Mian populations occupy and exploit a range of habitats; hunting provides most of the first class protein and gardens, predominantly of taro (which, Mian say, is "our bone"), most of their energy. Crude densities of this population of hunter–horticulturalists vary with altitude (from an average of less than 1 person per km^2 in the lower altitudes to an average of roughly 3 per km^2 in the highest altitudes), but subsistence practices make precise determination of the land used very difficult and not very useful. Clearly, though, Mian subsistence practices were highly land-extensive.

The overwhelming botanical feature of the Mian area is primary and very old secondary forest, which carpets the entire landscape, broken only by river courses, land-slips, sparsely distributed human settlements, and gardens. Nevertheless, there are important differences between the kinds of forest found in the various altitudinal zones, which affect the productive activities (and the histories) of its inhabitants. To summarize radically, gardening productivity under Mian technology generally declines with altitude, while hunting returns increase.[2]

Mian speak of those who occupy ancestral territories in the higher altitudes to the east and south as *am nakai* ("men of the house"), while those descended

---

2. There are two discernible seasons on the northern slopes of the central ranges that the Mian occupy: from April to November it rains heavily on most days and in the remainder of the year it rains even harder. In terms of the classifications meteorologists use, the area displays the lowest possible degree of seasonality, and although there is a statistically significant difference in the amount of rain that falls in the two seasons, there is no period—excepting the occasional drought—when the soil is unsaturated.

from migrants to the lower altitudes in the north and west are designated *sa nakai* ("men of the bush"). This distinction is also used evaluatively to suggest that the *am nakai* remain true to tradition in a way that the *sa nakai* do not. Accordingly its usage is more complex than a simple dichotomy might suggest: those in the middle altitudes regard themselves as *am nakai* in relation to those in the lower altitudes but will sometimes acknowledge that they are *sa nakai* relative to those higher up.[3]

A crucial feature of Mian social life is its smallness of scale. Prior to European contact (approximately 1950) the Mian applied no superordinate ethnonym to themselves (Gardner, 2004); the population of roughly 2,500 was divided between 22 cognatic descent categories, occupying roughly the same number of territories (some named groups occupied more than one territory, while others shared a territory). In addition, many territorial populations were divided between more than one settlement and almost all households had garden houses in which their members spent considerable time. The smallness of face-to-face networks increases in sociological significance when set in the context of the considerable distances between major settlements (usually several hours walk) and Mian preferences for local endogamy and sister-exchange marriage. Although the exigencies of sex ratios mean that local exogamy actually occurs in about 50% of marriages, variation across Mian territory is considerable. The sentimental ties between cross-sex siblings and the considerable distances between communities that make endogamy desirable also mean that exogamous marriage involves the couple in dual residence, which also runs at around 50%. Mian social organization presents, then, as a set of linked local clusters, within each of which social relations are, for most individuals, highly concentrated, yet which are highly permeable. Individual territorial mobility is significant and communities and networks are reconfigured steadily, even over the short to medium term.

Social life and political practice, accordingly, revolve around the maintenance of local communities. The number of folk rather than land limits the effectiveness of local groups and the well-being of communities. In Marx's terms, the limiting productive force is labor power rather than the means of production. Accordingly, and despite explicit values concerning patrifiliation, families are often drawn to what seem to be greener pastures elsewhere, for a shorter or longer period, or permanently.

In precolonial times, group mobility was also significant since settlements were subject to roughly cyclical rhythms. A group would pioneer an area, under the leadership of an impressive man and dwell in a single large, multihearth communal house, and a few garden cycles later, the community would be divided into smaller households units, sometimes dispersed across several hamlets. When hunting returns began to diminish, good garden land became harder

---

3. This distinction, its relation to the marked variation in the form and organization of (the pan Ok) male cult practices, and its sociological correlates framed Gardner's initial research (1975–1977).

to find and other aspects of the good life were judged to be on the wane, a territorial community (or, often, some portion of it) would cross a watershed to a new territory. Settlement patterns were not homogeneous throughout the Mian area, however. The lower altitude *sa nakai* communities tended to move more frequently, and sustain greater levels of dispersion for longer periods of time than *am nakai* groups.

Residential patterns were always connected to the fortunes and skills of locally charismatic leaders, which were subject to variation due to chance and to competition between them. Such competition was mostly incipient in that a family attracted by conditions in another settlement could have a significant impact on the relative size of the one it left (given average settlement size), but when it was between men of the same territorial community, it was often overt and could become bitter.

The factors outlined above underpin the peculiarly contingency-prone nature of Mian social life: intracommunity and intercommunity relations are susceptible to sudden disruption as a result of factors that are contingent with respect to the formal structure of those relations. Passions resulting from an illness or death that is attributed to sorcery, or from a slight and the festering sense of betrayal it produces, or a dramatic breach of a threshold in a simmering conflict can suddenly drive a section of a community to move elsewhere. And if the bonds of trust and loyalty that bind members of a primary community are in any case under strain (as they sometimes are if two men display the qualities expected of a leader), then such an event may split a whole community. Other factors countered this susceptibility to fission, but these are unevenly distributed across the Mian area. There were two important and interconnected factors. First, there is the involvement of a community in subregional cult practices, which entailed the joint initiation of boys and young men, a significant degree of dependence upon cult seniors in other settlements, and a general sense that the fates of component communities were bound up with one another. Cult elders had tremendous power with respect to communities and their leaders, as well as a personal and transcendental interest in maintaining their congregations. Thus, the power of cult seniors was particularly significant in those situations of conflict that might otherwise lead to community division. Someone (in living or spiritual form) was always thought to be responsible for the death of an adult, and political conflict, including armed violence, was frequent after a death (Gardner, 1987). Cult elders were crucial to limiting the severity of the consequences of this source of conflict. The second factor countering tendencies for settlements to divide involved warfare. The communities with the strongest commitment to cult were the *am nakai*, whose territories were closest to powerful (e.g., Telefol) enemies who raided and/or were raided by the Mian. Alliances, and the cordial relations these entailed, were therefore of greater significance to the high altitude than to the lowlands Mian.

The broad history of the Mian runs thus: groups and subgroups have been expanding into lower altitudes and different ecological zones for the last four or five generations. The impetus for this movement is intimately connected to the expansion of the Telefol from their salubrious central highland valleys (Craig and Hyndman, 1990). As different Mian groups migrated into new areas (some were pushed, some less directly induced to move), their relations with those groups that remained in the higher altitudes and with one another were transformed. The transformation of social networks, the effects of which are evident in the content and form of intergroup and intragroup relations, is a result of people's responses to their changed circumstances and the effects of these on local communities. Especially important here are the changes in (1) the social volume and social density of subpopulations (to use Durkheim's handy terms), (2) patterns of morbidity and mortality associated with malaria and other insect-borne parasites, (3) the productivity of subsistence that migration has brought about, and (4) the extent to which local communities take part in multicommunity cult practices. The situation of the Mian population in the 1970s indicated a cline in almost all of the parameters just listed: larger, more densely settled, and healthier populations in the higher altitudes, committed to the local variant of the pan Ok initiation cult and enjoying better agricultural yields, contrasted with smaller, less densely settled, less healthy populations whose agriculture was less productive and among whom the cult and its ritual activity had become attenuated, all in rough proportion to how much lower in altitude they were than the groups still living on ancestral territories.

We want to underline the fact that the distinction between the communities of the *am nakai* and those which have moved into new (lower altitude) areas in the last few generations, *sa nakai*, is not merely a matter of historical geography, nor is it purely an evaluative term. Through its reference to power and the authenticity of cult practices of the different segments of the population, it is relevant to behavioral differences of some sociological moment. As a male initiatory cult, which was held to be the source of the power sustaining both subsistence production and the moral strength and fertility of human beings that Mian life depended upon, cult practices and the status divisions and taboos that were central to them were aspects of quotidian life: relations between men and women, seniors and juniors, people and foods and places were all normatively rationalized in terms of the cult and subject to sanction by cult elders. The precolonial attenuation of cult practices among *sa nakai* made for quite profound differences in the quality of daily social life, which is why *am nakai* elders were so scandalized by what they saw as the apostasy of the lowlanders. And given that cult involvement also indexed the web of alliances relevant to the standing conflict between Mian, Telefol, and Atbal communities, we can appreciate why high-altitude elders spoke with dismay of the more fractious lowlands communities and the readiness with which they split or attacked one another (Gardner, 1981).

Those lowlands communities could not avoid being susceptible to ecological contingencies, including disease, accident, and interpersonal conflict.

Ever since colonial contact, for example, government officials have noted the disastrous effects of influenza on the Mian. While these are postcontact tragedies, they do illustrate the comparative vulnerability of small social formations to local catastrophes and are consistent with the presence of hyperreactive malarious splenomegaly (see below), a condition that would have pre-existed the advent of Europeans. Less dramatic, but still very important to the overall Mian picture, is the variation in relative demographic fortunes that small community size entails. As suggested earlier, changes of residence by small numbers of people can significantly alter the relative political position of a community. Group histories demonstrate that even apparently trivial events, such as the killing of a domestic pig by a dog or a hunting accident, can spark a major realignment of political affiliation as two or three families remove themselves elsewhere. But the most frequently encountered contingency, and the one most threatening to good order, is disease. Any death is the occasion for sorrow and anger, and the death of any adult is certain to produce very great anger and an accusation of sorcery. In the past, the death of an important man or woman was liable to produce a raid on another community or the death of someone in the deceased's community accused of sorcery.

We hope we have presented a *prima facie* case for the relevance of the epidemiology of malaria to the cultural anthropologist of the Mian.

Malaria among the Mian

Like most other parts of New Guinea's highlands fringes, Mian territory is characterized by a sparse human population with relatively poor health indicators. Health surveys here are few, and health facilities have always been basic and unreliably available. However, it is abundantly clear that general health is poor and premature mortality is alarmingly high. While causes of ill health are certainly multiple—none is of greater concern than malaria, the cause to which fevers are normally attributed in the absence of confirmatory tests by anyone treating illness here.

Our characterization of Mian malaria draws principally on the survey of the population we conducted in collaboration with the Papua New Guinea Institute of Medical Research (Attenborough et al., 1996, and other unpublished information), to our knowledge the only malariometric survey yet undertaken. This was a cross-sectional survey, consisting of a demographic interview, physical examination, and thumb-prick blood sampling for malarial parasitemia, covering all available and consenting Mian individuals from roughly 25 settlements, totaling 626 (of an estimated 962) across all ages and both genders, surveyed at four survey locations within the western and central parts of Mian territory. Refusal rate was negligible so that population coverage was essentially limited only by geography, with males somewhat more likely than females to travel from the remoter settlements to our survey locations.

The altitudinal range the Mian exploit is climatically and ecologically significant; although it lies entirely within the range where malaria occurs endemically in New Guinea, the altitudinal gradient in ambient temperature exerts some impact on the rate at which the life cycle of the *Plasmodium* parasite proceeds while inside the *Anopheles* mosquito, and hence on the dynamics of malaria transmission and epidemiology (Attenborough et al., 1997). The 1986 survey focused on the groups in the lower lying western and central portions of the territory, where earlier fieldwork had suggested that settlements were smaller, population densities lower, and health poorer, than in ancestral Mian territories. Even so, the altitudinal range covered by the survey was appreciable (150–1,000 m), and survey locations were chosen to maximize the representation of people normally resident at both ends of this range.

The individuals surveyed were predominantly young (41% under 15 years, 4% 50 years or over), and this shortfall of older people appears representative of the population. Approximately 37% were found to have malaria-positive blood slides at the time of the survey; 68% of infections were of *Plasmodium falciparum*, the most virulent of the human malarias. Malaria parasitemia rates varied strongly with age (peaking at 80% in 2–4-year-olds and declining steadily to 15% in adults, for all *Plasmodium* species) but not with gender. Similar findings apply to parasite density, indicating not only that young children were the most frequently infected members of the population, but also that they were also the most heavily infected. Even though the Mian in 1986 did have limited access to antimalarial measures, these results much more closely resemble baseline results from the Wopkaimin (a southern Mountain Ok people) in the Ok Tedi baseline survey in 1982–1983 than those from the 1986 re-survey of the Wopkaimin following four years of intervention associated with the Ok Tedi mine project (Lourie, 1987).

Spleen enlargement (splenomegaly), although it can have causes other than malaria, is generally attributed to malaria when population prevalence is high (Bruce-Chwatt, 1985). The Mian survey showed that splenomegaly was near-universal and frequently the degree of enlargement was very high. Strikingly, over 60% of every age group had a Hackett spleen Grade 3 or greater, a figure that rose to over 80% among 5-to 14-year-olds. No significant gender differences were found. Comparison with other surveys suggests that whereas the Mian in 1976 and the Wopkaimin in 1982 had similar splenomegaly levels, they had alleviated for the Wopkaimin by 1986 (consistent with malaria control measures) but had deteriorated somewhat for the Mian, most likely owing, we speculate, to a historical increase in the prevalence of risk factors. The high frequency of splenomegaly among Mian adults as well as children suggests that not only hyperendemic malaria (Bruce-Chwatt, 1985) but also hyperreactive malarious splenomegaly (Crane, 1986, 1989)—an atypical and disadvantageous immune response to recurrent malaria, associated with high risk of premature mortality from ill-defined immediate causes, probably including spleen rupture and intercurrent infection—are major health problems and probably the leading health problems, for the Mian. Their implied burden of ill health is overwhelming, individually and perhaps demographically too.

TABLE 16.1 Mian *P. falciparum* Parasitemia Rates (%) by Age Group and Altitude of Usual Residence, Sexes Combined, 1986

Age Group	<2 Years	2–9 Years	10–19 Years	20+ Years
N	38	135	144	309
Resident 600 m+ a.s.l.	41.2	40.9	42.2	11.5
Resident < 600 m a.s.l.	47.6	59.3	29.3	16.9
p value (χ^2 test)	N.S.	0.04	N.S.	N.S.

So, within the internally contrasted microcosm that is the Mian physical and sociocultural world, what local variation is there in their health? How does it articulate with the other kinds of variation, discussed earlier, between the *am nakai* and the *sa nakai*?

While there are limits to what can be inferred from a single cross-sectional survey, there do appear to be some meaningful relationships here. We take altitude to be a rough measurable proxy for the complex of correlated sociocultural differences summarized above.

Overall, we find, in a series of unpublished analyses of which some aspects are summarized in Table 16.1, that statistical relationships between altitude of residence and either malarial parasitemia or parasite density are neither strong nor entirely consistent. Parasitemia rates are high in both altitudinal groups: nonetheless there are patterns. For example, in all age groups but the 10-to 19-year-olds, parasitemia rates are higher in the lower altitude groups, whether the crude parasite rate (all *Plasmodium* species) or *P. falciparum* only is considered. The difference is statistically significant for *P. falciparum* at the 5% level only among 2- to 9-year-old children.

We found a more consistent, yet still not very strong, relationship between altitude and splenomegaly. Raw spleen grade was weakly negatively but significantly correlated with altitude in the 2- to 9-year-old and 20+-year-old age groups, and uncorrelated in the other age groups. Table 16.2 shows a cross-tabular summary of essentially the same relationship, assessed via the percentage of individuals with spleens of Grade 3 or greater. Again, the lower altitude group again emerges as the worst affected consistently from age 2 years onward and significantly in adulthood, although the association is almost swamped by the extreme prevalence of splenomegaly at all ages.

To this we may add altitude-related findings from a small-scale entomological survey run in tandem with the Mian malaria survey in some of the same locations. Proportions of anopheline mosquitoes carrying malaria circumsporozoite antigens diminished monotonically with altitude, from 170 to 650 m, with no anophelines captured at 1,000 m. This is a potentially important relationship

TABLE 16.2 Mian Splenomegaly (% Spleen Grades 3–5) by Age Group and Altitude of Usual Residence, Sexes Combined, 1986

Age Group	<2 Years	2–9 Years	10–19 Years	20+ Years
N	35	135	144	309
Resident 600 m+ a.s.l.	60.0	77.3	77.8	66.7
Resident < 600 m a.s.l.	60.0	85.7	82.8	77.5
p value (χ² test)	N.S.	N.S.	N.S.	0.04

complicated by variable mosquito abundance that is probably related more to local ecology than systematically to altitude (Attenborough et al., 1997). Even at 650 m, however, the observed malaria inoculation rate would be more than sufficient to sustain high human malaria transmission in the absence of accessible treatment services.

Running through these results are undramatic but recurrent signs that Mian people do indeed, as we had hypothesized, run an exacerbated health risk from malaria when they live in the lower lying portion of their lands. Are there reasons beyond the fact that even the upper end of the West Mian altitudinal range is not high enough to escape endemic malaria transmission, why this effect is not more powerful? There are probably a number answers to these questions.

Parasitemias may be transient and, especially among perennially exposed adults, there may be a strong stochastic element in who may happen to exhibit parasitemia at the time of a survey, even in the absence of treatment. When bed nets or malaria treatment is available, one of the sources is at a government station located at 180 m altitude above sea level (a.s.l.). Local ecological variation, for example, proximity to swamps favorable to mosquito breeding, no doubt plays a part. Our entomological survey showed that very significant variation in biting densities between villages only 1 km apart (as the mosquito flies) is possible. Varying availability of alternative hosts for the anophelines to bite, such as pigs, may play a part too. The landscape is steeply dissected, so that within short horizontal distances, certainly within those readily traveled by people and probably by anophelines too, there can be significant altitudinal variation. Even those based in higher altitude settlements can raise their exposure to night-biting mosquitoes through extended visits to gardens at lower altitude or to lower-lying settlements.

A more extensive survey than the 1986 one might be able to tease apart more fully these contributors to variability. One way further into this complex of ecological variables may be suggested from within our own dataset. If we classify villages according to their location either at or above the level of their local river, and examine again *falciparum* parasitemia and splenomegaly Grade 3+, we find the pictures shown in Tables 16.3 and 16.4. This new variable is

TABLE 16.3 Mian *P. falciparum* Parasitemia Rates (%) Sexes Combined, by Age Group and Village Situation of Usual Residence, 1986

Age Group	<2 Years	2–9 Years	10–19 Years	20+ Years
N	38	135	144	309
Resident above river level	37.5	44.4	40.5	10.7
Resident near river level	50.0	57.8	30.4	17.5
p value (χ^2 test)	N.S.	N.S.	N.S.	N.S.

TABLE 16.4 Mian Splenomegaly (% Spleen Grades 3–5) by Age Group and Altitude of Usual Residence, Sexes Combined, 1986

Age Group	<2 Years	2–9 Years	10–19 Years	20+ Years
N	35	135	144	309
Resident above river level	50.0	75.6	76.2	62.1
Resident near river level	66.7	86.7	83.3	80.1
p value (χ^2 test)	N.S.	N.S.	N.S.	0.001

not independent of altitude: there are fewer villages above river level in the lower altitudes. Again we see an almost consistent but not overwhelming trend in the direction expected, reaching statistical significance only in the case of splenomegaly among adults.

CONCLUSION

Although the altitudinal cline across which Mian are spread does not suggest that the risk of mortality and morbidity associated with malaria increases regularly or dramatically, in line with the sociocultural differences encoded in the Mian distinction between *am nakai* and *sa nakai*, the data indicate significant variations between the higher and lower altitudes overall, and make clear the generally large burden the disease imposes. They also underline the contingency-prone nature of social networks that this setting produces, as well as the extent to which interpretive dispositions that constitute part of the cultural fabric are integral to the production of that effect.

If malariometry is insufficient to explain the impact of the disease on local social networks in the lower altitudes, then a study that accounts for the interpretive practices of lowlanders, and the cultural representation of trust, envy, and enmity that thematize them may produce a more convincing account of the interaction between the epidemiology of the disease and the epidemiology of representations.

REFERENCES

Attenborough, R.D., Gardner, D.S., Gibson, F.D., 1996. Malaria and filariasis amongst the Mianmin of the highland fringes of Sandaun Province. Papua New Guinea: A report. Department of Archaeology and Anthropology, Australian National University, Canberra.

Attenborough, R.D., Burkot, T.R., Gardner, D.S., 1997. Altitude and the risk of bites from mosquitoes infected with malaria and filariasis among the Mianmin people of Papua New Guinea. Transactions of the Royal Society of Tropical Medicine and Hygiene 91, 8–10.

Bruce-Chwatt, L.J., 1985. Essential Malariology, second ed. Heinemann, London.

Clifford, J., Marcus, G.E. (Eds.), 1986. Writing Culture: The Poetics and Politics of Ethnography, University of California Press, Berkeley.

Craig, B., Hyndman, D. (Eds.), 1990. Children of Afek: Tradition and Change Among the Mountain-Ok of Central New Guinea. Oceania Monograph 40, Oceania Publications, Sydney.

Crane, G.G., 1986. Recent studies of hyperreactive malarious splenomegaly (tropical splenomegaly syndrome) in Papua New Guinea. Papua New Guinea Medical Journal 29, 35–40.

Crane, G.G., 1989. The genetic basis of hyperreactive malarious splenomegaly. Papua New Guinea Medical Journal 32, 269–276.

Gardner, D.S., 1981. Cult Ritual and Social Organisation among the Mianmin. Ph.D. thesis. Australian National University, Canberra.

Gardner, D.S., 1987. Spirits and conceptions of agency among the Mianmin of Papua New Guinea. Oceania 57, 161–177.

Gardner, D.S., 2004. The advent and history of Mianmin identity. In: Meijl, Toon van, Miedema, Jelle (Eds.), Shifting Images of Identity in the Pacific, KITLV Press, Holland.

Heintz, C., 2010. Cognitive history and cultural epidemiology. In: Martin, L.H., Sorensen, J. (Eds.), Past Minds: Studies in Cognitive Historiography., Equinox Press, London.

Lourie, J.A. (Ed.), 1987. Ok Tedi Health and Nutrition Project Papua New Guinea 1982-1986: Final report. Port Moresby and Tabubil, University of Papua New Guinea and Ok Tedi Mining Limited.

Robbins, J., 2004. Becoming Sinners: Christianity & Moral Torment in a Papua New Guinea Society. University of California Press, Berkeley.

Sahlins, M., 1976. Culture and Practical Reason. The University of Chicago Press, Chicago.

Sperber, D., 1996. Explaining Culture: A Naturalistic Approach. Blackwell, Oxford.

Chapter 17

Perceptions of Leprosy in the Orang Asli (Indigenous Minority) of Peninsular Malaysia

Juliet Bedford

Director, Anthrologica, www.anthrologica.com and
Research Associate, School of Anthropology, University of Oxford

INTRODUCTION

Orang Asli ("original man") is the generic name for eighteen distinct ethnic groups that collectively make up the indigenous minority of Peninsular Malaysia. While the term indigenous is both complex and highly contested and no universally agreed definition exists, the Orang Asli fulfill the key criteria to be regarded as indigenous according to the United Nations Working Group on Indigenous Populations (Kenrick, 2004; United Nations, 2007). Their minority status is undisputed. Numerically they make up a tiny proportion (0.58%) of the Peninsula's population (JHEOA, 2004). In 1991, their literacy rate was 30% compared with the national rate of 86%; in 2004, 76.5% of Orang Asli lived below the poverty line compared with 6.5% of other Malaysians; 45.7% of Orang Asli villages were classified by the government as underdeveloped; and 41.7% were located in interior regions of the country (Baer, 1999; Nicholas, 2000; JHEO, 2004; Nicholas and Baer, 2007).

There is widespread international recognition that indigenous peoples across the world have substantially lower than average standards of health for the nation state in which they reside (Stephens et al., 2006). Indigenous peoples have disproportionately high levels of communicable and vector-borne diseases and high levels of cancer, respiratory disease, stroke, and diabetes. They show increased morbidity and mortality levels compared to other population groups, a substantially lower life expectancy, and elevated infant and child mortality rates (Stephens et al., 2005).

Research into the standards of Orang Asli health in comparison to other Malaysians echoes this pattern. In 2004, the Orang Asli average life expectancy at birth was 53 years compared with the national average of 71.5 years, and their average infant mortality rate was 51.7 deaths per 1,000 births compared to

When Culture Impacts Health. http://dx.doi.org/10.1016/B978-0-12-415921-1.00017-8

193

the national average of 16.3 deaths per 1,000 births (JHEOA, 2004). The Orang Asli suffer from high incidence rates of tuberculosis and malaria; malnutrition is common; and levels of diabetes, hypertension, and cancer are increasing.

The incidence of leprosy in Orang Asli is also highly elevated compared to the national level and, according to the World Health Organization (2003), Malaysia eliminated the disease in 1994. In 2005 (the most recent complete data available), the Ministry of Health recorded the incidence rate in Peninsular Malaysia at 0.07 per 10,000, and for the Orang Asli, an incidence rate of 1.34 per 10,000. Only one previous publication deals with leprosy in this community (Kamaludin, 1997), and it reviews a 1994 survey of various groups, but provides scant data. Other works addressing Orang Asli health cite cases of leprosy only in passing. The research on which this chapter is based is the first anthropological study focusing on leprosy in the Orang Asli.[1]

The Department of Aborigines, now known as the Department for Orang Asli Development (*Jabatan Kemajuan Orang Asli Malaysia*; JAKOA, and before January 2011 as the Department of Orang Asli Affairs, *Jabatan Hal Ehwal Orang Asli*; JHEOA) has, since its formation in 1950, assumed responsibility for the "administration" of the Orang Asli with a mandate to assimilate the minority into mainstream Malaysia (JHEOA, 1961). Its medical division was established in 1953 as part of the "hearts and minds" campaign in which welfare measures were offered as an incentive for the community to side with the British administration against the communist insurgency during the Emergency period (1948–1960; Bedford, 2009).

This medical division remains the government's only health service provider that is organized according to ethnic criteria, and it is run with relative autonomy by the JAKOA, not the national Ministry of Health. The Orang Asli are, therefore, the only community in Malaysia to receive a discrete state-run medical service. The hub of the JAKOA medical division is Gombak Hospital, also known as the Orang Asli hospital, located on the outskirts of a northern suburb of Malaysia's capital, Kuala Lumpur. Orang Asli are permitted to receive free health care at any government clinic or hospital in the country, yet many travel long distances to seek treatment at Gombak as they regard it as "their" hospital. Patients report feeling less vulnerable seeking biomedical treatment at Gombak where they perceive risks associated with non-Orang Asli interaction to be reduced. Due to its orientation and location, however, the hospital is widely considered to be an isolated backwater of the medical profession in Malaysia. It is under-resourced in terms of funding, facilities, and staff, and the standard of health care offered often falls below that practiced in mainstream government hospitals.

---

1. The term Hanson's disease is favored in some recent literature. I use the term leprosy in line with the International Federation of Anti-Leprosy Associations and the World Health Organization. The term "leper" is, however, widely condemned as pejorative and stigmatizing and is now largely redundant. I use the phrase "leprosy patient" in reflection of the patients' self-identification.

Drawing on data gathered as part of a larger research project based at Gombak Hospital, which explored relations between the Orang Asli and the nation state through the lens of biomedical health care provision (Bedford, 2008), this chapter investigates the occurrence, treatment, and social presentation of leprosy in the Orang Asli, and discusses how, in light of their status as the indigenous minority of Peninsular Malaysia, leprosy assumes additional social configurations beyond its clinical manifestations.

METHODS

Data Collection

Research was conducted over a 9-month period (2004–2005) at Gombak Hospital and with the JAKOA medical division's mobile health teams and flying doctor service, visiting communities and rural clinics in the isolated interior of the country. Quantitative data were collated from JAKOA, the Ministry of Health, and from patient records at Gombak Hospital. Core empirical data were qualitative and gathered through a combination of methodological tools including in-depth interviews with key interlocutors (patients, community members, and health care professionals), focus group discussions, case studies and narratives, and direct and participatory observation. Open inductive qualitative methods ensured that multiple perspectives were considered and the quality of data gathered was maximized through triangulation. Participant observation was fundamental to the research, as it allowed insight into inconsistencies between actual and reported relations between Orang Asli patients and non-Orang Asli staff, which was a highly sensitive and political issue.

Detailed case studies were compiled of all leprosy patients admitted to Gombak Hospital during the research period ($n = 32$). A case study consisted of at least one in-depth interview with the patient, an interview with the patient's accompanying relative if possible, a detailed medical case history, documented treatment regime, and at least one briefing from the doctor managing the case.

For the in-depth interviews, a broad spectrum of research questions was designed and used as a semi-structured topic guide. Specific questions and probes were reviewed and refined during the research period in light of themes arising. The direction and content of each interview were determined by the key interlocutor and largely focused on issues they self-prioritized.

Interviews with patients and their accompanying relatives were conducted at Gombak Hospital, most often on the communicable disease ward, and were held in as much privacy as possible. At the start of each interview, it was made clear to the interlocutors that their participation was optional and voluntary, and would not affect any future referral or medical service required or received. Each interview lasted for approximately one hour. Audio recordings were not made. This helped foster a sense of trust and privacy and encouraged patients to speak more candidly than may otherwise have been possible.

Data Analysis

Preliminary analysis was conducted in-country throughout the research process. Detailed notes were compiled during every interview, and at the conclusion of each day were transcribed and annotated with initial comments. The interviews were conducted in Malay and translated into English. Sections of narratives were transcribed *ad verbatim*, translated, and back-translated and statements checked with the interviewee. All data, interview notes, and completed case studies were regularly reviewed.

The case studies were thematically analyzed at the end of the fieldwork period. Dominant themes were identified through the systematic sorting of data, labeling ideas, and phenomena as they appeared and reappeared. The emerging trends were critically analyzed according to the research objectives. Coding and analysis were iterative and by hand. A qualitative software package was not used.

Preliminary findings were discussed with the JAKOA medical division and other key stakeholders including the Selangor Public Health Department and the national Tuberculosis and Leprosy Control Unit of the Disease Control Division of the Ministry of Health. Their feedback was appropriately incorporated into the final analysis.

Ethical Considerations

The study was conducted in line with prevailing ethical guidelines to protect the rights and welfare of all participants. All data were kept confidential and anonymous. Overall permission for the research was granted by the Economic Planning Unit of the Prime Minister's Office in Malaysia. As no biomedical interventions were undertaken during the research, formal ethical consent was not required by Gombak Hospital or the JAKOA. Every effort was taken, however, to ensure that all those who participated in the research were given detailed information about its objectives and methods prior to their voluntary involvement. All participants gave their assent and were given the opportunity to seek clarification or ask questions at any time during the research.

CASE STUDIES

Due to space constraints, it was not possible to present the full qualitative analysis of the 32 case studies completed. Rather, the following excerpts from three longer case studies can be considered representative and illustrate the dominant themes of stigma, compliance, and responsibility discussed in the following sections.

Case Study 1—Itah

Itah had advanced lepromatous leprosy. He was 46 years old and had been first diagnosed in 1996. He had periodic treatment for one year due, he claimed, to an infrequent supply of medication. He had extensive anesthesia accompanied by anhidrosis and marked thickening of his facial skin. His anterior nasal spine had been destroyed resulting in a collapsed nose. His hands and feet were edematous with marked shortening and angulation of the digits on both hands. Itah had a quiet confidence and a large smile. His narrative was given on the ward in Gombak Hospital, sitting on the floor next to his bed as he flicked through the day's newspaper.

I have had leprosy for nine years. It began with pale patches. I had those for four years and then I started to lose the feeling. I think I was infected by my friend. There were three men in my village with the same illness. The other two have already passed away. My friend came to Gombak for treatment, but he came back to the village without finishing the medicine.

Before I came here, I went to a private clinic. They gave me injections for my illness. I have never been to Gombak for treatment before this year. The JOA [JAKOA] medical staff brought me to the hospital. I came with my family, but now they have all gone back to the village. It is better that they are in the village, then they can work.

At first I did not know what the patches were because they were bigger than normal [fungal] skin infections. But eventually I knew it was leprosy. I wanted to come to Gombak before to have treatment. But when the health teams went to the village, I was in the jungle working. I could not come by myself, I don't have transport. So it was very difficult. I was frightened, of course, this is normal. I could not come before. But now I do not have fingers, toes or my nose. There was no way I could come by myself. I do not feel angry. It is just one of those things, so I am sad. This [looks at his hands] only happened recently, about three years ago. I lost all sensation in my hands and feet. I had no feeling at all. But now with treatment, the feeling is coming back. Its ok, its not getting worse.

I miss my wife and children. I want to go home at the end of this month and take the medicine with me. I understand that I must keep taking it. I am worried my children will get this illness. But they have all been screened and are healthy. People in my village were worried when I became ill. They were worried they might get ill too. This is one reason I came for treatment.

Case Study 2—Tengah

Tengah was 36 years old when he came to Gombak with advanced lepromatous leprosy that had progressed untreated for 15 years. When he arrived in hospital transport, accompanied by his mother, he had severe malnutrition and a very low hemoglobin count. He was transferred to the central hospital in Kuala Lumpur for blood transfusions before starting multidrug therapy at Gombak for his leprosy. He was an inpatient at the hospital for 8 months.

Before he was brought to Gombak, the medical division had been aware of Tengah's deteriorating condition for many years. Whenever a mobile team visited his village, Tengah would hide in the surrounding jungle fringe, sometimes for days, until they had gone. Retreat or withdrawal from medical intervention, rather than confrontation, was a common tactic. Tengah's immediate community supported him and his family, and by so doing indirectly protected him from receiving treatment against his will. He eventually allowed himself to be brought to the hospital when his condition became too grave for his family to provide adequate care. Only then did he consider himself to be ill. When asked if he would have come for treatment when he first contracted leprosy had he known it would have arrested his condition, he smiled shyly and replied "probably not."

Case Study 3—Ana

Ana was diagnosed with lepromatous leprosy when she presented at the hospital in 2004 with widespread intense itchiness followed by the development of anesthetic patches on her face. After one month as inpatient, she absconded. Her husband perceived the treatment lacked efficacy as her symptoms were not markedly reduced. Over the following months, the medical division's mobile health teams tried to persuade her to return to the hospital and sent medication to her in the village.

Simultaneously, Ana's husband arranged for her to see a *bomoh* (traditional healer), believing the *bomoh* could more effectively treat his wife. When her condition continued to deteriorate despite the *bomoh's* interventions, the mobile team succeeded in persuading Ana to return with them to Gombak. In the interim, she had developed classic leonine features with pronounced thickening of the ear lobes, malar surfaces, and marked hair loss.

Four days after her readmission, her husband arrived at the hospital and insisted on taking Ana back to their village. He would not condone Ana's condition being treated in any way other than by his local *bomoh*. He sought to minimize interaction with the hospital and assiduously avoided the medical division and JAKOA authorities.

DISCUSSION

In Malaysia, the propagation of biomedicine is a sign of modernity legitimized by the rationale of the scientific. Biomedical health care is part of a comprehensive strategy of social transformation (Chee and Barracolough, 2007). In direct and meaningful ways, health care provision engages a specific discourse about states of modernity and progression versus states of underdevelopment and backwardness. Ethnicity remains the dominant ideological framework of contemporary Malaysia, and stereotypes are played out at Gombak hospital along ethnic lines of Orang Asli versus the nation state. In its very existence, Gombak perpetuates this discourse: it is the hub of a medical service for the indigenous minority and is distinct from mainstream health care. This dichotomy also influences the interpretation of disease and illness. Leprosy both represents and accentuates the divide: it has been characterized by some as a disease of the unclean, deviant, backward, or underdeveloped (Vaughan, 1991), and while it has been eliminated nationally, its incidence remains elevated among the Orang Asli.

High levels of stigma associated with leprosy are well documented, yet it is not universally stigmatized, and there have been recent calls for a more nuanced and less constrained interpretation of stigma and social exclusion in relation to the condition (Staples, 2011). There was no evidence to suggest that Orang Asli leprosy patients at Gombak Hospital had been stigmatized by or excluded from their village or community. Rather, patients described scenarios in which they remained fully integrated in their community. In the second case study, Tengah and his immediate family were supported both socially and financially by their community for a number of years. In the third case study, Ana was repeatedly taken back to the village by her husband who was distressed by admission to the hospital and preferred her to remain within the immediate confines of their community.

At Gombak Hospital there was no detectable change in behavior or attitude within the patient body toward a fellow inpatient with leprosy. Non-leprosy patients attached no particular significance to the condition, and interacted freely with the leprosy patients. The stigma that was evident came from the medical staff. For example, dental clinicians routinely refused to treat leprosy inpatients and other health care professionals sought to avoid work on the communicable disease ward. Studies have shown that doctors often display the highest levels of stigma toward individuals with leprosy, despite leprosy being one of the least contagious of human transmissible diseases (Scott, 2000; Arole et al., 2002). In light of this discrimination, Pfaltzgraff (2003) suggested that the problem of stigmatization should be considered from the perspective of the stigmatizer rather than the stigmatized.

Medical staff at Gombak stigmatized patients like Itah, Tengah, and Ana and labeled them noncompliant or uncooperative given their late presentation and history of defaulting treatment. As his narrative highlights in the first case study, Itah had been prevented from seeking sustained treatment by insurmountable logistical barriers involving transport and work patterns. Although he complied with the treatment regime while at Gombak, his late presentation and the fact that he had undergone inappropriate treatment earlier in his illness (injections at a private clinic) ensured that, in the eyes of the medical staff, his case history did not follow the preferred model of early detection, effective diagnosis, and successful treatment. His illness had progressed under the pressure of socioeconomic realities, where self-care took second place to daily survival. The discourse of compliance [Donovan and Blake, 1992; Donahue and McGuire, 1995; Ogden, 1999] broadly assumes that all patients are equally able to comply in the first instance, whereas in practice, as Farmer (1997) showed, "throughout the world, those least likely to comply are those least able to comply."

It was inconceivable to many medical staff at Gombak that Tengah had not sought treatment for his deteriorating condition. To them, his avoidance was irresponsible, even deviant. Within his framework of reference, however, his (non-)actions have a logical consistency. During the years prior to his admission, Tengah did not perceive himself to be ill, nor in need of treatment, because he was able to continue contributing to the social and economic life of his community. His case highlights the contest for medical knowledge: When is a person ill? When should they receive treatment? What treatment should they receive? Who should assume responsibility for it? What is the relationship between the clinical reality of a biomedical framework and the social reality of illness (of leprosy) as experienced by an Orang Asli patient?

Staples (2007) argued that for many leprosy patients, the medical cure of their illness that meant they were no longer infectious is socially irrelevant as many are "permanently rendered 'lepers' by what their corporeal appearance had come to signify." This was true of Tengah, whose severe physical impairments were, for the medical staff, a constant and magnifying reminder of his nonconformity and their lack of control. For Ana, the absence of immediate improvement with treatment at the hospital influenced the treatment-seeking behavior sanctioned by her husband. His dissatisfaction with treatment exacerbated his reluctance for her to be admitted to the hospital rather than remain in their own village. He did not want to deny treatment for his wife per se, but wanted to avoid biomedical treatment, preferring instead to engage the "traditional" health care of the *bomoh*. Undergoing treatment at Gombak Hospital necessitated crossing into a non-Orang Asli dominated environment that he understood in terms of the prevailing dichotomy of indigenous Orang Asli versus mainstream Malaysia. To him, Gombak and biomedical treatment represented diminished autonomy, generalized stigma, and the inherent threat of assimilation.

During my research, I was asked this by a Malay nurse:

Why are you interested in leprosy? Leprosy is an old disease. That is why the Orang Asli have it. They don't have new modern diseases like HIV and AIDS. There is no leprosy anywhere in Malaysia now, except in Orang Asli. Leprosy is appropriate for them.

It is explicit that the nurse's perception of leprosy as an old disease made it appropriate for the Orang Asli, in contrast to conditions that she associated with modernity and progression typified by HIV/AIDS. In India, Staples (2004) found that leprosy and leprosy patients were often regarded as "obstacles to development." Similarly, the Orang Asli are generally characterized within Malaysia as impediments to modernization. According to Nicholas (2000), "the state perceives that it cannot modernise effectively if it were to tolerate indigenous minority culture in its midst." Despite such opinions being common among medical staff, the notion of being doubly marginalized, of being in "double jeopardy" due to being Orang Asli and having leprosy, was widely denied by patients at Gombak Hospital (Morrison, 2000). To them, any additional stigma concerning their leprosy was normalized by its interpretation as typical anti-Orang Asli sentiment. As Waitzkin (1984) concluded, "the medical encounter is one arena where the dominant ideologies of a society are reinforced."

CONCLUSION

In the context of Gombak Hospital, leprosy is an illness where notions of responsibility, compliance, and stigma collide, and where experiences of health, illness, and treatment-seeking behavior are expressed along ideological and ethnic lines. In light of their status as the indigenous minority of Peninsular Malaysia, leprosy in the Orang Asli community assumes additional social configurations beyond its clinical manifestations.

Understanding these sociopolitical determinants of illness and the complexities around seeking and adhering to treatment enables us to better appreciate the context in which the delivery of health care functions. It is imperative for the effective design and implementation of health care programs that policies are properly contextualized, locally appropriate, and acceptable. It is not sufficient to have biomedical services in place and expect patients to attend and comply with treatment. Instead, we must focus on the interface between service delivery and uptake and find ways to maximize drivers that lead to positive treatment-seeking behavior while minimizing barriers that prevent it. With regards to leprosy, this would enable a move away from the problematic notion of elimination toward a more relevant and nuanced understanding of the condition and its treatment.

Reflections on Methodological Approach

One of the greatest hurdles in conducting this research was securing all necessary permissions from various branches of the Malaysian Government. Research with the Orang Asli is a highly sensitive issue in Malaysia for sociocultural, political, and religious reasons connected to issues of indigeneity and assimilation. Careful planning and substantial time were required to prepare adequately before the research could commence.

The research methodology proved effective and efficient as I was based at the hospital for an extended period of time and was able to build trusting relationships with both patients and staff through participant observation. Initially I was concerned that the patients and wider Orang Asli community would align me too closely with the JAKOA; however, I was able to establish a betwixt and between position. The patients grew to see me as a confidante and were encouraged by my overt interest in their community, while the medical staff regarded me as a health care professional working alongside them in a nonmedical capacity. In both cases, I was seen as being on "their side" yet somehow different, and this afforded me considerable insight into the workings of Gombak Hospital.

A limitation of the research design was that all of the leprosy patients I worked with were inpatients at Gombak Hospital. It would have been interesting to have also included people with leprosy who remained in the community and were not in treatment. Given the constraints of time and difficultly in identifying these potential interlocutors, particularly in the remote interior of the country, it was not possible during this research.

In qualitative research of this kind, issues of translation and interpretation can be problematic. I did an intensive course in Malay (the national language) before starting fieldwork and did not conduct interviews or record narratives until I was confident in my linguistic ability to do so accurately.

REFERENCES

Arole, S., Premkumar, R., Arole, R., Maury, M., Saunderson, P., 2002. Social stigma: a comparative qualitative study of integrated and vertical care approaches to leprosy. Leprosy Review 73, 186–196.

Baer, A., 1999. Health, disease and survival. Centre for Orang Asli Concerns, Malaysia.

Bedford, K.J.A., 2008. Gombak and its patients: Provision of healthcare to the Orang Asli (indigenous minority) of peninsular Malaysia. Unpublished D.Phil thesis. University of Oxford.

Bedford, K.J.A., 2009. Gombak Hospital, the orang asli hospital: government healthcare for the indigenous minority of Peninsular Malaysia. Indonesia and the Malay World 37, 23–44.

Chee, H.L., Barracolough, S., 2007. Health care in Malaysia: The dynamics of provision, financing and access. Routledge, London.

Donahue, J.M., McGuire, M.B., 1995. The political economy of responsibility in health and illness. Social Science and Medicine 40, 47–53.

Donovan, J.L., Blake, D.R., 1992. Patient non-compliance: deviance of reasoned decision-making? Social Science and Medicine 24, 507–513.

Farmer, P., 1997. Social scientists and the new tuberculosis. Social Science and Medicine 44, 347–358.

JHEOA., 1961. Statement of policy regarding the administration of the Orang Asli of Peninsular Malaysia. JHEOA, Kuala Lumpur.

JHEOA., 2004. Data Maklumat Asas. JHEOA, Kuala Lumpur.

Kamaludin, F., 1997. Strategies to overcome infectious disease among the Orang Asli—leprosy and tuberculosis. Paper presented at Emerging Trends in Infection. Second National Conference on Infection and Infection Control, Ipoh, Malaysia 14–16 March 1997.

Kenrick, J., Lewis, J., 2004. Indigenous peoples' rights and the politics of the term "indigenous." Anthropology Today 20, 4–9.

Morrison, A., 2000. A woman with leprosy is in double jeopardy. Leprosy Review 71, 128–143.

Nicholas, C., 2000. The Orang Asli and the contest for resources. International Workgroup for Indigenous Affairs, Copenhagen.

Nicholas, C., Baer, A., 2007. Health care for the Orang Asli: Consequences of paternalism and non-recognition. In: Chee, H.L., Barraclough, S. (Eds.), Health care in Malaysia: The dynamics of provision, financing and access, Routledge, London, pp. 119–136.

Ogden, J.A., 1999. Compliance versus adherence: Just a matter of language? The politics and poetics of public health. In: Porter, J.D.H., Grange, J.M. (Eds.), Tuberculosis: An interdisciplinary perspective, Imperial College Press, London, pp. 213–234.

Pfaltzgraff, R.E., 2003. Begging as a profession and dehabilitation among leprosy patients. Leprosy Review 74, 280–281.

Scott, J., 2000. The psychosocial needs of leprosy patients. Leprosy Review 71, 468–491.

Staples, J., 2004. Delineating disease: self-management of leprosy identities in south India. Medical Anthropology 23, 69–88.

Staples, J., 2007. Peculiar people, amazing lives: Leprosy, social exclusion and community making in south India. Orient and Longman, Delhi.

Staples, J., 2011. Interrogating leprosy stigma: why qualitative insights are vital. Leprosy Review 82, 91–97.

Stephens, C., Nettleton, C., Porter, J., Willis, R., Clark, S., 2005. Indigenous peoples' health—why are they behind everyone, everywhere? Lancet 366, 10–13.

Stephens, C., Porter, J., Nettleton, C., Willis, R., 2006. Disappearing displaced and undervalued: a call to action of indigenous health worldwide. Lancet 367, 2019–2028.

United Nations, 2007. Declaration on the Rights of Indigenous Peopleshttp://daccess-dds-ny.un.org/doc/UNDOC/GEN/N06/512/07/PDF/ N0651207.pdf?OpenElement.

Vaughan, M., 1991. Curing their ills: Colonial power and African illness. Polity Press, Cambridge.

Waitzkin, H., 1984. The micropolitics of medicine: a contextual analysis. International Journal of Health Services 14, 339–378.

World Health Organization, 2003. Overview and epidemiological review of leprosy in the WHO western and pacific region 1991–2001. World Health Organisation Regional Office of the Western Pacific, Manila.

Chapter 18

A Qualitative Exploration of Factors Affecting Uptake of Water Treatment Technology in Rural Bangladesh

Shaila Arman,[1] Leanne Unicomb,[1] and Stephen P. Luby[1,2]
[1]*International Centre for Diarrheal Disease Research, Bangladesh (ICDDR,B), Dhaka, Bangladesh,*
[2]*Director of Research, Centre for Innovation and Global Health, Stanford University, USA*

BACKGROUND

Although Bangladesh is the delta of two major waterways, the Ganges and the Brahmaputra, safe drinking water is in short supply due to the rapidly expanding population that increases the demand of ground and surface water, contamination from both agricultural and industrial activities, and the natural geological distribution of heavy metals. During the 1980s, Bangladesh achieved notable success in providing 95% of the rural population with shallow tube-wells as the primary source of drinking water to replace highly contaminated surface water (DPHE, 2011). At present, these tube-wells are the most common source of drinking water in rural Bangladesh (WHO, 2007). However, about 40% of the tube-wells are contaminated with fecal organisms (Islam et al., 2001; Luby et al., 2008a). Previous studies have shown no reduction in the incidence of diarrheal diseases through this improved source of drinking water (Sommer and Woodward, 1972; Levine et al., 1976; Khan et al., 1978). In addition to microbial contamination, arsenic was also identified in tube-well water in the early 1990s (Smith, 2000). Iron is another metal present in most tube-wells in Bangladesh, although it does not have adverse health consequences. Even if many of the tube-wells are contaminated with arsenic and microbial contamination, most people in Bangladesh do not believe they get sick from this source of drinking water. One study found that only 21% of Bangladeshi people believed that their drinking water could sometimes make their family ill (Gupta et al., 2008).

Improving microbiological quality of water can prevent waterborne diseases (Mintz et al., 1995; Quick, 1999; Clasen et al., 2007) . To address the issue of unsafe drinking water and related diseases, several groups have attempted to promote point

When Culture Impacts Health. http://dx.doi.org/10.1016/B978-0-12-415921-1.00018-X

of use (POU) water treatment as an effective inexpensive approach to protect house-holds (Mintz, 1995; Sobsey, 2008). During the past decade, many government and non government organizations (NGOs) in Bangladesh have introduced and pro-moted POU water treatment technologies focused on the removal of either arsenic or microbial contamination. However, in Bangladesh and elsewhere, these technol-ogies have not been widely adopted and have failed to achieve high rates of regular use (Luby et al., 2006; Gupta et al., 2008; PATH, 2008; DuBois et al., 2010).

Economic, social, cultural, and environmental factors all influence human behavior related to the uptake of new behaviors or technology. Many public health interventions that have focused on safe drinking water have not achieved sustained use in the past because existing practices, ideas, and preferences of the target pop-ulation were not taken into account. Understanding why earlier efforts were not successful can provide insights on how to develop effective interventions. There-fore, we conducted this anthropological study to understand the factors affecting the uptake of POU water treatment technologies in rural Bangladesh.

RESEARCH PROCESS

For our study, we purposively chose two rural villages located in southwest-ern Bangladesh—a flat plain land area where people have similar types of occupations and houses and eat the same food. They also used similar sources of drinking water, primarily from hand-pumped shallow tube-wells similar to other plain areas in Bangladesh (Figure 18.1). Previously, many of the tube-wells in both villages had been tested by the Government of Bangladesh inspectors and were found to be contaminated with variable levels of arsenic and iron. These tube-wells were marked with a red color by Government

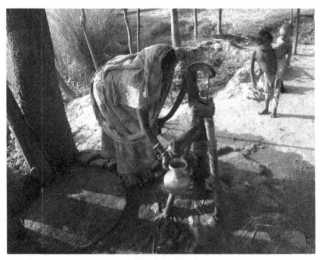

FIGURE 18.1   A woman collecting drinking water from a tube-well

inspectors to indicate they were contaminated. To provide arsenic-free water, government officials recommended that new tube-wells should be more than 150 m deep (DPHE, 2011).

In 2008, a local NGO, the "NGO Forum for Drinking Water and Sanitation, Bangladesh," implemented a project to promote both household and community-based water treatment technology for arsenic removal. The NGO Forum sold 60 arsenic-removal commercial filters (SONO, ALCAN, and READ-F) to individual households in these two villages on a first-come, first-serve basis at a subsidized price, with payment on installments (Figure 18.2a,b).

From April to May 2009, the study team enrolled mothers of children over the age of 5 who were primarily responsible for water handling, whose household income was less than $70 a month (5,800 Bangladesh Taka), and who were willing to participate in the study. The study team enrolled 20 informants from these two villages, including 10 mothers who had experience using the NGO-promoted arsenic-removal filters, and 10 who had no experience using any kind of water treatment technology (Table 18.1).

The research team consisted of four members, including an anthropologist as the lead researcher, all of whom had training and experience in collecting qualitative data. We used an in-depth interview guideline to explore issues linked to the study aim, including location of water sources, water collection and storage practices, perceptions of their water quality and what safe water is, waterborne diseases, and experience with filter use. These interviews, in Bengali, lasted 45 to 90 minutes and were recorded with a digital audio recorder. After the interview we transcribed the recordings into Bengali verbatim using MS Word, before uploading text onto the qualitative data analysis software, Atlas-ti version 5.2. We then used a code list that had been prepared according to the objectives of the study. We summarized the findings of each code in English, and then examined the similarities, differences, and connections between each factor.

Local Water Context

Tube-well water that had variable levels of heavy metal such as arsenic and iron was the main source of drinking water. The other sources of water for our rural informants were ponds and rivers, which were also used for cooking; bathing; and washing cattle, clothes, and utensils. Informants reported that most of their tube-wells were only 60–80 m deep, which did not meet the government's recommendation, and that they could not afford to dig a new tube-well deep enough to meet the recommendations. As one woman informant said:

Although it is with red mark, we drink from this tube well. Many people said establishing a long pipe with it will allow us to get better (arsenic free) water, but I could not do so due to lack of money. I am continuing drinking from this tube well. Sometimes we went to neighbors house to collect arsenic free water as their tube well is with green mark, but our children don't go. When they felt thirsty they instantly drink from our tube well.

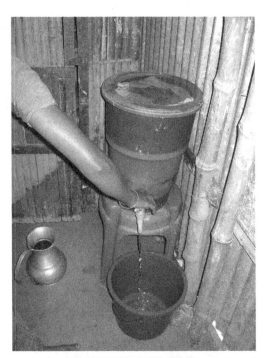

FIGURE 18.2a   ALCAN filter

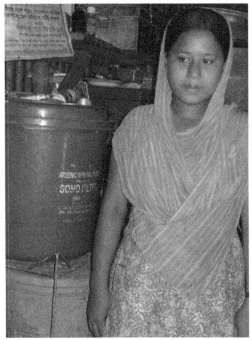

FIGURE 18.2b   SONO filter

TABLE 18.1 Sociodemographic Data of Informants with <5,000 Taka Monthly Income

Sociodemographic data		Users	Nonusers	Total N = 20
Age (years)	21–30	7	8	15
	31–40	2	2	4
	41–50	1	—	1
Education	Illiterate/can sign	4	7	11
	Class 1–5	3	3	6
	Class 5–10	3	—	3
Occupation of household head	Tenant peasant	3	2	5
	Rickshaw/van puller	2	1	3
	Bus driver/helper	2	2	4
	Day laborer	2	3	5
	Cook	—	1	1
	Honey seller	1		1
	Teacher		1	1

Factors Affecting the Use of the Arsenic-Removal Filter: Barriers and Motivators

Informants identified several barriers to regular use of the arsenic-removal filters including: water-storing practices and preferred attributes in drinking water, perception of safe water and tube-well water quality, perceptions of waterborne diseases, perception of the cause of diarrheal diseases, and knowledge and experience with the water treatment technologies.

Each of these factors is elaborated on in the following section.

Water-Storing Practice and Preferred Attributes of Drinking Water

Informants did not habitually store drinking water. Instead, they collected it directly from the tube-wells for immediate consumption. This is because tube-wells were mostly located in their courtyard; for those who did not have their own tube-well, the closest tube-well was within 10 minutes' walking distance. They preferred to drink freshly collected tube-well water due to its cool temperature. They perceived that stored tube-well water had a strong unpleasant taste of iron, compared with freshly collected tube-well water. Informants who did not have a functioning tube-well in their households told us that they

collected water from their neighbors' tube-wells. Although these people sometimes stored drinking water, they also preferred to drink freshly collected
drinking water.

Perception of Safe Water and Tube-Well Water Quality

Our informants associated "safe water" with its source, taste, and color, not
with germs or pollutants. Most expressed a positive attitude toward the quality of their tube-well water, despite the arsenic and iron contamination. Even
those users of arsenic-removal filters who were positive about the filter mentioned they liked water direct from the tube-well more than filtered water. They
referred to tube-well water as "good water" (*bhalo pani*). They preferred drinking unfiltered tube-well water because it originated underground, and, as it was
covered all the time, it was not exposed to dirt as pond or river water would be.
As one of our housewife informants said:

> Tube-well water is safe. Ours was installed with a long pipe. If the pipe of the tube well is
> long then the water is good, no arsenic is there. It also stays covered .... Can we get safer
> water than this source? No.

Perception of Waterborne Diseases

Most of our informants mentioned cold, fever, skin disease, stomach upset,
and cholera as waterborne diseases. However, none of our informants mentioned arsenic poisoning and they did not recognize it as a serious health
hazard. This could be because symptoms do not immediately become visible.
Within their life experience, our informants could not directly link drinking
arsenic-contaminated tube-well water to any adverse health outcome. One
woman expressed her attitude toward arsenic contamination in tube-well
water as

> I am not having any problem in drinking water from a red marked tube-well. And I do not
> know whether illnesses will occur now or in future. For example, if I drink the water today
> and if the illness will occur five days later then how will I realize this has occurred due to
> today's water consumption? I will not be able to realize it.

Perception of the Cause of Diarrheal Diseases

Diarrheal diseases were perceived to be natural, easily curable, and not serious.
Treatment cost of these diseases was also cheap to our informants. Our informants had their own definition of diarrhea such as "watery loose stool" (*patla
paikhana*) and thought that getting diarrhea was related to eating stale food, not
drinking unsafe water. As one woman said;

> Loose stool occurs from food items.... say for example, foods can get exposed to flies when
> these remain uncovered, that apart, filth can fall on these food items.... people also get
> loose stool if they take stale (bashi) food.

Knowledge and Experience with Water Treatment

Many of our informants mentioned they knew about water treatment methods such as water boiling, sieving with a strainer, and using alum potash (*fitkiri*) in turbid water. However, they only treated water with alum potash during a flood before using and or knowing about the arsenic-removal filter. Women reported boiling water to give to their children when they were ill, perhaps illustrating that they perceived boiled water as medicine, rather than as a preventive measure.

During our study period none of our user informants were current users of water filters. They had all stopped using filters due to a variety of technical barriers including the slow flow of filtered water, the time required to clean the filters, and difficulties in reassembling the parts. After the NGO stopped its promotion, users could not continue to use this technology as spare parts were not available.

In our explorations, we also identified several motivators, or reasons why people started using the arsenic-removal filters and at least initially continued to do so, including: the option to pay through installment, the filter's ability to remove iron from tube-well water, and the filter's use as a water storage vessel.

Option to Pay through Installment

Our informants perceived that the arsenic-removal filters were of good value as they were low cost, available with an installment payment plan, and easier and less expensive than digging a deeper tube-well. Those who did not get the opportunity to pay by installment reported that they would welcome it.

Filter's Ability to Remove Iron from Tube-Well Water

Although our user informants purchased the filters to remove arsenic form tube-well water, most also appreciated the filters' ability to remove iron. Our informants did not like the taste of iron in drinking water. They also reported that iron content in water gave food, utensils, and clothes an unwanted reddish tint. For these informants, the good taste and removal of iron color was as much a motivator as the capacity to remove arsenic. This could be because arsenic is not visible and causes no immediately observable health outcome.

Filter's Potential Use as a Water Storage Vessel

The filter could also be used as a water storage vessel. It was convenient and saved time for family members when collecting water. Additionally, for children under 5 who were not strong enough to operate a hand pump, the filter allowed them to draw their own water from the filter whenever they were thirsty.

DISCUSSION

Findings from this anthropological study identified a number of factors that prevented uptake of the arsenic removal filter. In addition to the usual practices of water collection, storage, and use, their perceptions regarding safe water and waterborne diseases, and technical and supply issues restricted the filters' uptake and sustainable use. People from this low income rural community made decisions based on their direct experiences and changed their behavior only when they perceived an advantage to doing so. A key factor in community members' continuing to drink tube-well water, despite its arsenic contamination, is that they liked the taste, freshness, and coolness of it. Using the arsenic-removal filters destroyed all the preferred attributes of tube-well water. Research conducted in Guatemala, Kenya, and India also found that taste, color, and temperature of treated water were all cited as barriers in using the water-treatment technologies (PATH, 2008; Luby et al., 2008b; DuBois et al., 2010). In this rural context, water-treatment technologies that do not require storage might be a more popular solution. Additionally, our informants' perception and knowledge of safe water and microbial contamination of tube-well water also limited filter use. In this community, where arsenicosis is not perceived as a serious health hazard, and where people are not aware of microbial contamination of tube-well water, high uptake of a POU technology that is not recognized as having any advantages is unlikely.

As found in previous studies in Bangladesh (Blum and Nahar, 2004) our data also highlighted that as diarrheal diseases were not perceived to be serious, and treatment was available and affordable in the local market, our informants were less interested in spending money to prevent diarrheal diseases. They tended to go to a nearby pharmacy or grocery shop for medicine or oral rehydration solution to treat diarrheal diseases. They reasoned that purchasing medicine was much cheaper than purchasing water-treatment technology.

Our findings suggest that for future water interventions in rural Bangladesh using health issues as a motivator might not be effective. Along with the above-mentioned practices and perceptions regarding water management and water-related diseases, technical difficulties, such as the poor durability of the hardware, inconvenience of use, and unavailability of spare parts limited the uptake of POU water treatment technology at the household level. A previous study of a different water-treatment technology in rural Bangladesh reached a similar conclusion (Gupta et al., 2008). As establishing a new tube-well with a deeper pipe was not affordable for most of our informants, promotion of low-cost arsenic-removal filters in this context could be successful, especially if the technology was distributed through easy payment installments and spare parts were available in the market. In contrast, a difficult technology that requires spare parts and ongoing investment is not likely to succeed.

Despite these barriers some factors could still act as motivators toward promoting drinking safe water in theses rural communities. As most of our informants in this rural community did not have the habit of storing drinking water, the women offered several advantages to using the filter as a container that could make household water management easier, including having to fetch water less often, and their children having easier access to it. Although the women like the taste of cool, fresh water from tube-wells, which they considered "clean water," they did not like the presence of iron in the water. If a filter could remove iron to make water taste better and prevent the reddish stain while simultaneously removing arsenic and microbes, uptake could be higher.

ACKNOWLEDGMENT

We thank the study participants for their time, Fazlul Kader Chowdhury and Md. Al Mamun for help conducting the research, and Dorothy Southern for her support in guiding and editing this manuscript. The International Centre for Diarrheal Disease Research, Bangladesh, acknowledges with gratitude the U.S. Agency for International Development for supporting this study.

REFERENCES

Blum, L.S., Nahar, N., 2004. Cultural and social context of dysentery: implications for the introduction of a new vaccine. Journal of Health, Population and Nutrition 22, 159–169.

Clasen, T., Schmidt, W.P., Rabie, T., Roberts, I., Cairncross, S., 2007. Interventions to improve water quality for preventing diarrhoea: systematic review and meta-analysis. British Medical Journal 334, 782–785.

DPHE, Arsenic contamination and Mitigation in Bangladesh. Department of public health engineering, Bangladesh, http://www.dphe.gov.bd/index.php?option=com_content&view=article &id=96&Itemid=104. (accessed on 26.09.11.).

DuBois, A.E., Crump, J.A., Keswick, B.H., Slusker, L., Quick, R.E., Vulule, J.M., Luby, S.P., 2010. Determinants of Use of Household-level Water Chlorination Products in Rural Kenya, 2003–2005. International Journal of Environmental Health Research and Public Health 7, 3842–3852.

Gupta, S.K., Islam, M.S., Johnston, R., Ram, P.K., Luby, S.P., 2008. The chulli water purifier: acceptability and effectiveness of an innovative strategy for household water treatment in Bangladesh. The American Journal of Tropical Medicine and Hygiene 78, 979–984.

Islam, M.S., Siddika, A., Khan, M.N., Goldar, M.M., Sadique, M.A., Kabir, A.N., Huq, A., Colwell, R.R., 2001. Microbiological analysis of tube-well water in a rural area of Bangladesh. Applied and Environmental Microbiology 67, 3328–3330.

Khan, M., Mosley, W.H., Chakraborty, J., Sardar, A.M., Khan, M.R., 1978. Water sources and the incidence of cholera in rural Bangladesh. Scientific Report No. 16. Cholera Research Laboratory, Bangladesh.

Levine, R.J., Khan, M.R., D'Souza, S., Nalin, D.R., 1976. Failure of sanitary wells to protect against cholera and other diarrhoeas in Bangladesh. Lancet 2, 86–89.

Luby, S.P., Agboatwalla, M., Painter, J., Altaf, A., Billhimer, W., Keswick, B., Hoekstra, R.M., 2006. Combining drinking water treatment and hand washing for diarrhoea prevention, a cluster randomised controlled trial. Tropical Medicine and International Health 11, 479–489.

Luby, S.P., Gupta, S.K., Sheikh, M.A., Johnston, R.B., Ram, P.K., Islam, M.S., 2008a. Tubewell water quality and predictors of contamination in three flood-prone areas in Bangladesh. Journal of Applied Microbiology 105, 1002–1008.

Luby, S.P., Mendoza, C., Keswich, B.H., Chiller, T.M., Hoekstra, R.M., 2008b. Difficulties in bringing point-of-use water treatment to scale in rural Guatemala. The American Journal of Tropical Medicine and Hygiene 78, 382–387.

Mintz, E.D., Reiff, F.M., Tauxe, R.V., 1995. Safe water treatment and storage in the home: a practical new strategy to prevent waterborne diseases. The Journal of the American Medical Association 273, 948–953.

PATH, July 2008. Project Brief. Findings from investigation of user experience with household water treatment and storage products in Andhra Pradesh, India.

Quick, R.E., Venczel, L.V., Mintz, E.D., Soleto, L., Aparicio, J., Gironaz, M., Hutwagner, L., Greene, K., Bopp, C., Maloney, K., Chavez, D., Sobsey, M., Tauxe, R.V., 1999. Diarrhea prevention in Bolivia through point of use disinfection and safe storage: a promising new strategy. Epidemiology and Infection 122, 83–90.

Smith, A.H., L. E, Rahman, M., 2000. Contamination of drinking-water by arsenic in Bangladesh: a public health emergency. Bulletin of the World Health Organization 78(9), 1093–1103.

Sobsey, M.D., S. C, Casanova, L.M., Brown, M.J., Elliot, M.A., 2008. Point of use household drinking water filtration: a practical, effective solution for providing sustained access to safe drinking water in the developing world. Environmental Science and Technology 42, 4261–4267.

Sommer, A., Woodward, W.E., 1972. The influence of protected water supplies on the spread of classical-Inaba and El Tor-Ogawa cholera in rural East Bengal. Lancet 2, 985–987.

WHO, 2007. Country health system profile: Bangladesh, New Delhi, India.

Chapter 19

Anthropological Approaches to Outbreak Investigations in Bangladesh

Shahana Parveen,[1] Rebeca Sultana,[1] Stephen P. Luby,[1,2] and Emily S. Gurley[1]

[1]ICDDR,B, Dhaka, Bangladesh, [2]Director of Research, Centre for Innovation and Global Health, Stanford University, USA

BACKGROUND

Bangladesh encounters a variety of disease outbreaks each year. Such an outbreak is defined as the occurrence of rapid or sudden increase of more cases of disease than normally expected within a specific place or group of people who might have common exposure over a given period of time (Gordis, 2004). Over the past decade, at least eight major different disease outbreaks, including emerging infectious diseases and toxic outbreaks, have affected the economic and social lives of Bangladeshi people and increased the public health burden (Faruque et al., 2003; ICDDRB, 2008, 2009a,b, 2011; Brooks et al., 2009; Luby et al., 2009; Homaira et al., 2010b) in this densely populated country of 157 million people in a 144,000 km^2 area (BBS, 2010).

The Institute of Epidemiology, Disease Control, and Research (IEDCR) of the Bangladesh Government has the mandate to lead the response to these outbreaks. Since 2002, icddr,b (International Centre for Diarrhoeal Diseases Research, Bangladesh), has been providing technical assistance to support IEDCR in outbreak investigations and response.

During a highly fatal (75% case fatality) outbreak caused by Nipah virus (NiV) in 2004, anthropologists were first invited to join the clinicians, epidemiologists, and microbiologists and/or a laboratory investigation team, as the epidemiological investigation suggested person-to-person transmission (Gurley et al., 2007; Blum et al., 2009). There was little information about behavioral practices that might contribute to risk factors for person-to-person transmission, so the outbreak investigation team requested the anthropological team to explore the local perceptions of the illness and caring practices provided for NiV-infected patients (Blum et al., 2009).

When Culture Impacts Health. http://dx.doi.org/10.1016/B978-0-12-415921-1.00019-1

Since then, anthropological investigations conducted by anthropologists and sociologists have been a key part of the work of the multidisciplinary investigation team. Anthropological investigations have complemented epidemiological and clinical investigations by using an explanatory model (Kleinman, 1980) to describe the illness, symptoms, exposures, causal explanation, and behaviors that are associated with the outbreak, which has helped the investigation team to understand the broader or specific context of the outbreak. The investigations are now strengthened by examining the outbreak from a more holistic perspective, with insights from the technical expertise of each of the multiple disciplines.

Anthropological investigations of outbreaks in Bangladesh use conventional qualitative data collection tools and techniques, including in-depth interviews, formal and informal discussions, and more general observations. In some situations investigators also use participatory rapid assessment, such as social mapping, mobility mapping, and time line exercises. The application of a particular tool or technique depends on the nature, magnitude, and context of a particular outbreak. During an outbreak, structured questionnaires are used to find the exposures associated with the outbreak, but there is a very limited scope for obtaining sufficient details of these exposures with this technique. In contrast, qualitative tools capture detailed illness and exposure histories related to illness, which can offer complementary understanding of the cultural context of these exposures. One of the major benefits of applying these qualitative data collection techniques is that they can elicit responses about the behaviors or exposures seen as taboo or stigmatized by the community, but related to the outbreak. The behavioral practices often contribute to the development of a hypothesis about the mode of transmission, which is subsequently tested as part of the epidemiological investigation (Gurley et al., 2010). This chapter describes the steps that anthropology researchers from icddr,b and IEDCR followed during an outbreak investigation and the contribution that this process brings to the overall response to broader public health effort.

Example from a Nipah Virus Encephalitis Outbreak Investigation

In Bangladesh over the past decade, Nipah virus (NiV) has caused 10 outbreaks of severe febrile encephalitis in humans. The two most common pathways of NiV transmission in Bangladesh are as follows: (1) from a natural reservoir of NiV fruit bats (*Pteropus giganteus*) to humans through drinking contaminated raw date palm sap and (2) from person-to-person, which can occur from close contact with respiratory secretions and other bodily secretions of highly infectious NiV patients (Chadha et al., 2006). In Bangladesh, raw date palm sap is a delicacy that is drunk during the winter season (Nahar et al., 2010). Therefore, each winter people who consume contaminated raw sap may be at risk for infection with this virus. After exposure to this virus, a person may develop symptoms within 6–11 days (Hossain et al., 2008).

The anthropological contribution to outbreak investigation was well illustrated in an NiV outbreak in 2007, when seven people were affected and three of them died. As part of the public health response approved by the Government of Bangladesh, the preliminary epidemiological investigations identified that the male index case (the first case of the outbreak) and his wife died before any biological specimens were collected, but five other subsequent cases had confirmed IgM antibodies to NiV detected by ELISA (Homaira et al., 2010a). The epidemic curve and primary exposure histories of the infected cases suggested that there was a possibility of person-to-person transmission. After the third death of this outbreak, the affected community became very frightened. In the typical societal structure of rural communities in Bangladesh, it is customary for neighbors and relatives to frequently visit a person who is sick. But during this NiV outbreak, many of the residents of the affected village and adjacent villages stopped visiting households of sick or deceased cases. The adjacent villagers also put a barricade at the entrance of the outbreak village to restrict the movement of affected community residents. The challenge for the anthropology team was to build good rapport with the residents of the outbreak community while investigating person-to-person and other possible exposures to develop a causal explanation of the outbreak.

The anthropology team conducted in-depth interviews with the surviving cases, family members, relatives, and friends of patients who died, to collect illness histories and to understand their levels of exposure to NiV. The team also interviewed the date palm sap harvester of the outbreak village to know his sap collection history and selling locations in the previous weeks in the outbreak area. The team conducted informal discussions with the neighbors and friends of dead and surviving cases, and also conducted a social mapping exercise with the help of community residents that produced a map of the area that located the proximity of household cases, the presence of date palm trees, date palm sap selling points, and existing bat roosts in the outbreak area.

From several in-depth interviews with family members, researchers learned that the index case had a shop in the local village market where a vendor brought raw date palm sap. Researchers located this sap-selling place in the local village market from the social mapping exercise. From the interviews and informal discussions, researchers identified one friend who also had a shop in that local market, adjacent to the index case's shop. Researchers then interviewed the friend to explore the exposures of the index case while he was in the local market. The friend said that the index case purchased raw sap from that vendor and drank it 15 days before the onset of his illness. This exposure was also reported by friends and colleagues during subsequent data collection for the epidemiologic case-control study.

After collecting a detailed illness history and exposure history of the index case, the anthropology team used in-depth interviews with surviving cases, and relatives and friends of cases to understand the chain of person-to-person transmission. We explored the care giving practices and level of contacts/exposures of each person with cases during their illness. To follow up the team also cross checked this information in several group discussions with relatives and friends.

In-depth interviews revealed that the wife and sister in-law of the index case cared for him throughout his five-day illness at home and in the hospital. They fed him, cleaned him, sponged his body, and wiped the saliva and froth from his mouth. His wife also shared the same bed with him throughout his illness. On the third day of his illness, a cousin and a friend took him to a local village doctor on a motorbike. On their way to the doctor's office, the friend was driving the bike, the index case was in the middle, and the cousin was sitting and holding him from his back. On the fourth day of the index case's illness, the friend and the cousin again took him to a local pharmacy on a motorbike again using the same sitting arrangement. On their way back home the index case had a severe cough and breathing difficulty, so he laid his head on his friend's shoulder. When he returned home, his condition deteriorated and temperature increased so his relatives and friends admitted him to the local subdistrict hospital. On his way to the hospital, his wife, brother, sister in-law, cousin, and a neighbor accompanied him in the microbus. In the hospital, the doctor administered intravenous saline and gave him two tablets to swallow. After he was admitted, his wife's sister, brother in-law, and a friend visited him and tried to feed him and comforted him by touching his head and forehead. On the fifth day he deteriorated and was first taken to a local clinic and from there was shifted to the district level government hospital by the same microbus used earlier. During that time his level of consciousness decreased. A total of seven relatives and friends accompanied him in the microbus. When they arrived at the district hospital, the microbus driver carried the index case over his shoulder to the hospital trolley. Altogether, more than 15 relatives and friends provided care and had contact with the index case during his illness. Out of them, six people developed illness between 7 and 13 days after their contact/exposure and two of them died. None of these six cases drank raw date palm sap in the 14 days before their illness.

Comments

The anthropological investigation in this outbreak provided the specific context in which person-to-person NiV transmission occurred. Epidemiology effectively summarizes risk exposures, for example, "close contact with a person with encephalitis," but it is the details of the in-depth interviews that describe the context that suggests how the virus was likely transmitted and what type of contact needs to be avoided or actions taken to prevent such transmission.

During any outbreak with human fatalities like NiV, affected communities typically become frightened, tense, and/or stigmatized. The investigation team attempted to build good rapport with residents of this affected community from the beginning. This key principle of anthropological data collection (Bernard, 2005; Hahn and Inhorn, 2009) eventually changed the understanding about the occurrence of the disease and paved the way for further investigative activities. For example, the index case's family was stigmatized because community residents perceived that he was infected by acquired immune deficiency syndrome (AIDS) because he drank local alcohol, used marijuana, and used to visit sex workers. In the course of the investigation the team visited households of both dead and surviving cases, talked intensely with their family members, and further explained the possible routes of transmission of this disease. All of these activities influenced the residents, changing their understanding that the index case and his wife were affected by NiV, not AIDS.

The detailed exposure and contact histories helped to identify the appropriate proxy respondents for deceased and very sick cases. Based on the in-depth understanding of the affected community, the anthropology team contributed to the development of appropriate language for the case-control questionnaire to ensure its acceptability to the community residents, so that participants did not feel offended or stigmatized by any question. Ultimately, this generated more valid information for the identification of the risk factor for this outbreak.

Example from a Pufferfish Poisoning Outbreak Investigation

Over the past two decades Bangladesh has sporadically experienced pufferfish poisoning outbreaks in humans. Pufferfish, globally known as blowfish or globefish, belong to the Tetraodontide family and contain a water-soluble and heat-resistant neurotoxin that when a person ingested can block the sodium channel of nerve tissues, ultimately paralyzing muscles and causing death (Chew et al., 1983; Benzer, 2007).

The toxin concentration in the fish is higher in liver, gallbladder, intestines, gonads, and and/or skin, but muscles are usually less poisonous (Chew et al., 1983; Ahasan et al., 2004). The toxicity in different marine species and freshwater species varies with sex, season, and geographical variation (Lee et al., 2000). There are 13 species of pufferfish found in Bangladesh; two of them are only known to live in freshwater and the rest live in the ocean (Zaman et al., 1997; Diener et al., 2007). Not all available species of pufferfish are fatally toxic; some species contain only a little concentration of toxin (Lee et al., 2000).

During 2008, several outbreaks of pufferfish poisoning occurred in Bangladesh. The first three consecutive outbreaks occurred from April to June. In response to the first two outbreaks, investigators conducted epidemiological investigations that focused on the onset of illness, signs and symptoms, exposure history, local availability of the fish, knowledge about its toxicity, treatment received, and the outcome of the illness. In these outbreaks, 28 people experienced illness after ingesting pufferfish and 10 (36% fatality rate) of them died. Epidemiologic investigations identified that all people intoxicated in the first two outbreaks consumed pufferfish and developed illness between 30 minutes and 3 hours. People involved in these outbreaks consumed this variety of fish for the first time and most were unaware of its toxicity. Only a few of them knew that this fish can contain some toxin, but none was aware of the risk of fatality (Homaira et al., 2010b).

During the third outbreak, the investigation team noted that all the outbreaks occurred in noncoastal areas, but were attributed to marine species pufferfish. Several questions arose in regard to these outbreaks including: Why were there so many outbreaks occurring in a short time frame? Was there any specific reason for the outbreaks to occur away from coastal areas? Was this fish routinely available in the local market? Were people aware of the level of pufferfish toxicity? As answers to these questions require a broader perspective than just identifying immediate risk factors, a team of anthropologists conducted an in-depth exploration of these issues using the tools and perspectives of this discipline, which is particularly effective when exploring an outbreak.

The anthropology team conducted in-depth interviews and group discussions with the people who developed illness, people who consumed this fish but did not develop any symptoms, their family members, and residents of the outbreak community. The team learned that people of the affected community had previous experience with eating small freshwater pufferfish without any toxic reaction. They locally called this fish *tepa*; it was commonly available in their village river and local water bodies, and they enjoyed its delicious taste. They had never heard that any varieties of this fish were dangerous to eat. People of the affected community said that the larger marine variety of pufferfish had been transported to their local fish market on the day of the outbreak, possibly from the coastal part of the country. Community residents were unfamiliar with the appearance of larger marine pufferfish. When it became available in their local market, they bought this marine species based on their previous pleasant experiences with the small freshwater variety. Other types of fish of similar weight might cost more than $1.50/kg, but the pufferfish was available in the market for ~$0.50/kg. Some purchasers reported that because of inflation in cost of daily necessary goods, the relatively lower cost of a "larger size" pufferfish increased its appeal to customers at the fish market.

Women in this outbreak community described in their interviews that when preparing small freshwater pufferfish, they always removed the intestines, liver, gallbladder, gonads, and lips, but never discarded the skin and head. Then they boiled the flesh with the skin and head of this fish with spices to make a curry. For larger marine pufferfish the affected families followed the process they used for other big fish: they removed the intestines and gallbladder, but then cooked the flesh with the skin, liver, eggs, and head together with spices. During preparation of a special pufferfish dish with bare hands, a cook from one of the affected families tasted it by touching her finger to her tongue. Approximately 20 minutes later she developed tingling sensations and heaviness in her tongue, coldness in her limbs, and dizziness. She died within an hour. Two families who cooked only the fillet of pufferfish did not become ill. Perhaps this was due to a very low concentration of toxins in the flesh of the marine pufferfish. However, these two families told us they were not aware of its toxicity, they traditionally learned to fillet small pufferfish from elder family members.

To explore the availability and trade of marine pufferfish, the team then visited Cox's Bazar, one of the main fishing ports on the Bay of Bengal coast. They talked with deep-sea fishermen, wholesalers, and dry fish makers to explore their practices related to catching and selling of this fish and their perception and knowledge about puffer toxicity. At first the anthropology team observed the central fish depot market where fishermen brought boatloads full of fish to sell to the wholesalers. Based on the interactions/trade between fishermen and wholesalers and businessmen, the team identified fishermen for group discussions and in-depth interviews. The fishermen told us that they catch pufferfish in their nets along with other commercially important fish. They consider pufferfish as "low category" fish and usually do not sell or consume it as they know it is poisonous. Sometimes if they can catch a large quantity of pufferfish, such as 20–30 kg, they sell it to wholesalers who then sell it to the dry fish preparers. The anthropology team observed one of these sales and tracked down some wholesalers for interview. Subsequently the team followed the clues related to pufferfish uses provided by wholesalers and selected the next informants—the dry fish preparers.

The wholesalers and dry fish preparers mentioned that pufferfish are routinely used to make dried fish products for animal and human consumption. During dry fish processing all the viscera, including the liver, gallbladder, intestines, and eggs are removed, leaving only the head, skin, and flesh to dry under the sun. The dry fish preparers perceived that only the gallbladder and eggs contain the toxin and therefore, removing them intact makes the fish safe to eat. These dried pufferfish are distributed to other parts of country where they are used as poultry feed, and they are also consumed by some indigenous group people. However, these fishermen and wholesalers told us that when there is a plentiful catch of marine pufferfish, some businessmen occasionally distribute the fresh fish to noncoastal parts of the country, where people are unfamiliar with the appearance of larger marine variety, are more likely to purchase it.

Comments

The anthropological investigation in this outbreak identified the sociocultural factors necessary to understand these repeated toxic outbreaks. The in-depth exploration gave insight about how existing practices related to the preparation and cooking of pufferfish and lack of awareness about its toxicity resulted in fatalities among community residents. Our investigation underscored that previous pleasant experiences of consumption of small freshwater pufferfish had influenced people to buy this fish even though they were unfamiliar with the marine species' appearance. Additionally, this large size fish, at a lower price, increased its appeal to the community residents. The recent increase in food prices, including the Bangladesh staples of rice and wheat, in 2008 may have increased the attractiveness of the pufferfish (ADB, 2008).

DISCUSSION

In outbreak investigations in Bangladesh, the contributions of anthropological investigations have been established. Anthropological investigations provide multidisciplinary teams with insights about the broader context by thoroughly describing illness histories, exposure histories, local interpretations of illnesses, caring practices, and health-seeking and help-seeking behaviors (Trostle, 2005) in a particular culture. The in-depth exposures and contact histories can often contribute to the identification of appropriate proxy respondent for a case-control study, as was done during the 2007 NiV outbreak (Homaira et al., 2010a).

During tense outbreak situations, anthropologists spend extensive time interacting with residents of affected communities, both individually or in a group and listening to them carefully. This approach helps the investigative researchers to establish trust with local residents, paving the way for broader investigative activities by the team. It opens a channel for communicating sound information regarding the outbreak and steps the community can take to reduce their risk.

During acute outbreaks there is a need to provide immediate communication messages to control or prevent the further spread of the disease. As local interpretations of the illness often differ from the biomedical paradigm, an anthropological approach can help in developing compelling preventive messages, which is vital for uptake and for designing long-term prevention strategies. During the NiV outbreaks in 2004 when the outbreak community perceived the cause as supernatural (Blum et al., 2009) or in 2007 when they thought it was AIDS, the preventive messages that were developed without incorporating local causal explanations were not convincing for communities. Thus, the anthropological approach bridges the gap between the local interpretation and biomedical paradigm to make the prevention messages meaningful for the affected communities to follow.

The anthropological findings from the pufferfish poisoning investigation suggested that dissemination of awareness messages on a large scale in the communities and in the market areas about the variety of species of pufferfish available and the varying toxin distribution in these fish could prevent future fatal intoxication. Considering the broader social and economic context of the raising business of both dry and fresh pufferfish and their impact in the public health, this anthropological investigation also urged the design and implementation of an explanatory study to explore the supply and distribution chain of this fish across the country.

REFERENCES

ADB, 2008. Asian Development Outlook 2008 Update. http://beta.adb.org/publications/asian-development-outlook-2008-update, Vol. 2011. Asian Development Bank.

Ahasan, H.A., Mamun, A.A., Karim, S.R., Bakar, M.A., Gazi, E.A., Bala, C.S., 2004. Paralytic complications of puffer fish (tetrodotoxin) poisoning. Singapore Medical Journal 45, 73–74.

BBS, 2010. Statistical Year Book of Bangladesh-2009. Bangladesh Bureau of Statistics.

Benzer, I., 2007. Toxicity, Tetrodotoxin. eMedicine, pp. 1–8.

Bernard, H.R., 2005. Research Methods in Anthropology: Qualitative and Quantitative Approahes, fourth ed. AltraMira, Walnut Grove, CA.

Blum, L.S., Khan, R., Hahar, N., Breiman, R.F., 2009. In-depth assessment of an outbreak of Nipah encephalitis with person-to-person transmission in Bangladesh: implications for prevention and control strategies. The American Journal of Tropical Medicine and Hygiene 80, 96–102.

Brooks, W.A., Alamgir, A.S., Sultana, R., Islam, M.S., Rahman, M., Fry, A.M., et al., 2009. Avian Influenza Virus A (H5N1), Detected through Routine Surveillance, in Child, Bangladesh. Emerging Infectious Diseases 15, 1311–1313.

Chadha, M.S., Comer, J.A., Lowe, L., Rota, P.A., Rollin, P.E., Bellini, W.J., Ksiazek, T.G., Mishra, A., 2006. Nipah virus-associated encephalitis outbreak, Siliguri, India. Emerging Infectious Diseases 12, 235–240.

Chew, S.K., Goh, C.H., Wang, K.W., Mah, P.K., Tan, B.Y., 1983. Puffer fish (Tetrodotoxin) poisoning: clinical report and role of anti-cholinesterase drugs in therapy. Singapore Medical Journal 24, 168–171.

Diener, M., Christian, B., Ahmed, M.S., Luckas, B., 2007. Determination of tetrodotoxin and its analogs in the puffer fish Takifugu oblongus from Bangladesh by hydrophilic interaction chromatography and mass-spectrometric detection. Analytical and Bioanalytical Chemistry 389, 1997–2002.

Faruque, S.M., Chowdhury, N., Kamruzzaman, M., Ahmad, Q.S., Faruque, A.S., Salam, M.A., Ramamurthy, T., et al., 2003. Reemergence of epidemic Vibrio cholerae O139, Bangladesh. Emerging Infectious Diseases 9, 1116–1122.

Gordis, L., 2004. Epidemiology. Elsevier Saunders, Philadelphia.

Gurley, E.S., Montgomery, J.M., Hossain, M.J., Bell, M., Azad, A.K., Fiaz, M.A., Islam, M.R., Molla, M.A., et al., 2007. Person-to-person transmission of Nipah virus in a Bangladeshi community. Emerging Infectious Diseases 13, 1031–1037.

Gurley, E.S., Rahman, M., Hossain, M.J., Nahar, N., Islam, N., Sultana, R., Khatun, S., Uddin, M.Z., et al., 2010. Fatal outbreak from consuming Xanthium strumarium seedlings during time of food scarcity in northeastern Bangladesh. PLoS One 5, e9756.

Hahn, R.A., Inhorn, M.C., 2009. Anthropology and Public Health: Bridging Differences in Culture and Society, second ed. Oxford University Press, New York.

Homaira, N., Rahman, M., Hossain, M.J., Epstein, J.H., Sultana, R., Khan, M.S., et al., 2010a. Nipah virus outbreak with person-to-person transmission in a district of Bangladesh, 2007. Epidemiology and Infection, 1–7.

Homaira, N., Rahman, M., Luby, S.P., Rahman, M., Haider, M.S., Faruque, L.I., et al., 2010b. Multiple outbreaks of puffer fish intoxication in Bangladesh, 2008. The American Journal of Tropical Medicine and Hygiene. 83, 440–444.

Hossain, M.J., Gurley, E.S., Montgomery, J.M., Bell, M., Carroll, D.S., Hsu, V.P., et al., 2008. Clinical presentation of nipah virus infection in Bangladesh. Clinical Infectious Diseases 46, 977–984.

ICDDRB, 2008. Outbreak of mass sociogenic illness in students in secondary schools in Bangladesh during. July-August 2007, Health and Science Bulletin Vol. 6, ICDDR, B, Dhaka, pp. 6–12.

ICDDRB, 2009a. Cutaneous anthrax outbreaks in two districts of North-Western Bangladesh. August-October 2009a, Health and Science Bulletin Vol. 7, ICDDR, B, Dhaka, pp. 1–8.

ICDDRB, 2009b. Outbreak of hepatitis E in a low income urban community in Bangladesh. Health and Science Bulletin Vol. 7, ICDDR, B, pp. 14–20.

ICDDRB, 2011. Outbreak of mild respiratory disease caused by H5N1 and H9N2 infections among young children in Dhaka, Bangladesh, 2011. Health Science Bulletin Vol. 9, ICDDR, B, pp. 5–12.

Kleinman, A., 1980. Patients and Healers in the Context of Culture: An Exploration of the Border-land between Anthropology, Medicine and Psychiatry. University of California Press, Berkeley.

Lee, M., Jeong, D.Y., Kim, W.S., Kim, H.D., Kim, C.H., Park, W.W., et al., 2000. A Tetrodotoxin-Producing Vibrio Strain, LM-1, from the Puffer Fish Fugu vermicularis radiatus. Applied and Environmental Microbiology 66, 1698–1701.

Luby, S.P., Hossain, M.J., Gurley, E.S., Ahmed, B.N., Banu, S., Khan, S.U., et al., 2009. Recurrent zoonotic transmission of Nipah virus into humans, Bangladesh, 2001–2007. Emerging Infectious Diseases 15, 1229–1235.

Nahar, N., Sultana, R., Gurley, E.S., Hossain, M.J., Luby, S.P., 2010. Date Palm Sap Collection: Exploring Opportunities to Prevent Nipah Transmission. Ecohealth 7, 196–203.

Trostle, J.A., 2005. Epidemiology and culture. Cambridge University Press, New York.

Zaman, L., Arakawa, O., Shimosu, A., Onoue, Y., 1997. Occurrence of paralytic shellfish poison in Bangladeshi freshwater puffers. Official Journal of the International Society on Toxinology 35, 423–431.

Chapter 20

Post-Disaster Coping in Aceh: Sociocultural Factors and Emotional Response

Rebecca Fanany and Ismet Fanany

School of Humanities and Social Sciences, Deakin University, Burwood, Victoria, Australia

The 2004 Indian Ocean tsunami led to an unprecedented level of international aid to affected areas. The Indonesian province of Aceh, which had recently emerged from a long period of conflict, received much of this aid as its inhabitants were viewed as suffering from a double blow of trauma resulting, first, from civil strife and, second, from natural disaster. For this reason, many international programs offered counseling and psychological support for victims. Many of these programs were not successful, however, and a majority of victims did not appear to react to their situation in the ways anticipated. This chapter describes the coping response of tsunami survivors in Aceh in the context of their culture, society, and religion, including their perception of its causes and how this perception influenced their emotional state following the event.

The research reported here is based on visits to Aceh made in 2006 and 2010 at which time in-depth interviews were conducted with members of the provincial government, nongovernment agencies involved in the reconstruction efforts, and members of the public who experienced the tsunami firsthand. The original aim of these interviews was to elicit information about effects of the disaster on various social institutions and the need for capacity building in relation to reconstruction. Through the interview process, however, a strong theme relating to coping, at both the individual and community level, began to emerge, and an expanded interview protocol based on the methodologies of resilience (see Hall and Zautra, 2010) was developed and used to build the conceptualization of disaster described here. Material from the interviews was supplemented by a systematic search of print and new media to form a picture of public discourse following the tsunami.

BACKGROUND

On December 26, 2004, a large undersea earthquake caused a tsunami that impacted the Indian Ocean coastal regions of South and Southeast Asia resulting

When Culture Impacts Health. http://dx.doi.org/10.1016/B978-0-12-415921-1.00020-8
225

in significant damage and loss of life. One of the most severely affected areas was the Indonesian province of Aceh located at the northern tip of the island of Sumatra. Aceh, whose population was approximately 4 million, is inhabited by a number of Indonesian ethnic groups and is almost entirely Muslim. Sometimes nicknamed "The Veranda of Mecca," Aceh is religiously conservative and fundamentalist and, when the tsunami occurred, had already begun to express these views in its local laws. A large-scale program of government decentralization, which resulted in Regional Autonomy and devolution of responsibility for a wide range of public functions to the regions, became law in 2001. Regional Autonomy also gave new momentum to the Free Aceh Movement (GAM), which had been in a state of rebellion against the Indonesian government since the 1970s. This movement, which advocated independence for Aceh, enjoyed wide public support by the 1990s. Following the tsunami, however, both sides declared a cease-fire and resolved to end the conflict. In 2005, a peace agreement gave Aceh special autonomy status and mandated the withdrawal of most of the Indonesian troops in exchange for the disarmament of GAM.

The effects of the Indian Ocean tsunami have been discussed extensively in the literature, but much of this research has concerned physical reconstruction of infrastructure and institutions and has also documented aid efforts and the role of international organizations in rehabilitation programs. Comparatively little attention has been paid to the emotional response of disaster survivors. Several authors have addressed the psychological distress observed in some individuals immediately following the tsunami (see, e.g., Aitken, 2005; Carballo et al., 2006; Souza et al., 2007), but these discussions have simply noted a need for counseling or commented that the issue requires further study. There has been, to date, no study of the strategies employed by tsunami victims to return to a normal life nor has the question of emotional resilience been considered from their point of view. Work on emotional resilience has been limited to inferences drawn from observations of affected groups (e.g., Carballo et al., 2005; Wilson, 2007; UNSCAP, 2008). This chapter will consider the question of emotional resilience among tsunami survivors in Aceh in the context of their culture, society, and religion, with reference to their perception of the causes of the disaster and the way in which this view influenced their emotional state following the event. Using their narratives as a way to elucidate their psychosocial perspective, survivor reactions in Aceh will be contrasted with the Western understanding of post-traumatic stress such as might be expected in individuals following an event of this type.

THE CONCEPTUALIZATION OF TRAUMA

Guidelines and manuals developed by organizations like CARE, the Red Cross, the World Health Organization, the Global Development Group, and many others all assume that natural disaster survivors must be traumatized and are likely to suffer from post-traumatic stress disorder (PTSD). PTSD, which emerged as a separate disease category in the 1980s, encompasses aspects of several previously observed conditions, including shell shock, combat stress, and delayed stress syndrome (Young, 1995). It has been suggested, however, that PTSD is really a politicosocial response to a particular event in certain individuals or groups (Summerfield, 1999) and does not represent a universal condition (Von Peter, 2008). In fact, cross-cultural application of the concept of PTSD has been widely criticized (see Kleinman, 1988; Summerfield, 1999; Littlewood, 2000; Mezey and Robbins, 2001), specifically whether the Western, medical conceptualization of mental trauma, which is taken to derive from individual experience, reflects the range of social, historical, and group dynamics that shape response to events like natural disasters or political conflict (see Eisenbruch, 1991; Watters, 2001; de Jong et al., 2003; Von Peter, 2008).

Nonetheless, the Western medical conceptualization of PTSD and emotional distress following natural disasters and other extreme events has tended to form the basis of international aid programs following disasters around the world. The World Health Organization (2005), for example, suggests that PTSD is to be expected in individuals who have suffered internal displacement; survived disasters; or have been affected by war, genocide, or terrorism. This reflects the idea that certain events must lead to mental distress, regardless of how this is expressed, because it is presupposed that there are experiences no human being would be able to cope with without suffering trauma. This contrasts with a statement by the American Refugee Committee (2005) about the tsunami that noted a high level of acceptance by survivors, which was assumed to be a result of their strong religious beliefs. For many of the aid agencies involved, this observation proved confusing in light of their expectations and was further confounded in Aceh by the rejection of their assistance by disaster survivors (see, e.g., Huda et al., 2007; Telford and Cosgrove, 2007; Perlez, 2005; ABC News, 2006). One important reason for the apparent unacceptability of aid was a lack of understanding about how survivors conceptualized their own mental health and the role of sociocultural factors in their understanding of the disaster.

ISLAM IN ACEH

Adherence to Islam is a characteristic feature of identity as a member of the Acehnese ethnic group. The Acehnese people are native to the northernmost part of Sumatra and speak a local language that is linguistically related to Malay. They make up approximately 50% of the province's population, with the remainder being Javanese, Gayo, Alas, and other ethnicities. In total, about 99% of the population is Muslim (BPS, 2009). The province's full name, *Nanggroe Aceh Darussalam*, reflects both Acehnese culture and Islamic influence, and local scenery is characterized by the presence of mosques in every settlement, large or small. Other manifestations of Islamic culture and society include the widespread wearing of Islamic dress, the use of Arabic script on buildings and in political and public information campaign slogans, decorative art resembling those of the Middle East, and more recently the implementation of *syariah* (Islamic) law at the local level.

Islam seems to have come to Aceh with traders; was adopted peacefully by choice, rather than imposed by force; and incorporates many elements of Sufi beliefs (McAmis, 2002). Sufism represents the inner, mystic dimension of the religion and places strong emphasis on hospitality, ritualized acknowledgement of God, and divine determinism (Howell, 2001). In Aceh, these elements of belief form the core of individual and group response to disaster and tragedy. An Acehnese proverbial saying derived from the Quran states that, in times of trouble, people should "hold fast to the rope of God."

SURVIVOR UNDERSTANDING OF THE TSUNAMI

Almost without exception, the Acehnese public ascribed the 2004 earthquake and tsunami to an act of God. Unlike in the West, to the people of Aceh, an act of God is not random and without clear cause. Such events are believed to be caused deliberately for reasons known to God and that may be deduced by humans. That is, while the Acehnese believe that it is not possible for people to understand or know God's plan for them, they may be able to discern certain aspects of God's intent and to respond to them through religious and moral actions.

Following the tsunami, it was obvious to many people in Aceh that laxity in their own moral and religious attitudes had caused the disaster. To many, the evidence suggesting this was overwhelming and was easily visible where mosques had been spared while every other building around them was washed away by the tidal wave. This occurred in Banda Aceh, Lampuuk, Baet, Kaju, Meulaboh, and many other areas and was reported by the media across the region (see, e.g., ChannelNewsAsia, 2005). Many residents who sought refuge in mosques survived the tsunami, further strengthening the idea that the disaster was a form of divine commentary on the community's religious behavior. A number of observers, including several from international aid agencies, saw a more prosaic explanation for this phenomenon, which they ascribed to the fact that mosques tended to be more strongly built because of their social importance and were frequently located at the highest point available as a sign of reverence. Survivors often accepted this judgment, saying that these facts were equally a sign of God's participation in the affairs of humans as surely it was He who caused people to build their mosques in this way and in these locations.

To many people in Aceh, the need for a divine warning in the form of a tsunami was a result of a perceived slackening of religious observance and declining moral standards that came about because of a number of factors. These included the long period of conflict with the government of Indonesia, which distracted the public from its religious life; a growing interest in material objects and corresponding weakening of traditional communal institutions; and the increasingly secular nature of the public sphere, possibly as a result of integration into Indonesian national culture. In other words, the tsunami was viewed as a divine pronouncement about the social change that had been observable for some time and that had accelerated in recent years. This verdict seemed to be overwhelmingly negative to the majority of those affected.

One woman, who served as chair of the provincial branch of a national Islamic women's organization, expressed this general idea in a very personal and vehement manner. She recounts watching television at her home in Banda Aceh on Christmas Eve 2004 and being shocked to find a national Christmas variety program was being broadcast by the Aceh affiliate of TVRI, the Indonesian national television station. She was affronted, as this program contained references to the religious nature of the holiday even though it also featured entertainment acts of a secular nature. She says that, seeing the program, she prayed to God, asking that He just destroy the world if even Aceh was now showing Christmas programming to its Muslim population. The next day, the tsunami struck; this woman and one of her daughters took refuge on the second floor of the house. As the building began to fill with water and she realized they were going to die, she changed her mind and began to pray that God would save them. The water receded after a time, sparing the woman and her daughter but killing another of her children as well as many friends, relatives, and colleagues. When interviewed after the disaster, this survivor was convinced both her prayers had been answered and was proud to relate this story of what she believes is God's direct response to her prayers. She seems to feel no internal conflict at the idea that, if she is correct, her prayers were directly responsible for the deaths of hundreds of thousands of people in her town and elsewhere, as well as widespread destruction across the region.

While extreme in nature and more personal, this survivor's perception of the disaster is by no means unique in Aceh. A majority of survivors have the same sort of view about their importance to God and see the tsunami as a reasonable warning about their behavior. While they, of course, feel the loss of loved ones, property, livelihood, and cultural institutions, they believe that this was their fate (*takdir*) and there is no point fighting God's will. A similar response is often seen among religious Muslims elsewhere in Indonesia as a response to natural disasters, such as in Padang, West Sumatra, which experienced a large and very destructive earthquake on September 30, 2009.

Interestingly, some elements of the Muslim community in Indonesia outside of Aceh also ascribed a divine origin to the tsunami and agreed that it was triggered by the behavior of the Acehnese. They observed, however, that the Acehnese were extremely arrogant about the quality of their religious observance and piety, and the tsunami was a warning from God to be more humble and stop placing themselves above the rest of the Indonesian Muslim community (see, e.g., Miftach, 2004). Some Indonesian bloggers even suggested the reason so many young people were killed by the tsunami was because their excessive religious zeal would lead them to become terrorists in the future, and God wished to prevent this before it happened (see, e.g., derkeiler.com).

Generally, there was wide agreement among the public in Aceh that the tsunami had been a warning sent by God and that the appropriate response required rebuilding and reestablishing their culture and society but also introspection focusing on their own behavior and attitudes in the context of Islamic law and theology. It was this understanding that led to the rejection of foreign aid that came from organizations thought to have a "Christianizing" mission or that seemed to impose requirements that were incompatible with traditional social patterns and lifestyle. The issue of missionary activity (*Kristenisasi*) in Aceh has been widely discussed in Indonesia and led directly to demands by the Acehnese public that certain aid agencies be expelled from the region (see Artawijaya et al., 2006, for complete documentation of this issue as it was discussed in the Indonesian media).

SURVIVOR RESPONSE TO THE TSUNAMI

Because of the widespread perception of the tsunami as a manifestation of divine will and a warning to the public about its religious and moral conduct, survivors overwhelmingly did not experience the emotional distress and trauma reaction that would have been expected in a Western setting and for which relief agencies had prepared. In fact, survivors were observed to be surprisingly resilient given the scope of the disaster and level of loss and did not feel in need of any kind of psychological support. Perceptions of need centered on housing, the means of making a living, and being reunited with friends and family members in an attempt to return to a normal life. This is not to suggest that individual survivors were not distressed at all, but the level of emotional disturbance seemed to be well within the capacity of sufferers, as well as the community, to absorb.

In this context, it is worth considering how some affected individuals compared the emotional and psychological impact of the devastation caused by the tsunami and that resulting from armed conflict with the Indonesian army. A high-ranking provincial government official, for example, noted that, while the loss of life and material damage associated with the tsunami was many times greater than the conflict, the trauma and emotional impact of the conflict was much greater than that of the tsunami. He could accept what he saw as the wrath of God but not the cruelty of other human beings. He also found he could easily understand that God might warn or even punish the Acehnese with such a disaster and believed that God always acted in their best interest. The Indonesian army, however, clearly did not, and he wondered why there had been no counseling available during the conflict when some Acehnese might have needed it. He did not comprehend why foreign aid providers, in particular, insisted on offering this service when the Acehnese were not overly distressed. Similar views were expressed repeatedly by many individuals and illustrate the depth of the Acehnese belief in God's will and their acceptance of even extremely severe events that they attribute to this cause.

The importance of community in the emotional response and ability of tsunami survivors to adapt cannot be ignored. Malay culture tends to be highly sensitive to social norms; a very high premium is placed on consensus and conformity, and it is generally not considered desirable to stand out or go against the group. An interesting example of this attitude was found in the town of Lampuuk, which was almost totally destroyed (except for its mosque) by the tidal wave. One of the most pressing needs of survivors in this area following the disaster was housing. They quickly formed a group to represent the interests of all residents and began negotiating with aid agencies for assistance replacing their lost dwellings. Eventually, the residents' committee decided to accept aid from the Turkish Red Crescent. After long delays and a number of setbacks during which survivors had to live in emergency accommodation, all 700 promised dwellings were ready for occupation in April 2007. Even though many houses had been available long before this and there had been serious disagreements about how the rehousing process should be handled, the Lampuuk survivors all waited to move in until everyone could be accommodated because of their desire to preserve their community structure and maintain the traditional orientation of their village. Even after the new houses were ready, many remained empty as the residents preferred to live in groups and chose to occupy certain houses only. Many of them lost all or most of their family members and did not want to live in relatively empty houses or by themselves. This reaction is typical in the Malay world where, in times of trouble, support networks based first on extended family ties and then on community or group affiliation serve as the main social structure in coping with the situation. In better times when more opportunities are available, this behavior is not usually seen, with individuals tending to act in their own interests. The reversion to a group mentality fostering mutual dependence among individuals who are related through family or geographical ties is a major emotional strategy among the Malay that serves to promote emotional resilience and support a return to normal life.

Despite the importance of traditional social structures in adjusting to post-disaster reality, in most cases the first institution the Acehnese turned to was religion, no doubt because of its importance in driving group experience and encouraged perhaps by the survival of many mosques, as noted above. As a religious significance was ascribed to the tsunami itself, it seemed appropriate to most survivors that the solution to their dilemma be sought in religion as well. To most of them, this meant restoring the means of religious observance and a moral lifestyle as quickly as possible, on both a personal as well as community level.

The cognitive rationale for this centered on the idea of *takdir*, that their fate was to experience and survive the tsunami, just as it was the destiny of others to die at this time. As their fate represented God's decision for them and was part of His overall plan for creation, there was no point in opposing an inevitable outcome.

Similarly, many survivors felt there was no reason to be distraught beyond a manageable emotional response to loss, because this type of reaction amounts to doubting God's judgment about the proper unfolding of events. This kind of rationale is often employed by Indonesian Muslims in other contexts and provides considerable support, which results in the commonly observed resilience of individuals as well as communities in the Malay world. This reaction tends to be genuine and is not generally a suppression of distress; the individuals involved do not believe themselves to be experiencing unusual stress as their attribution of events to a divine source and resulting acceptance of them makes such a reaction unnecessary in their eyes. It was for this reason that counseling efforts offered to tsunami victims in Aceh were met with such dissatisfaction and rejection (see, e.g., Miller, 2005; World Health Organization, 2006; Zulkarnain, 2006), and survivors were particularly adamant about the inappropriateness of these services.

For this reason, for survivors of the tsunami in Aceh, the experience often served to renew their interest in religious practice and identification. It is worth noting, however, that outward expressions of faith—such as attendance at religious services and events, modes of dress, fasting at appropriate times, and so on—are not necessarily an indication of personal feelings or beliefs, but these visible aspects of religion were considered extremely important following the tsunami as part of the new, reconstructed society in Aceh. The widely held view that it was necessary to restore Islamic culture and institutions in the region meant, to many people, that this would have to include conformity to certain aspects of religious practice in daily life. If people were not inclined to conform to more rigorous social norms, many survivors felt it would be appropriate to require such behavior by law.

As a result, there has been a strong and undeniable trend toward and demand for the implementation of *syariah* (Islamic) law in Aceh in the years since the tsunami. This movement began prior to that event, around the time Regional Autonomy took effect in 2001, but gained momentum following the disaster. *Qanun*, as *syariah* laws are referred to in Aceh, have been passed by the Regional Parliament as allowed by Indonesian Law No. 11 of 2006 on Governance in Aceh. Most recently, *qanun* have mandated severe punishment (public lashing, imprisonment, punitive fines) for offenses like homosexuality, adultery, rape, and pedophilia that are seen as detrimental to the public's morals. Earlier rulings addressed Islamic dress for women, mandatory completion of the five daily prayers, fasting during Ramadan, mandatory almsgiving, and prohibition of gambling and alcohol. Although these new rulings have been heavily criticized in the Indonesian media, especially in the context of what has been viewed as bizarre punishment for moral offenses, several of Aceh's political parties have taken the implementation of Islamic law as their main platform issue and have enjoyed considerable public support (Kompas, 2009). Despite the fact that laws with penalties of this kind are foreign to Indonesia's legal system, many people in Aceh are anxious that their region become an "Islamic state" by implementing the *qanun*.

Returning to the issue of need in the Acehnese community following the Indian Ocean tsunami, it is apparent that the perceptions of survivors about their own mental and emotional needs, as well as the type of aid that was most required, were very much at odds with those of international donors and aid agencies who based their expectations on a model of response derived from Western experience. The rejection of aid by survivors is more understandable in the context of their religious views and interpretation of the meaning of the event. The unacceptability of certain types of aid offered was a direct result of the lack of understanding about how these survivors conceptualized their own emotional state, their needs, and the central role religion and other sociocultural factors played in their experience. Generally, the effects of religion, culture, social structure, and traditions on health in this cultural group have not been well researched, despite the importance of Islamic beliefs in shaping ideas about health and emotional response. Islam is a central aspect of Malay identity and part of the policy making and cultural environment in Indonesia and other parts of Southeast Asia (see Masyhur, 1989; Rahardjo, 1993; Saidi, 2001).

This suggests that further research is needed into the role Islamic beliefs play in emotional response, distress reactions, coping, and resilience in Indonesia. This will further elucidate the difficulties experienced in the implementation of Western counseling approaches as part of aid efforts in Aceh and elsewhere in Indonesia and will provide insight that can be used to make such programs more effective in the future. This will further provide a means by which the psychosocial conceptions of non-Western disaster survivors can be better understood and addressed in an appropriate manner.

A reflection on the research process and methodology suggests that the in-depth interviewing used for this study was a valuable tool for eliciting survivor understanding of the meaning and nature of the Indian Ocean tsunami. The people of Aceh were very willing to talk about their experiences and share their perceptions of the event. However, it would not have been possible to collect meaningful data without fluency in Indonesian on the part of the researchers or without extensive knowledge of traditional and modern culture in Indonesia, including an understanding of Indonesian Islam. This highlights a dilemma in conducting research in non-Western cultures, where English-speaking investigators often make use of local interpreters or assistants. This approach means that any information goes through several levels of interpretation between the source and the researcher, and the kind of cultural insight that can be obtained through language use itself (word choice, nuances, and connotations of phrases) is likely to be lost. Additionally, this research strongly suggested that Western paradigms may be a poor fit in explaining the experience of non-Western societies, a well-known situation but one that has been difficult to implement in actual practice and that may limit the usefulness of findings and their future applications.

ACKNOWLEDGMENT

The fieldwork reported here was supported by a Deakin University OSP grant received in 2010 by Dr Ismet Fanany.

REFERENCES

ABC News 2006. Tsunami Survivors Ditch Aid Agency. April 14, 2006. Available at ABC News http://www.abc.net.au/news/stories/2006/04/14.

Aitken, A., 2005. Psychosocial support for tsunami survivors. Bereavement Care 24, 15.

American Refugee Committee, 2005. Post-Tsunami Rapid Psychosocial Needs Assessment Interview of 78 People in Ramong and Phang Nga Provinces. ARC, Minneapolis, MN.

Artawijaya, Bastoni, H.A., Mulyatman, E., 2006. Serambi Mekkah Dihempas Tsunamai, Diterjang Kristenisasi. Liputan Langsung Wartawan Sabili, Qalammas, Jakarta.

BPS Badan Pusat Statistik, 2009. Statistik Nanggroe Aceh Darussalam. BPS, Banda Aceh Available at, http://aceh.bps.go.id/.

Carballo, M., Heal, B., Hernandez, M., 2005. Psychosocial aspects of the tsunami. Journal of the Royal Society of Medicine 98, 396–399.

Carballo, M., Heal, B., Horbaty, G., 2006. Impact of the tsunami on psychosocial health and wellbeing. International Review of Psychiatry 18, 217–223.

ChannelNewsAsia, 2005. "Miracle" Mosques Defy Tsunami Onslaught. Available at, http://www.channelnewsasia.com/stories/afp_asiapacific/view/125438/1/.htm.

de Jong, J.T., Komproe, I.H., van Ommeren, M., 2003. Common mental disorders in postconflict settings. Lancet 36, 2128–2130.

Eisenbruch, M., 1991. Southeast asian refugees. Social Science and Medicine 33, 673–680.

Hall, J.S., Zautra, A.J., 2010. Indicators of Community resilience. What Are They, Why Bother? In: Reich, J.W., Zautra, A.J., Hall, J.S. (Eds.), Handbook of Adult Resilience, The Guilford Press, New York and London, pp. 350–376.

Howell, J.D., 2001. Sufism and the indonesian islamic revival. The Journal of Asian Studies 60, 701–729.

Huda, K., Yamamoto, N., Maki, N., Funo, S., 2007. Rehabilitation of urban settlements in the early reconstruction stage after a tsunami: a case study of banda aceh municipality in indonesia. Journal of Asian Architecture and Building Engineering 6, 103–110.

Kleinman, A., 1988. Rethinking Psychiatry: From Cultural Category to Personal Experience. Free Press, New York.

Kompas, 2009. Syariah jadi Isu Utama: Kampanye Dari Pintu ke Pintu. Kompas, Jakarta. March 17, 2009. Available at, http://bisniskeuangan.kompas.com/read/xml/2009/03/17/09452622/syariah.jadi.isu.utama.

Littlewood, R., 2000. Introduction. Cultural Psychiatry and Medical Anthropology: An Introduction and Reader. In: Littlewood, R., Dein, S. (Eds.), Athlone Press, London.

Masyhur, A. (Ed.), 1989. Teologi Pembangunan: Paradigma Baru Pemikiran Islam, LKPSM-BU-DIY, Yogyakarta.

McAmis, R.D., 2002. Malay Muslims: The History and Challenge of Resurgent Islam in Southeast Asia. Wm. B. Eerdmans Publishing, Cambridge, UK.

Mezey, G., Robbins, I., 2001. Usefulness and validity of post-traumatic stress disorder as a psychiatric category. British Medical Journal 323, 561–563.

Miftach, A., 2004. Pengajian Tauhid Wahdatul Ummah. Front Persatuan Nasional. December 31, 2004. Available at, http://persatuan.web.id/?p=127.

Miller, G., 2005. The tsunami's psychological aftermath. Science 309, 1030.

Perlez, J., 2005. Indonesia Rejects UN's Aid for Aceh. International Herald Tribune April 20, 2005.

Rahardjo, D.M., 1993. Islam dan Pembangunan: Agenda Penelitian Sosial di Indonesia. In: Muzani, S. (Ed.), Pembangunan dan Kebangkitan Islam di Asia Tenggara, PT Pustaka LP3ES, Jakarta, pp. 1–24.

Saidi, A., 2001. Hubungan Agama dan Negara: Sebuah Rekonstruksi Kebijakan. Kebijakan Kebudayaan di Masa Orde Baru, LIPI & The Ford Foundation, Jakarta.

Souza, R., Bernatsky, S., Reyes, R., de Jong, K., 2007. Mental health status of vulnerable tsunami-affected communities: a survey in aceh province, indonesia. Journal of Traumatic Stress 20, 260–269.

Summerfield, D., 1999. A critique of seven assumptions behind the trauma programs in war-afflicted areas. Social Science and Medicine 48, 1449–1462.

Telford, J., Cosgrove, J., 2007. The international humanitarian system and the 2004 indian ocean earthquake and tsunamis. Disasters 31, 1–28.

UNSCAP. United Nations Economic and Social Commission for Asia and the Pacific (2008) Enhancing Community Resilience to Natural Disasters: Lives of Children and Youth in Aceh. UNSCAP, Bangkok.

Von Peter, S., 2008. The experience of "Mental trauma" and Its transcultural application. Transcultural Psychology 45, 639–651.

Watters, C., 2001. Emerging paradigms in the mental health care of refugees. Social Science and Medicine 52, 1708–1718.

Wilson, J.P., 2007. Culture, Trauma and the Treatment of Post-Traumatic Syndromes: A Global Perspective. In: Marsella, A.J. et al., (Eds.), Ethnocultural Perspectives on Disaster and Trauma, Springer, New York, pp. 351–375.

World Health Organization, 2005. Manual for the Community Level Worker to Provide Psychosocial Care to Communities Affected by the Tsunami Disaster. WHO, New Delhihttp://www.searo.who.int/LinkFiles/List_of_Guidelines_for_Health_Emergency_community_level-workers.pdf.

World Health Organization, 2006. WHO Recommendations for Mental Health in Aceh. WHO, Genevahttp://who.or.id/eng/contents/aceh/aceh/WHO_Recommendations_Mental_Health_Aceh.pdf.

Young, A., 1995. Harmony of Illusions: Inventing Posttraumatic Stress Disorder. Princeton University Press, Princeton, NJ.

Zulkarnain, 2006. Client Values in the Counselling Process. Prosiding Persidangan Antarabangsa Pembangunan Aceh. pp. 117–123, Universiti Kebangsaan Malaysia, Bangi December 26-27, 2006.

Methodological Lessons

Chapter 21

The Positioning of Indigenous Australians as Health Care Recipients

Jill Guthrie[1] and Maggie Walter[2]
[1]National Centre for Indigenous Studies, Australia National University, Canberra, Australia,
[2]School of Sociology and Social Work, University of Tasmania, Tasmania, Australia

INTRODUCTION

One's position within Australia's socioeconomic, racial, and cultural hierarchies shapes how we "be" in our social world. Our way of "being"—our ontology—envelops our understanding of the world and of how others "be." It also shapes how we "do" our practice of being as people and as professionals. Health professionals tend to occupy the dominant position on all hierarchies, often while working directly with people who differ from them racially and culturally. From this dominant position, it can be hard to grasp that what is for them racially and culturally "normal" may not equate to what is "natural." The tendency in any society, including our own, to conflate normal with natural is what gives racial and cultural hierarchies their form and power.

The everyday operations of Australia's socioeconomic, racial, and cultural hierarchies have health consequences for Indigenous Australians. By comparing the socioeconomic and demographic positioning of Indigenous and non-Indigenous Australians, we explore how the dominant "being" and "doing" of those who operate and control the health system impact Indigenous Australians. The ramifications of the ontological chasm between the two are then demonstrated in what happens, or not, around the seemingly straightforward task of collecting Indigenous status data for health statistics.

INDIGENOUS SOCIOECONOMIC POSITIONING

While most Indigenous Australians are urban or regional dwellers, and approximately one-quarter reside in remote locations, Indigenous Australians share low socioeconomic positioning. Table 21.1 shows the geographic diversity, yet positional similarities of Perth (urban), Dubbo

When Culture Impacts Health. http://dx.doi.org/10.1016/B978-0-12-415921-1.00021-X

TABLE 21.1 Indigenous and Non-Indigenous Socioeconomic Positioning by Location

Indicator	Dubbo Indigenous	Dubbo non-Indigenous	Perth Indigenous	Perth non-Indigenous	Maningrida* Indigenous
Median age	17	37	20	36	20
Owner/purchaser	34	64	38	68	6
Renter	62	34	55		90
Household with 6+ usual occupants	11	3	12	3	92
Educated to year 12	16	34	21	49	5
Postschool qualifications	12	31	13	36	3
In education for 18–24 years	12	27	14	39	NA
Unemployment rate	22	5	16	4	16
Labor market participation rate	56	67	51	64	44
Median weekly individual income	$306	$463	$327	$515	$209

*Non-Indigenous population of Maningrida is too small for valid statistical comparison.
Source: Derived from Australian Bureau of Statistics (2006) Census data.

(regional), and Maningrida (remote). Across locations there are demographic and socioeconomic consistencies for Indigenous Australians: conversely, little similarity between Indigenous and non-Indigenous Australians in the same locations. Indigenous Australians are younger and negatively positioned on socioeconomic indicators; Indigenous home ownership in Perth and Dubbo is half that of non-Indigenous, Indigenous Australians are twice as likely to live in public housing, and overcrowding is at least four times non-Indigenous rates—in Maningrida levels are much starker. Indigenous Australians have comparatively low proportions of Indigenous Australians with postschool qualifications and of youth in full-time education. Similarly, despite record low levels of unemployment generally, Indigenous Australians across locations experience high unemployment and low labor market participation. Indigenous median income across locations is also well below that of the non-Indigenous population. Critically, while overtime data indicate small gains in some areas in relative rather than absolute terms, Indigenous Australia's level of social and economic disadvantage appears to be static at best (Walter, 2008).

As shown, albeit briefly, most Indigenous and non-Indigenous Australians reside in different realms. Most Anglo-Australian health professionals are of middle-class background, a milieu often preventing any significant interaction with Indigenous Australians, either professionally or nonprofessionally. For example, while Sydney has Australia's largest Indigenous population, this is concentrated in suburban corridors (e.g., the southwest of Sydney), with over half occupying the lowest quartile by socioeconomic advantage and over 80% occupying the city's least advantaged half, findings that are mirrored for other Australian locations (Atkinson et al., 2010). Less than 10% of non-Indigenous Australians mix regularly with Indigenous Australians, with the likelihood of interaction decreasing by higher levels of income, education, and urbanness (Walter, 2010). This "everyday life" segregation means that most non-Indigenous health professionals are unlikely to "know" Indigenous Australians, except as patients, policy problems, or data sources. The socioeconomic positioning of Indigenous Australians ensures their disproportionate presence in mortality and morbidity data. Indigenous health is core business in Australia. Health professionals are therefore likely to work with Indigenous Australians regularly and are likely to know about these dire statistics. However, "knowing about" is not the same as "knowing." The social positioning of most health professionals almost ensures an ontological gulf between how they "be" and how their Indigenous patients "be."

We contend that, first, health professionals inhabit spaces that are culturally and socially separate from Indigenous Australians and second, this divide often results in less-than-ideal outcomes for Indigenous Australians. Our central premise is not that health professionals should know more about Indigenous Australians (although this also would be positive), but that a prerequisite for health professionals working with Indigenous Australians is that they understand *their own* social and cultural positioning and, more critically, assumptions and value systems emerging from these. Such assumptions and value systems are integral to professionals' health practices, and inform (possibly subconsciously) their interactions with, judgments about, and treatment of Indigenous Australians.

ASKING THE INDIGENOUS STATUS QUESTION

Our arguments derive from a broader doctoral research that explored the experiences of families of Indigenous children hospitalized in the Australian Capital Territory (ACT). The ACT, covering approximately 2,400 km^2, is located about 300 km southwest of Sydney and 655 km northeast of Melbourne. Among research methods used were analysis of hospital separation data, interviews with 13 Indigenous and non-Indigenous health professionals, 15 Indigenous and non-Indigenous parents having contact with the ACT public hospital system, and analysis of clinical records for their 21 Indigenous children for the years from 2000 to 2005 (comprising 107 emergency department and 47 inpatient occasions, representing 154 opportunities for ascertaining Indigenous status). Analysis of hospital separation data showed that 335 of 2,212 (15%) occasions of care were inaccurate in terms of Indigenous identification (Guthrie, 2012). A reference group comprising Indigenous and non-Indigenous Australians reviewed and interpreted initial findings. Excerpts from selected parents' and health professionals' interviews follow. In the doctoral study, the two notions of the "3-Is" and "manifestly Indigenous" as an interpretive device were coined and explored: these are also described below (Guthrie, 2009).

The 3-Is: Identification, Identifiability, and Identity

The 3-Is—identification, identifiability, and identity—together with the notion of *manifestly Indigenous* are separate yet inextricably linked concepts, each difficult to explain independently of the others. The juxtaposition of the 3-Is is borne out in studies documenting the unreliability of Indigenous status data in health settings including hospitals (Barton, 1998; Jackson-Pulver et al., 2003; Adams, et al., 2004; Australian Institute for Health and Welfare, 2005; Lovett, 2005) highlighting slow progress in this public policy area including in the ACT (Australian Bureau of Statistics and Australian Institute of Health and Welfare, 2005).

Identification

"Identification" refers to (the administrative task of) being asked the Indigenous identifier question. It is understood and accepted that in order to relate to and interpret others, we use cues to inform ourselves about others' characteristics. Any relevance of these observations is often overlooked because once any differences or similarities are registered, they are typically taken for granted as simply being the way things are (Link and Phelan, 2001). This "taken for grantedness" can extend to how health professionals inform themselves about Indigenous Australians. This notion can be seen as the relationship Heidegger described as that of the individual to their "lifeworld," expressing the idea that individuals' realities are influenced by the world in which they live (Lopez and Willis, 2004). A health professional might perceive someone as *manifestly Indigenous* because that person accords with certain characteristics in terms of their (the health professional's) preconceived ideas about appearance and/or behaviors of Indigenous Australians (This concept is discussed in the next section). This is not to suggest that mentally aligning appearance and behaviors with preconceptions is inherently wrong or racist: stereotyping plays an important role in social interactions by allowing us to categorize and simplify the vast amounts of information our brain receives (Westen et al., 2006). Rather, stereotyping is a means by which, in Heideggerian terms, we "make sense of the world in which we live" (Lopez and Willis, 2004), a sophisticated and often helpful way of engaging appropriately with others. Indigenous and non-Indigenous people do this. Prejudice, on the other hand, involves prejudging another person according to group membership and stereotypes associated with that group; it is not just an opinion or belief, but an attitude associated with a wide range of often negative emotions (Westen et al., 2006). The activity of stereotyping becomes problematic when, as part of health service provision, health professionals apply their own *manifestly Indigenous* criteria about whether a person is Indigenous, and document it (or not) accordingly.

Knowing a person's Indigenous status can have various implications for their health care. In the doctoral study, qualitative analysis revealed that some children were *never* identified as Indigenous in hospital records and hence never counted in Indigenous data collections. Being asked the Indigenous identifier question was important to parents Rosie and Mick:

Rosie:

. . . it must be ascertained so all the necessary social supports are established. They should [always ask the Identifier question], because it gives them an idea of the family dynamics. . . . things like, Do they have support?

Mick:

. . . but his cultural identity wasn't asked. . . . medically, there are things within our community and Indigenous kids that they could have looked for, but because the question wasn't asked . . . Especially through Emergency—most of our community go through there.

Mick's narrative shows his unwillingness to challenge the fact that his son's Indigenous status was not sought. An interpretation of this may be that Mick was "opting out" of revealing his son's status while his son's medical fate was uncertain: that only when his son's condition improved was Mick prepared to challenge the system by stating that the Indigenous status information had not been correctly collected, by which time he may have been confident of no repercussions arising for him or his child, either from his challenging (i.e., power relationships between Mick as health consumer and the health system), or because they were, in fact, Indigenous (i.e., racism on the part of the health professional).

Identifiability

"Identifiability" refers to how *manifestly Indigenous* a health care recipient is according to a health professional's subjective assessment of how that person accords with certain characteristics in terms of preconceived ideas about appearance and/or behaviors of Indigenous Australians. For Rachel, the effect of health professionals invoking their own identifiability assessments is illustrated. Rachel's interpretation of the fact that her son's Indigenous status was not recorded highlights an inconsistent systemic approach to ascertainment of Indigenous status:

Rachel:

It is interesting that this time I wasn't asked what [son's] status was but that it was still recorded as "NOT Aboriginal and/or Torres Strait Islander." I'm curious as to whether the person who spoke to me when he was in emergency made an assumption based on the colour of my skin [and] that my child couldn't have possibly been Indigenous as she actually didn't see [my son].

In terms of stereotypical attributes, Kelly's identifiability was not clear to health professionals. She was challenged about her Indigenous identification, seemingly because she was not *manifestly Indigenous* to them:

Kelly:

I'm sick of getting that thing "You don't look Aboriginal." I get that sometimes.

It is also important to consider the situation of a health professional deliberately choosing *not* to inform themselves of a patient's Indigenous status. An interpretation of this situation is that health professionals may intrinsically feel that they are not skilled enough to properly engage with and care for an Indigenous patient or family and would rather not confirm that gap in their knowledge and skills, a point suggested by a reference group member when discussing the poor recording of Indigenous status on hospital records:

Reference group member:

. . . it is not an undercount if the patient does not identify as Indigenous when properly asked.

The important words in this assertion are, "when properly asked." We acknowledge that "properly asking" *everyone* who engages with the hospital system about their Indigenous status has resource implications. It is no small undertaking. Nonetheless, understanding by health professionals of the need to consistently ask the Indigenous status question, and of the implications of that information collection, is essential.

Identity

Identity refers to a person's sense of him- or herself in terms of their Indigenous status. Indigenous identity is a fraught concept that must be considered from the perspective of non-Indigenous Australians' uncomfortable historical relationships with Indigenous Australians. This is at the heart of why identifiability and identification are challenging.

Depending on the manner in which the Indigenous identifier information is sought, an Indigenous Australian can experience either feeling "questioned" (a stressful, negative emotion) or "heard" (an affirming, positive emotion). Obviously, the latter is optimal. For many parents therefore, the fact that the Indigenous identifier question is *not* asked, means they do not feel heard. Unless and until there is dialog, at many levels, about these complex issues, Indigenous identity for data collection purposes will remain subject to institutional racism and a fraught area of public policy and practice.

Manifestly Indigenous

Manifestly Indigenous is a term that was coined and utilized as an interpretive device in the doctoral study. As a phenomenon it appears to operate in the space between a health professional ascertaining a health care recipient's Indigenous status, and their *"knowing"* (somehow) that a recipient is Indigenous. It accounts for how health professionals might make subjective assumptions about a health care recipient's characteristics and behaviors in terms of whether, subjectively, the recipient meets the health professional's criteria for "being Indigenous." Health professionals seem to find it difficult to ask a person's Indigenous status often *not* because it will offend people who are (manifestly) Indigenous, but rather because it will offend "manifestly *non*-Indigenous" recipients (who may or may not in fact be Indigenous). To this end, some Indigenous Australians are expected to engage in conversations regarding their health care that are begun with the health professional exclaiming, *"You don't look Aboriginal!,"* such as described earlier by Kelly.

Often people, including health professionals, will not ask a question they do not know the answer to. This could explain why health professionals are prepared to ask about personal hygiene habits, biological details, sexual practices, drug taking, substance abuse, and other sensitive activities, yet many seem uncomfortable about asking Indigenous status. Notwithstanding that everyone *should* be asked their Indigenous status, directly asking the Indigenous status question is often avoided. As expressed in their interviews, many parents regard it as important that Indigenous status is properly ascertained and acknowledged. For them, it not only increases the possibility that appropriate services are received, but it can indicate an understanding by health professionals of underlying health and social conditions for Indigenous Australians.

Of the 154 opportunities for ascertaining Indigenous status in the hospital records examined, only 4 resulted in *complete* ascertainment for that child's whole hospitalization history. This raises curiosity on two levels: could incorrect or intermittent ascertainment be a product of either ambivalence about or active resistance on the part of individual health professionals to asking the Indigenous status question, arising from a patient's *manifestly Indigenous* appearance? Or could it possibly represent reluctance by Indigenous patients to identify on any given occasion? Some non-Indigenous health professionals interviewed stated that the rationale for collecting Indigenous status data is that it is purely "for statistical purposes only." Interestingly, all *Indigenous* health professionals interviewed believed there is a need for knowing a person's Indigenous status.

Supposing that ascertainment of Indigenous status is consistently and systematically sought in the hospital setting, there is, nonetheless, a qualitative difference between two rationales for ascertainment; one is for statistical purposes and the second is gathering this information in order to care for a person in a culturally appropriate way. It is apparent that some health professionals (as illustrated below) subjectively assess a person's identifiability, with many indicating how they "make sense" of their observations, not necessarily for the purposes of administrative recording of Indigenous status, but certainly in Heideggerian lifeworld terms.

(Health professional) Fran:

… sometimes it's extra obvious [that a person is Indigenous].

(Health professional) Helen:

… [if a person] looks like a migrant, or they look Aboriginal, that's how they get treated.

(Health professional) Linda:

I have to say I haven't seen an awful lot of Aboriginal people over here.

(Health professional) Penny:

… if I have a patient who either looks Aboriginal, like their typical characteristics are Aboriginal, or their demeanour appears to have some Aboriginality … [then] ….

and finally (Health professional) Ken:

… apart from those who look to be Aboriginal, and I'll then enquire, Are you?

Another example was illustrated by (health professional) Ken remarking on how often he hears the claim,

Ken:

… But there's no Aboriginal people in the ACT!

(Health professional) Sally's strategy for dealing with a situation where she somehow *knows* that a health care recipient is Indigenous—arguably applying by her manifestly Indigenous criteria—even when that person has not identified Indigenous, was to indicate to them that the information gained through asking the Indigenous identifier question is "for statistical purposes only," suggesting that simply having these data in a database is benign and more palatable than having the information for any other reason.

Replicating the approaches of these health professionals who demonstrated that they apply their own *manifestly Indigenous* criteria, and combining these with subjective observations, in the doctoral study, 15 of the interviewed parents were described as *manifestly Indigenous*. Observations of the *manifestly Indigenous* status of parents were then juxtaposed against the accuracy of the record of their child's Indigenous status to investigate to what extent the individual parent's *manifestly Indigenous* characteristics predicted the accuracy of hospital records in terms of a child's Indigenous status. Based on this analysis, the contention was that generally for *manifestly Indigenous* parents, their child's Indigenous status is accurately ascertained and recorded. Further, where parents had the combined attributes of being manifestly Indigenous and were agreeable and did not challenge the authority of the system, health professionals were usually comfortable with them, and indeed, keen to be seen to be interacting with them (a *manifestly Indigenous* family) appropriately and respectfully. Conversely, where parents had the combined attributes of being *manifestly Indigenous* but were not generally agreeable and perhaps challenged the authority of the system, this often became a trigger for invoking the services of the Hospital Aboriginal Liaison Officer (HALO). The HALO reflected on such a situation:

HALO:

Often I don't think [staff] would know [that many of the patients are in fact Indigenous]. It depends on who you're talking about. I think a lot of the times, unless there's a problem, if a patient isn't causing any problems, then they don't [get in touch with the HALO]. If they're [Indigenous patients] causing problems, then they would get onto us, otherwise it wasn't an issue for them, we wouldn't hear from them.

In addition, it appeared that for "non-manifestly Indigenous" parents, the Indigenous status of their children was generally not consistently and accurately ascertained and recorded. Where a parent was articulate or challenged the authority of health professionals their hospital experience was generally less pleasant if they did not conform to expected norms of being "Indigenous." For parents Kirsty and Dan, both *manifestly Indigenous*, a note on their file regarding their "dysfunctional" home situation may have been an additional subtle indicator to other health professionals that this was indeed an Indigenous family. Parent Rosie, not *manifestly Indigenous*, represented the counter-example: the Indigenous status of both her children was mostly correctly documented. However, during interviews Rosie was comfortable with her Indigenous identity and spoke openly about it. There was no ambiguity on her part about her Indigenous identity. It may be that during interactions with health professionals she asserted her Indigenous identity. She therefore allowed the system, as represented by the health professionals working in it, to "get it right."

CONCLUSION

We have argued that there is a qualitative difference between the two rationales for ascertainment of Indigenous status, namely that one is for "statistical purposes" and the other is for staff to be aware of a person's Indigenous status in order to provide culturally appropriate health care. The concept of *manifestly Indigenous* appears to operate in the space between these two activities. The identification of children of *manifestly Indigenous* parents is generally accurately ascertained and recorded, especially where parents do not challenge the authority of the system and health professionals are comfortable with them. However, health professionals are less likely to accurately ascertain and record the status of Indigenous children of a non-manifestly Indigenous parent, and are less comfortable dealing with *manifestly Indigenous* Australian parents if that parent is perceived as difficult.

It is important that health professionals engaging with and caring for Indigenous Australians are aware of the sociopolitical context within which Indigenous Australians are operating and to be aware that interactions may be imbued with that sociopolitical context. In the absence of properly articulated policies and well-understood protocols for ascertaining Indigenous status information from *everyone*, engaging with the health and hospital system, the challenge of improving the currently poor reliability of Indigenous status data will continue.

The constant turnover of patients and staff in hospitals underlines the fact that new relationships between the patient and health professional need to be established on almost every occasion. There is a need, therefore, for consistent ascertainment of Indigenous status and for health professionals to always inform themselves of a person's Indigenous status.

REFERENCES

Adams, K., Kavanagh, A., Guthrie, J.A., 2004. Are you aboriginal and/or torres strait Islander? improving data collection at breastscreen victoria. Australian and New Zealand Journal of Public Health 28, 124–127.

Atkinson, R., Taylor, E., Walter, M., 2010. Burying indigeneity: the spacial construction of reality and aboriginal Australia. Social and Legal Studies 19, 311–330.

Australian Bureau of Statistics, 2006. Census data by location, Canberra.

Australian Bureau of Statistics, 2005. Australian Institute of Health and Welfare, The health and welfare of Aboriginal and Torres Strait Islander people. ABS, Canberra 2005.

Australian Institute for Health and Welfare, 2005. Improving the data quality of Indigenous identification in hospital separations. AIHW, AIHW, Canberra.

Barton, M., 1998. Quality of data on aboriginal hospitalisation. Aboriginal and Islander Health Worker Journal 22, 10–11.

Guthrie, J.A., 2009. An exploration of the experiences of families of Indigenous children hospitalised in the Australian Capital Territory. School of Public Health and Community Medicine. University of New South Wales, Sydney.

Guthrie, J.A., 2012. Estimating the magnitude of potentially avoidable hospitalisations of Indigenous children in the Australian capital territory: some methodological challenges. Australian Aboriginal Studies Journal 92–97.

Jackson-Pulver, L.R., Bush, A., Ward, J., 2003. Identification of Aboriginal and Torres Strait Islander women using an urban obstetric hospital. Australian Health Review 26, 19–25.

Link, B.G., Phelan, J.C., 2001. Conceptualizing stigma. Annual Review of Sociology 27, 363–385.

Lopez, K.A., Willis, D.G., 2004. Descriptive versus interpretive phenomenology: their contributions to nursing knowledge. Qualitative Health Research 14, 726–735.

Lovett, R., 2005. ACT public hospital staff attitudes concerning Indigenous origin information and estimating Indigenous under identification in ACT public hospital admission data: Masters of Applied Epidemiology thesis. National Centre for Epidemiology and Population Health. Australian National University, Canberra.

Walter, M., 2008. Lives of diversity: Indigenous Australians. Occasional paper 4/2008 Census Series # 2. Australian Academy of the Social Sciences, Canberra.

Walter, M., 2010. The politics of the data: how the statistical Indigene is constructed. International Journal of Critical Indigenous Studies 3, 45–56.

Westen, D., Burton, L., Kowalski, R., 2006. Psychology: Australian and New Zealand edition. John Wiley & Sons, Milton, Queensland.

Chapter 22

Capturing the Capitals: A Heuristic for Measuring the "Wealth" of New Zealand Children in the Twenty-First Century: An Application to the Growing Up in New Zealand Longitudinal Cohort

Vivienne Ivory,[1] Susan Morton,[2] Johanna Schmidt,[2] Te Kani Kingi,[3] and Polly Atatoa-Carr[2]

[1]*University of Otago, Wellington, New Zealand,* [2]*University of Auckland, New Zealand,* [3]*Massey University, Wellington, New Zealand*

INTRODUCTION

A "WEALTHY" ENVIRONMENT?

Optimal child development and well-being are dependent on many factors both within the child and in their multiple environments (Maggi et al., 2010). One useful way of conceiving how environments might contribute to child outcomes is to consider the "wealth" that is potentially available to children in their everyday lives. As a theoretical construct, wealth is commonly recognized to include multiple forms of resources that are potentially available from a variety of settings or locations (Williams Shanks, 2007). Yet empirical measures of wealth are often restricted to household-based financial resources. Incorporating broader measures of wealth into studies of child development and well-being requires collecting rich data that account for the complexity of children's lived environments with a strategy that is systematic and manageable. Doing so is particularly valuable when projects attempt to bring together disciplines and cultural perspectives while managing priorities for data collection. This chapter presents a strategy developed for the measurement of wealth as part of the Growing Up in New Zealand study.

Growing Up in New Zealand is a cohort study of New Zealand children from prior to their birth until they are 21 years old. It incorporates both life course and socioecological frameworks and aims to capture the dynamic inter-actions between children and their multiple environments accumulated over time (Morton et al., 2012b). At birth, the cohort comprised 6,846 children and is broadly generalizable to current births in New Zealand on the basis of ethnicity and markers of socioeconomic status. The children's mothers and their partners have taken part in three face-to-face interviews, and additional infor-mation is obtained through short telephone interviews with the mothers and through linkage to routinely collected health data. The project is multidisci-plinary, and information is collected relating to six key overlapping research domains relevant to child development: family and whānau, societal context and neighborhoods, education, health and well-being, psychological and cognitive development, and culture and identity. Woven through the domains are themes relating to Māori, Pacific, European, and Asian ethnic identity. For an overview of the study design, see Morton et al. (2012b). Results from the antenatal and nine month data collection waves are available in Morton et al. (2010, 2012a), respectively.

Growing Up in New Zealand requires the coordinated collection of data across the overlapping domains to best reflect the conceptual framework of the study and the particular cultural and historical context of New Zealand. As illustrated in Figure 22.1, the study's overarching framework proposes that children's development, health, and well-being over time are situated at the intersections of a broad range of influences that are at varying proximity to the child (Morton et al., 2012b). Studies with such a broad scope face consid-erable challenges designing data collections that are both comprehensive and feasible. Capturing access to and utilization of a range of resources (economic and otherwise) is recognized as critical to understanding child outcomes and is therefore an overarching concern of the entire study crossing all domains. We wanted to know what a wealthy environment might mean across cultures and settings, and how various cultural and social forms of resources may (or may not) supplement economic resources, notably by going beyond primarily house-hold economic factors.

Robustly measuring wealth in such a complex and comprehensive way requires extensive data that can be onerous to collect; establishing household levels of material wealth alone typically requires that surveys include detailed information on household composition, income levels and source, assets and debts, and so on. Therefore we wanted to formulate a strategy that focused our attention on developing measures that were *sufficient* for examining pathways to positive child outcomes within the data collection capacity of the wider study. In many instances, this meant utilizing measures that were relevant across plural domains within Growing Up in New Zealand so as to optimize the utility of the data collected within the study. A heuristic approach has been recommended in cases such as ours where researchers are faced with the problem of "how [to] link both conceptually and methodologically, such a huge and varied inventory of information" (Frohlich et al., 2007, p. 300).

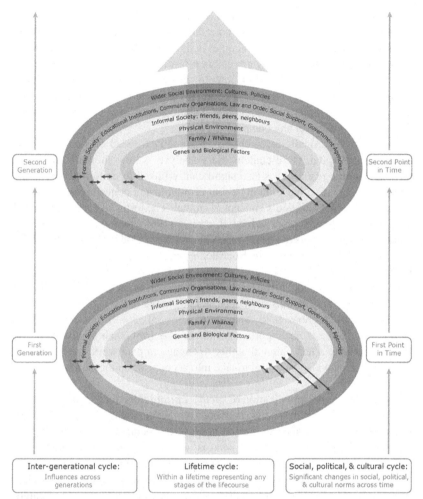

FIGURE 22.1   Conceptual framework for understanding child development in Growing Up in New Zealand.

Such an approach also allows researchers to identify the gaps for new data collection.

Forms of Wealth

Wealth has conventionally been measured in terms of the economic and/or material resources accumulated at the individual or household level (Williams Shanks, 2007). For example, research investigating the socioeconomic determinants of child outcomes frequently uses variables such as household income (Williams Shanks, 2007; McCurdy et al., 2010), home ownership (Barker and

Miller, 2009), and car ownership (Von Rueden et al., 2006) as indicators of the underlying construct of family or household wealth. Accumulated economic wealth (over and above current income) is thought to be particularly beneficial to health through the buffering effects such resources can provide during times when immediate income is inadequate to meet needs (Pollack et al., 2007). Williams Shanks (2007) found that child development is more strongly associated with overall household economic resources (or "long economic status") than income poverty at any one point.

Although historically research has specifically focused on financial forms of economic capital, more contemporary analysis is now showing that access to noneconomic resources is also significantly linked to child outcomes. As a means of integrating our thinking about economic and noneconomic resources we call on Pierre Bourdieu's concept of capital. The forms of economic, social, and cultural capitals proposed by Bourdieu (1986) have been identified as potentially relevant to a variety of child outcomes (Jaeger and Holm, 2007; Christensen, 2011). Briefly, in Bourdieu's terms, *economic capital* concerns both material "assets," and the means to acquire them (Bourdieu, 1986). Measures of economic capital have included assets such as owning a home (Barker and Miller, 2009), pensions and debts, and economic buffers such as insurance, car ownership, and household capacity (Currie et al., 2008). Because engaging in the labor force is an important means of acquiring such assets, observing factors that may affect parental ability to engage in paid work (such as access to child care) can also be useful to take into account when measuring economic capital.

Bourdieu's conceptualization of *social capital* refers to the social resources or "credits" linked to social networks or membership of social groups (Bourdieu, 1986). It takes account of not just the social networks that children and their families are part of but what is accessed through them; in Jaegar's terms "gainful social networks" (Jaeger and Holm, 2007). For example, participation in social networks can provide access to social support, as well as useful information (Carpiano, 2006). While this can seem relatively straightforward, care must be taken to avoid approaching the measurement of social capital from an ethnocentric or class-specific perspective (Shortt, 2004). For example, it has been argued that the reduction in membership of formal associations, clubs, and organizations is evidence of a "decline in the engagement of citizens within their communities" (van Deth, 2003), and hence a decrease in the possession of social capital within those communities. However, this focus on more "conventional" indicators of social capital may fail to recognize specific cultural contexts (De Silva et al., 2007). We wanted to take into account the ways in which social capital may be understood differently within Māori culture. For example, European understandings are that social capital operates outside the family context, while for Māori social capital rests on extended family relations. Māori understandings of social and cultural capital are also so closely linked that the two concepts are virtually inseparable (Statistics

New Zealand, 2001). A further reason for thinking carefully about the measurement of social capital is the presence of relatively recent migrant groups in New Zealand. Macpherson and Macpherson's (1999) studies of migrant Samoans in the 1960s and 70s found that they were frequently both geographically and occupationally concentrated, resulting in the formation of Samoan enclaves within large cities such as Auckland. These social groups have continued to provide security and potential stores of capital for new migrants who are unfamiliar with the ways of hegemonic New Zealand culture (Macpherson and Macpherson, 1999).

As conceptualized by Bourdieu, *cultural capital* is demonstrated through competence in and knowledge of "legitimized/dominant" activities (Bourdieu, 1986). Educational qualifications and occupational status are widely used as indicators of competency in societal-level institutions (Christensen, 2011). Engagement in certain activities has been used to measure cultural capital, including visiting museums and reading (Jaeger and Holm, 2007), or participating in so-called "high culture" practices deemed "worthy" by the dominant culture such as attending the theater or opera (Christensen, 2011). Our interest specifically focuses on practices, preferences, and competencies that may contribute specifically to child well-being, for example, the ability to engage effectively with organizations such as the health sector and social welfare systems. A challenge for measuring cultural capital in an increasingly diverse society such as New Zealand is defining what counts as the dominant culture, as well as what would demonstrate "competence" in it. Given that over 40% of the cohort in Growing Up in New Zealand are expected to identify with more than one ethnicity (Morton et al., 2010), there may well be multiple legitimate cultures operating successfully to provide wealthy environments for children. Measuring cultural capital over time will allow observation of how access to different cultures impacts on children.

Jaeger and Holm (2007) demonstrated that a family's social and cultural capital can significantly affect how educational opportunities are utilized for the children of the family. With respect to health outcomes, Christensen found that parental cultural capital is associated with healthier weights in their children, arguing that "parental perceptions and practice are embodied in the habitus of the children, which disposes them to continue certain forms of practice on healthy living, dietary intake, physical activity and body formation" (Christensen, 2011, p. 474). Borgonovi's (2010) longitudinal work illustrated that, even when controlling for childhood circumstances such as physical and mental health status, socioeconomic disadvantage, and parental engagement, social capital remains significantly associated with health outcomes.

As well as identifying individual forms of capital, authors such as Lee (2009) and Jaeger and Holm (2007) demonstrated the value of Bourdieu's multiple capitals by positioning economic forms alongside other types of resources. Their examinations of the interaction between various capitals demonstrated how a combination of stressors, support, and beliefs combine to result in specific child outcomes. Adopting such a multifactorial approach can allow research to tease out the ways in which, for example, socioeconomic status (economic capital) and competence in cultural activities (cultural capital) interact with and reinforce each other.

Locations of Wealth

Socioecological approaches such as that employed by Growing Up in New Zealand (see Figure 22.1) highlight the importance of accounting for multiple environments and the interactions between them when thinking about health and well-being (Dahlgren and Whitehead, 1991; Morton et al., 2012b). One useful way of thinking about how different environments contribute to child outcomes over time is to conceptualize these environments as locations of wealth resources. Put simply, how wealthy are the various environments that are part of a child's life in their early years? Starting closest to the child, crucial resources can be "located" within parents or primary caregivers. As noted above, parental employment status and education levels are consistently used as indicators of the wealth available to children. Wealth located at the slightly wider scale of the child's residential household can include household income and home ownership (Williams Shanks, 2007), material goods (e.g., washing machines; Christensen, 2011), social resources (e.g., useful social connections; Christensen, 2011), and cultural goods and practices (e.g., reading to children; Dunt et al., 2011), all of which may contribute to the child's wealth environment.

Beyond the household, access to similar resources can also come from family not living in the child's home, notably nonresident parents and extended family. For example, instrumental and social support from extended family may counteract household-level hardship by providing goods, child care, and supportive advice (Woody and Woody, 2007), as well as links to useful social networks (Webber and Huxley, 2007).

Wealth may also be available to the child through more distal locations. A wealthy neighborhood environment can provide "opportunity structures" (Baum and Palmer, 2002) for residents who support well-being, for example, by providing sites for social connection and physical activity. Witten et al (2003) identified factors such as local parks, pedestrian infrastructure, amenities, and social spaces as contributing to a supportive neighborhood environment for parenting. Neighborhoods can also provide access to quality schools that can increase the chances of positive educational outcomes for the child (Croft, 2004).

Other environments that may or may not be in the immediate neighborhood can contain possible sources of capital for children. Child care and educational institutions have the potential to influence child outcomes based on the multiple resources they provide to children. Engagement with community-based organizations such as churches, charities, interest groups, and peer groups (such as parent support groups and friends) can be potential sources of capital for children and their families (Leventhal and Brooks-Gunn, 2001). Institutions such as social services can also provide income assistance and housing support if families are able to access them (Maggi et al., 2010).

Pinkster and Fortuijn (2009) emphasized the need to investigate the contribution of one environment (such as the neighborhood) alongside others (such as the household). They found that parents manage the risks associated with living in a disadvantaged area, for example, by driving to "safer" or "better" schools elsewhere, and restricting where children can play. Alternatively, Jack (2006) highlighted the potential role for wealthy neighborhood settings to counteract household disadvantage by providing a supplementary source of resources, such as quality play spaces. But proximity does not necessarily equate to availability; household factors may make the utilization of neighborhood resources difficult if accessing them is restricted by factors such as cost, transport, or cultural barriers (Jack, 2006). In recognition of the potential influence such settings may have on child outcomes, longitudinal studies are now incorporating neighborhood environments into data collection through measures of parental perception of their local environment (e.g., Edwards, 2006; Carter et al., 2009) and linked objective measures (e.g., Cohen et al., 2008).

A Heuristic for Measuring Wealth

Faced with the quantity and diversity of potential wealth indicators suggested above, we clearly needed a strategy to prioritize the ongoing data collection related to wealth. We employed a heuristic approach that helped us systematically consider forms of wealth potentially relevant to children's everyday lives. To do this, we developed a matrix that incorporates the socioecological basis of the study as a whole and the multiple forms of wealth we seek to measure in the societal context domain. Taking a functional approach we ask at each intersection in the matrix if we can identify whether children "possess" capital by having access to resources that may contribute to their development and well-being, and whether that access can be quantified in terms of poverty or affluence. We could then prioritize the measurement of components of wealth based on the relative importance of a given location or capital for child outcomes at each developmental stage, and practical factors such as the availability of measurement tools and the consideration of the needs of multiple domains within any one data collection wave. As noted previously, making the most of the resources at our disposal and minimizing respondent burden are optimized by the utilization of measures that are relevant across domains wherever possible. For example, effective home heating is of concern to the health and well-being domain because of links between inadequate heating and child health (Free et al., 2010), but adequate means of heating (or the resources to provide this) can also be considered to be part of the wealth available to the child within his or her home.

Based on the conceptual model underlying the study (see Figure 22.1) we identified key locations distinguished by social and physical boundaries, ranging from parents and immediate households (including extended family and nonrelatives living in the child's house), to family outside the child's house (e.g., nonresident parents, extended family) and informal groups (e.g., community groups, neighborhoods, commercial work and interest groups, peer groups), through to the more distal formal institutions (e.g., schools, churches, local and central government). We operationalize the economic, social, and cultural capitals as specific resources that contribute to child development and well-being.

Translating into Study Design

Table 22.1 illustrates the matrix of "capitals" and "locations" that has been used to formulate the "ideal" measurement of wealth, with the three forms of capitals in rows, and columns representing the locations, from the most proximal on the

TABLE 22.1 Wealth Matrix of Forms of Capital and Locations

	Locations				
Capitals	Parent	Family (within household setting)	Wider family (supra- household)	Informal social institutions	Formal institutions
Economic: assets and the means to acquire them	Household assets: • The means to acquire them • As a measure of wealth • As a means of accessing nonhousehold wealth			• Presence/absence of nonhousehold assets • Characteristics of non-household assets • Contribution to child's environment	
Social: networks and the goods that come via them	Identify the social settings to which parents and child are connected Identify how those connections bring resources to the child's environment		Significant nonhousehold social ties and settings Settings characteristics Resources/goods that come from them	Parent and child con-nections to institu-tions and resources that are therefore accessed	
Cultural: compe-tence in given activities	Parent "compe-tency" and status indicators Norms and values	Family participation in cultural practices and social institutions		"Availability" of cultural and social institutions to child	

left, to relatively distal institutions on the right. At each intersection of a capital and location we ask the following:

- What resources are important for child development and well-being in this location?
- How do we measure them, taking into account presence, quantity, quality, and degree of child access and utilization of resources?
- When is the optimal time to measure and/or are multiple measurements required across time?

Populating the matrix can begin at any point. It can start with the constructs under investigation, or from the tools that are potentially available. Gaps will quickly become apparent because the construct is less relevant to a capital or location, because there are no tools currently available, or because there is limited capacity to measure everything. Table 22.2 provides examples of how the matrix has been populated with the constructs and measurement tools that have been used in the initial data collection waves within Growing Up in New Zealand, and which might be employed in order to measure the wealth available to cohort children.

Economic capital located within the child's household includes assets and parental characteristics associated with their acquisition. Assets include housing tenure and characteristics of the house that capture the material quality relevant to child well-being, such as heating sources and safety features. We include indicators of the ability to acquire assets such as the nature of parental employment, as well as access to and utilization of child care given its importance for engaging in employment. The role of the family outside of the child's household is recognized by using measures of instrumental assistance such as child care, as well as material flows between households.

Moving beyond the child's household and family takes our attention to resources located in settings such as neighborhoods and institutions. Using measurement tools that can be linked via address data, a child's neighborhood can be characterized as more or less wealthy in terms of available area-level resources (e.g., health-promoting resources such as "'green space," health services, food environments, and sociocultural amenities such as libraries, early childhood centers, or schools; Pearce et al., 2006). Small area-level indicators of deprivation (Salmond et al., 2007) and/or material wealth could also act as proxies for household-level wealth, for example, aggregate measures of house value. Child and family interactions with neighborhood resource environment can also be identified (Panter et al., 2009; Dahl et al., 2010). As well as measuring parental perception of neighborhood safety and quality, the utilization of resources within the neighborhood can be assessed as an indicator of how dependent children might be on local resources (e.g., using the child's primary health care address data to determine location).

Some resources are potentially available through settings that are not necessarily neighborhood based. Early childhood education can provide alternative

TABLE 22.2 Populating the Matrix: Constructs and Tools from the Initial Data Collection Waves of Growing Up in New Zealand That Can Be Utilized to Measure Forms of Capital and Locations of Wealth

		Locations		
Capitals	Parent	Family (within household setting)	Wider family (supra-household)	Informal social institutions and settings (including neighborhood)	Formal institutions
Economic	Employment status Hours worked and schedule Job security Child-care use (to enable workforce participation)	Income Food and housing security: living standards Material assets: housing tenure, housing quality, value, and location Physical environment: crowding household amenities and resources (e.g., transport) Child-care arrangements Modes of accessing non household resources, e.g., Internet access	Material assistance; income contribution to and from other households Assistance with child care (to support parental employment)	Quality of the neighbor-hood physical & material environment—resources, deprivation Linked measures of neighborhood resources, deprivation, and environ-mental Child's access, and utilization of local and nonlocal physical and material resources Perceived quality of resources Sources of support (material, instrumental)	Social assistance packages; income and housing assistance, contact with organizations, utilization of child care

TABLE 22.2 Populating the Matrix: Constructs and Tools from the Initial Data Collection Waves of Growing Up in New Zealand That Can Be Utilized to Measure Forms of Capital and Locations of Wealth—*Cont'd*

Capitals	Parent	Family (within household setting)	Wider family (supra-household)	Informal social institutions and settings (including neighborhood)	Formal institutions
			Locations		
Social	Membership of "groups"—formal, informal: relationship status, workforce participation in communities, cultural groups, family groups Resources that come via membership—social and instrumental support, child-related information	Membership of organizations and social settings: workforce participation, family participation in communities, cultural groups, extended family groups	Extended family social ties with child and family Source of information on child rearing, expert advice Source of support (material, emotional, instrumental)	Neighborhood and other community participation Source of information on child rearing, expert advice; source of support (material, emotional, instrumental), whether local or nonlocal Quality of neighborhood social environment (social cohesion); perceived and objective measures	Membership of and engagement with organizations: Are they a source of information and/or support? Source of "expert" information on child-rearing and health-related practices

Continued

TABLE 22.2 Populating the Matrix: Constructs and Tools from the Initial Data Collection Waves of Growing Up in New Zealand That Can Be Utilized to Measure Forms of Capital and Locations of Wealth—*Cont'd*

Capitals	Parent	Family (within household setting)	Wider family (supra-household)	Informal social institutions and settings (including neighborhood)	Formal institutions
Cultural	Parent social status indicators: education qualifications and occupational status Language skills Knowledge of and engagement in culture (mainstream and traditional)	Norms and values around childrearing and well-being Participation in forms of recreational and cultural activities and events, holidays, events, cultural practices related to birth/early childhood Reading, singing, story-telling to child Health practices: physical activity, immunization, pregnancy-related nutrition changes, child's diet	Norms and values around child-rearing and well-being Educational histories Cultural histories; ties to place, language skills, traditions carried across generations	"Match" with key social settings: sense of belonging to community, language skills, acculturation Barriers to engagement with social institutions (e.g., community-based groups, parenting, and interest groups)	Barriers to engagement with organizations (e.g., preschool, health care, churches, state and local government facilities), such as cost, transport, closed membership, language skills Culturally appropriate engagement with child-care and health services: knowledge of where to access health services, access to preferred maternity care, participation in preschool

Locations

environments to supplement economic capital in the home (e.g., providing quality play equipment and learning experiences), and charities or community groups can provide subsidized access to resources such as car seats and toys. At a much wider societal scale, state sector institutions can contribute to child outcomes by providing income and housing assistance (among others), reflecting policy environments.

Social capital located within the child's household requires measurement of both parent-specific and general household engagement with groups and networks, and the resources available through that engagement. Indicators of group membership include parents' relationships with partners and peers, and their participation in workplace and community groups. Resources arising from parental participation in social networks can include social support, information on child-rearing practices and health, and information on how to access other resources, such as "good" preschools, places to shop, or safe playgrounds.

Extended family living outside of the child's household may contribute social capital–based resources. For example, grandparents may provide support to the child's household, including assistance such as household goods, helping out, social support, and information. Beyond the family, engagement in informal groups such as community groups and child-specific support groups can be a means of accessing support and assistance. While not typically regarded as part of a social network, we wanted to recognize that parent's engagement with formal institutions is an important source of support in the form of "expert" advice and information.

The potential *cultural capital* accessible to a child may be approached in a number of ways. Children may benefit from parental "competence" in key societal institutions, as indicated by educational and occupational status. Parental English-language proficiency and literacy can be an indicator of the ability to engage effectively with informal settings such as neighborhoods, as well as with formal organizations such as the health or education sector. On the other hand, non-English language skills may be an important indicator of competency in non-Western cultures in New Zealand. Within the household, parents and family members may hold preferences for certain goods and activities and have beliefs about child development, parenting, and the role of the child in the family, all of which may be reflected in everyday child-related activities. To observe a wide range of practices we can collect information about behaviors such as reading, singing, and telling stories to children; participation in events and activities; diet; and preventive measures such as immunization.

Outside of the household, we are interested in how children and their families engage with various institutions. Parents may belong to a range of communities and report various degrees of belonging to key settings such as the neighborhood. Effective engagement may be dependent on skills such as language and being able to access information to get income or housing assistance, for example. Organizations and groups, whether formal or not, may also have "rules" of access that result in restricted engagement, for example, membership may be dependent on invitation, payment, or geographical location (e.g., school zones). Membership of such groups can rest on having the cultural capital to know the "right" groups to belong to, as well as appropriate behaviors within those groups.

DISCUSSION

The utility of a heuristic such as this to assist with the measurement of wealth in Growing Up in New Zealand is threefold. First, it makes visible the breadth of resources that potentially contribute to a wealthy environment for children in their early years. The matrix approach draws attention to multiple forms of wealth and their differing locations. This has meant that the societal context domain has been able to utilize tools and measures that have been implemented across the whole study for various purposes, rather than just focusing on those tools *specifically* related to wealth measurement. From a practical point of view the heuristic also helps us manage the complexity of measuring wealth by prompting us to prioritize what is important *and* manageable at any given data collection point. Some matrix points may become more crucial at a particular point in time (e.g., educational experiences of grandparents might be less relevant early in a baby's life but may be pertinent at five years if they influence a child's school entry experience). Others, such as income and employment status, may need to be assessed repeatedly. It is also clear that collecting data for some matrix points may be more problematic. For example, while the intergenerational transmission of cultural capital within the extended family is of particular interest in New Zealand, there are limited empirical tools capable of accounting for cultural diversity and the multiple ways in which cultural capital might be transferred from one generation to the next—a gap we are addressing.

When trying to populate the matrix we realized that in some instances no tools were appropriate or available to measure the construct of interest. As a consequence the heuristic drove the development of new tools, or the creative use of proxies or other data sources to "fill in" a critical matrix point. For example, rather than directly measuring neighborhood environments we could use address data to link individual observations with previously developed indirect measures such as measures of neighborhood social environments (Ivory et al., 2011). Sometimes it was not possible to find an acceptable alternative, prompting us to think through the implications of not being able to collect data for a given matrix point at this particular data collection. Thus we had a good sense of what was being measured (and why) as well as what could not be captured within our study.

Second, the heuristic prompted us to consider how to collect data that will allow examination of interaction between forms of capital, and between different locations. For example, affluence can often be necessary to gain access to private schools that provide not only the type of education that allows one to adopt the more powerful positions in society (cultural capital), but also the social capital that results from being embedded in the connections that are typified in the concept of the "old boy's network." This becomes cyclical across generations, as these positions allow one to readily afford to send one's children to the same schools.

The potentially negative aspects related to noneconomic forms of capital also need acknowledgement, particularly in relation to social capital. Shortt (2004) noted that the potential for strong social ties to lead to the exclusion of outsiders, restrictions on individual freedoms, and expectations for reciprocation may lead to excessive demands on some group members, which can be a problem if there are limited financial resources. However, while reciprocation may indeed be a "burden," Webber and Huxley (2007) also showed that the *potential* for reciprocation is a crucial indicator of the willingness of individuals to utilize the social capital that they may have access to. These findings suggest that it is not just engagement in social networks per se that may be beneficial, but that researchers also need to take into account the nature of the engagements and the goods arising from them.

From a translational perspective, more fully assessing the range of wealth available to children will allow us to examine components of child-related wealth and how policy might contribute to the improvement of child outcomes in contemporary New Zealand. In particular, collecting information on child and family engagement with formal institutions alongside other settings will facilitate examination of when and how government assistance is effective for promoting well-being, as well as identifying those who miss out.

Finally, use of Bourdieu's capitals allows understanding of the ways in which children's access to forms of capital can shape outcomes through the concept of "habitus" (Christensen, 2011). Bourdieu advanced the concept of habitus to describe the relationship between social structure and practice in different domains of an individual's life, including the economic, political, social, and cultural (Bourdieu, 1986). A focus on habitus, as expressed through practice, allows for the understanding of how the life of the individual is embedded in a particular social context or "field," thus ameliorating the tendency of traditional epidemiological approaches to assume that "risk"—for example, living an "unhealthy lifestyle"—can be resolved at an individual level (Cockerham, 2005). Understanding practice as occurring at the intersection of structure and agency allows for a better appreciation of how individuals make choices that are both enabled and constrained by their social position, and by the history of experience that has brought them to this social position. "Practice—everyday activities—is therefore shaped *both* by the habitus, which *disposes* people to act in particular ways, *and* by the availability of various types of capital in different fields" (Gatrell et al., 2004, p. 248).

The habitus of the child can be thought of as the "outcome" of the measures outlined in this chapter, in that the economic, social, and cultural forms of wealth accessed throughout their childhood shape how they develop into adolescents and adults. At the same time, this habitus can be an intermediate variable, as it is the child's habitus that will, to a significant extent, shape how they live the rest of their lives and hence is integrally linked to life chances in adulthood. Over time, the combined data collected will allow us to describe how particular configurations of economic, social, and cultural capitals in various settings shape what is possible in a child's life, and to examine the consequences for child health and well-being across the life course.

CONCLUSION

Researchers are increasingly attempting to incorporate the complexity of factors contributing to child outcomes in to their studies. Yet this presents methodological challenges to manage the richness and quantity of data that may be required. Within the Growing Up in New Zealand study we have used the example of wealth to present a heuristic approach that makes visible the complexity of measuring a wider conception of wealth, while prompting systematic and pragmatic data collection over multiple data collection waves. By placing cultural factors alongside social and economic processes we hope that the data collected over time will improve our ability to examine how they interact to explain observed patterns of health and disease.

REFERENCES

Barker, D., Miller, E., 2009. Homeownership and child welfare. Real Estate Economics 37, 279–303.

Baum, F., Palmer, C., 2002. "Opportunity structures": urban landscape, social capital and health promotion in Australia. Health Promotion International 17, 351–361.

Borgonovi, F., 2010. A life-cycle approach to the analysis of the relationship between social capital and health in Britain. Social Science & Medicine 71, 1927–1934.

Bourdieu, P., 1986. The forms of capital. In: Richardson, J. (Ed.), The Handbook of Theory and Research for the Sociology of Education, Greenwood, Westport, CT, pp. 241–258.

Carpiano, R.M., 2006. Toward a neighborhood resource-based theory of social capital for health: can Bourdieu and sociology help? Social Science & Medicine 62, 165–175.

Carter, S., Williams, M., Paterson, J., Iusitini, L., 2009. Do perceptions of neighbourhood problems contribute to maternal health? Findings from the Pacific Islands Families study. Health & Place 15, 622–630.

Christensen, V.T., 2011. Does parental capital influence the prevalence of child overweight and parental perceptions of child weight-level? Social Science & Medicine 72, 469–477.

Cockerham, W.C., 2005. Health lifestyle theory and the convergence of agency and structure. Journal of Health & Social Behavior 46, 51–67.

Cohen, D.A., Inagami, S., Finch, B., 2008. The built environment and collective efficacy. Health & Place 14, 198–208.

Croft, J., 2004. Positive choice, no choice or total rejection: the perennial problem of school catchments, housing and neighbourhoods. Housing Studies 19, 927–945.

Currie, C., Molcho, M., Boyce, W., Holstein, B., Torsheim, T., Richter, M., 2008. Researching health inequalities in adolescents: the development of the Health Behaviour in School-Aged Children (HBSC) Family Affluence Scale. Social Science & Medicine 66, 1429–1436.

Dahl, T., Ceballo, R., Huerta, M., 2010. In the eye of the beholder: Mothers' perceptions of poor neighborhoods as places to raise children. Journal of Community Psychology 38, 419–434.

Dahlgren, G., Whitehead, M., 1991. Policies and strategies to promote social equity in health. Institute for Futures Studies, Stockholm.

De Silva, M.J., Huttly, S.R., Harpham, T., Kenward, M.G., 2007. Social capital and mental health: a comparative analysis of four low income countries. Social Science & Medicine 64, 5–20.

Dunt, D., Hage, B., Kelaher, M., 2011. The impact of social and cultural capital variables on parental rating of child health in Australia. Health Promotion International 26, 290–301.

Edwards, B., 2006. Views of the village: parents' perceptions of their neighbourhoods. Family Matters 74, 26–33.

Free, S., Howden-Chapman, P., Pierse, N., Viggers, H., 2010. More effective home heating reduces school absences for children with asthma. Journal of Epidemiology & Community Health 64, 379–386.

Frohlich, K.L., Dunn, J.R., McLaren, L., Shiell, A., Potvin, L., Hawe, P., Dassa, C., Thurston, W.E., 2007. Understanding place and health: a heuristic for using administrative data. Health & Place 13, 299–309.

Gatrell, A.C., Popay, J., Thomas, C., 2004. Mapping the determinants of health inequalities in social space: can Bourdieu help us? Health & Place 10, 245–257.

Ivory, V.C., Collings, S.C., Blakely, T., Dew, K., 2011. When does neighbourhood matter? Multilevel relationships between neighbourhood social fragmentation and mental health. Social Science & Medicine 72, 1993–2002.

Jack, G., 2006. The area and community components of children's well-being. Children and Society 20, 334–347.

Jaeger, M.M., Holm, A., 2007. Does parents' economic, cultural, and social capital explain the social class effect on educational attainment in the Scandinavian mobility regime? Social Science Research 36, 719–744.

Lee, C.Y.S., Anderson, J.R., Horowitz, J.L., August, G.J., 2009. Family income and parenting: the role of parental depression and social support. Family Relations 58, 417–430.

Leventhal, T., Brooks-Gunn, J., 2001. Changing neighborhoods and child well-being: understanding how children may be affected in the coming century. Advances in Life Course Research 6, 263–301.

Macpherson, C., Macpherson, L., 1999. The changing contours of migrant Samoan kinship. In: King, R., Connell, J. (Eds.), In Small Worlds, Global Lives: Islands and Migration, Pinter, London and New York, pp. 277–291.

Maggi, S., Irwin, L.J., Siddiqi, A., Hertzman, C., 2010. The social determinants of early child development: an overview. Journal of Paediatrics & Child Health 46, 627–635.

McCurdy, K., Gorman, K.S., Metallinos-Katsaras, E., 2010. From poverty to food insecurity and child overweight: a family stress approach. Child Development Perspectives 4, 144–151.

Morton, S.M.B., Atatoa Carr, P.E., Bandara, D.K., Grant, C.C., Ivory, V.C., Kingi, T.R., Liang, R., Petersen, E., Pryor, J., Reese, E., Robinson, E.M., Schmidt, J.M., Waldie, K.E., 2010. Growing Up in New Zealand: a longitudinal study of New Zealand children and their families. Report 1. Before we are born. Growing Up in New Zealand, Auckland.

Morton, S.M.B., Atatoa Carr, P.E., Grant, C.C., Lee, A.C., Bandara, D.K., Mohal, J., Kinloch, J.M., Schmidt, J.M., Hedges, M.R., Ivory, V.C., Kingi, T.K.R., Liang, R., Perese, L.M., Peterson, E., Pryor, J.E., Reese, E., Robinson, E.M., Waldie, K.E., Wall, C.R., 2012a. Growing Up in New Zealand: a longitudinal study of New Zealand children and their families. Report 2: Now we are born. Growing Up in New Zealand, Auckland.

Morton, S.M.B., Atatoa Carr, P.E., Grant, C.C., Robinson, E.M., Bandara, D.K., Bird, A., Ivory, V.C., Kingi, T.K.R., Liang, R., Marks, E.J., Perese, L.M., Peterson, E.R., Pryor, J.E., Reese, E., Schmidt, J.M., Waldie, K.E., Wall, C., 2012b. Cohort Profile: growing Up in New Zealand. International Journal of Epidemiology.

Panter, J.R., Jones, A.P., van Sluijs, E.M.F., Griffin, S.J., 2009. Attitudes, social support and environmental perceptions as predictors of active commuting behaviour in school children. Journal of Epidemiology & Community Health, jech.2009.086918.

Pearce, J., Witten, K., Bartie, P., 2006. Neighbourhoods and health: a GIS approach to measuring community resource accessibility. Journal of Epidemiology & Community Health 60, 389–395.

Pinkster, F.M., Fortuijn, J.D., 2009. Watch out for the neighborhood trap! A case study on parental perceptions of and strategies to counter risks for children in a disadvantaged neighborhood. Children's Geographies 7, 323–337.

Pollack, C.E., Chideya, S., Cubbin, C., Williams, B., Dekker, M., Braveman, P., 2007. Should health studies measure wealth? A systematic review. American Journal of Preventive Medicine 33, 250–264.

Salmond, C., Crampton, P., Atkinson, J., 2007. NZDep2006 Index of Deprivation. Department of Public Health. University of Otago, Wellington.

Shortt, S.E.D., 2004. Making sense of social capital, health and policy. Health Policy 70, 11–22.

Statistics New Zealand, 2001. Framework for the measurement of Social Capital in New Zealand. Statistics New Zealand, Wellington.

van Deth, J.W., 2003. Measuring social capital: orthodoxies and continuing controversies. International Journal of Social Research Methodology 6, 79–92.

Von Rueden, U., Gosch, A., Rajmil, L., Bisegger, C., Ravens-Sieberer, U., 2006. Socioeconomic determinants of health related quality of life in childhood and adolescence: results from a European study. Journal of Epidemiology & Community Health 60, 130–135.

Webber, M.P., Huxley, P.J., 2007. Measuring access to social capital: the validity and reliability of the Resource Generator-UK and its association with common mental disorders. Social Science & Medicine 65, 481–492.

Williams Shanks, T.R., 2007. The impacts of household wealth on child development. Journal of Poverty 11, 93–116.

Witten, K., Exeter, D., Field, A., 2003. The quality of urban environments: mapping variation in access to community resources. Urban Studies 40, 161–177.

Woody, D., Woody, D.J., 2007. The significance of social support on parenting among a group of single, low-income, African American mothers. Journal of Human Behavior in the Social Environment 15, 183–198.

Chapter 23

Cultural Consensus Modeling of Disease

Stanley Ulijaszek

Institute of Social and Cultural Anthropology, University of Oxford, UK

INTRODUCTION

Cultural Consensus Modeling (CCM) is an analytical technique that can be used to estimate cultural beliefs and the extent to which people share them (Weller, 2007). Cultural beliefs include values and perceptions that reflect health- or illness-promoting practices. The method was elaborated in the 1980s following the emergence of cognitive anthropology as a sub-discipline (Romney et al., 1986). It is similar to the knowledge, attitudes, and practice (KAP) model, which uses standardized survey questionnaires that have correct answers according to biomedical theory, and answers are evaluated relative to these. CCM can be used to determine knowledge and attitudes similarly to the KAP model, but without relating answers to any yardstick. With respect to health and disease, it has been used to investigate beliefs about disease contagiousness (Romney et al., 1986; Ruebush et al., 1992; Romney, 1999), knowledge, and attitudes about chronic disease and obesity (Chavez et al., 1995; Weller et al., 1999; Ulijaszek, 2007) and health care in clinical settings (Smith et al., 2004).

CCM seeks to group individuals according to common understandings or beliefs that come from them, rather than by imposing categories that may or may not be valid. Often it is assumed that cultures or groups share common values, differing from those of other groups. As a set of learned and shared beliefs and behaviors, culture has a normative component that groups are viewed to embody and are therefore important to understand. However, not all members of a group are likely to conform to the norm, while different groups may share some or many common values. CCM can tease out some of these similarities and differences. In this chapter, CCM is described, and then illustrated using examples from studies of understandings of diabetes causation, symptomatology, and management, and breast cancer risk among different groups in the United States and Latin America.

When Culture Impacts Health. http://dx.doi.org/10.1016/B978-0-12-415921-1.00023-3

THE METHOD

CCM is based on the jury theorem of collective competence of society and uses factor analysis to identify similarity of views and distribution of cultural knowledge concerning an issue or set of issues within groups, a society, or population (Romney et al., 1986; Weller, 1987). It works on the assumption that widely shared information shows high concordance among individuals. This method can identify agreement within and across groups with a set of norms, values, and understandings concerning an issue of importance, which is measured as cultural competence (CC). CCM has good validity with sample sizes as small as 4 where there is a high level of social homogeneity surrounding the issue in question, and as high as 17 when only half of a group have shared values (Romney et al., 1986). This makes it a good technique for a small-scale study. Sample size can be determined using initial assumptions concerning CC, the statistical confidence level (CL) expected, and the level of accuracy with which subjects are expected to respond to questions. CC is the extent to which all subjects in a group can understand and classify the questions in hand similarly. The statistical CL is set according to the proportion of between-subject difference in questionnaire response that is free from error due to the administration of the questionnaire. For example, if CL is set at 0.95, there would be an expectation that 95% of all answers would be free from error due to administration of the questionnaire. Sample size can be determined at a range of CLs, although levels of 0.95 and above should be sought. Accuracy is the extent to which any particular subject, if faced with the same question repeatedly, will answer it in the same way. A value of 0.95 means that subjects would answer the same questions the same way 19 times out of 20. Levels of accuracy, confidence, and CC should be set according to the needs of any particular study, although values of 0.95, 0.95, and 0.5 for the three variables, respectively, can be taken as default settings. Sample size calculations setting accuracy at 0.95 are presented in Table 23.1.

The greater the expected CC, the lower the sample size needed. If an acceptable outcome of a planned study is that over half of subjects should share the same values for the issues under investigation, then expected minimum CC can be set at 0.5. If a higher level of concordance is expected, then a higher expected minimum CC could be set, leading to a smaller sample size requirement. If for a particular study the CL and accuracy were both set at 0.95 and expected minimum CC was set at 0.5, then the sample size required per group would be 17. If there were one group involved in a study, the overall minimum sample size required would be 17. If the study involved a comparison of two groups or more, then a minimum of 17 subjects per group would be required. Balance is required between assumptions about expected minimum CC when determining sample size for a study, and the CC estimated by the study itself. If the sample size were based on expected minimum CC greater than 0.5, then the CC calculated from the study data would need to be greater than 0.5. If it were lower than this, inferences from the data would be based on inadequate sample size.

TABLE 23.1 Minimum Sample Sizes at Varying CLs and Different Expected Minimum Levels of Cultural Competence, Setting Accuracy at 0.95

Confidence level	Expected Minimum Cultural Competence					
	0.4	0.5	0.6	0.7	0.8	0.9
0.90	25	17	10	6	6	4
0.95	26	17	11	6	6	4
0.99	34	23	14	9	7	4
0.999	42	29	17	10	8	5

Source: Adapted from Romney et al., 1986.

CCM involves three stages of analysis: (1) identification of significant issues relating to the topic of enquiry, (2) determination of the values attributed to those issues, and (3) determination of CC and cultural consensus within the group or groups under investigation. The method lends itself to the study of groups that may be representative of a society or culture, specific social or ethnic groups, users of specific types of health services, or individuals suffering or being at risk of a specific disease or disease category. The first stage of the process can be carried out by literature review, interview, questionnaire, or focus group, while the second involves quantification of attitudes and beliefs about issues salient to the topic in hand. The third stage involves statistical manipulation using factor analysis. All CC scores should fall between zero and one, with no negative scores, as a minimum threshold for asserting that there is a single factor solution. Cultural consensus is identified by the ratio of component one to component two of principal component analysis; the value must exceed three to comply with criteria for consensus (Romney et al., 1986). The higher the ratio between eigenvalues one and two, the greater the agreement among the group and the greater is the cultural consensus. If cultural consensus is achieved, shared values are represented by component one of principal components analysis. Examples of CC and cultural consensus calculations and their interpretation are given in the next section.

CULTURAL CONSENSUS, CULTURAL COMPETENCE, AND DISEASE

The two examples presented here illustrate ways in which CCM has been used to generate CC and cultural consensus values that can identify differences in understandings of diabetes causation, symptomatology and management, and breast cancer risk among groups of questionable heterogeneity or homogeneity in the United States and Latin America. In the first example, the question that is addressed is "are all Latin American populations homogeneous in their understandings of diabetes?" In the second example, the question is "do Latin American populations differ from Anglo-Americans and clinicians in their understandings of breast cancer risk?"

There is a high prevalence of diabetes among people of Latin American origin in the United States (Engelgau et al., 2004), and in Latin America (Barcelo et al., 2003). There is also considerable heterogeneity of place of origin and background of so-called Hispanic populations in the United States. According to the U.S. Census Bureau, the terms "Hispanic" or "Latino" refer to persons who trace their origin or descent to Mexico, Puerto Rico, Cuba, Spanish-speaking Central and South America countries, or other Spanish cultures. Origin can be considered as the heritage, nationality group, lineage, or country of the person or the person's parents or ancestors before their arrival in the United States (United States Census Bureau, 2012). Populations and groups may also vary according to their nation, place of residence, and socioeconomic position. Is it therefore legitimate to bundle together all Hispanic and Latin American groups with respect to their understandings of diabetes causation, symptomatology, and management? Weller et al. (1999) asked this question when applying CCM to beliefs about diabetes in four different Latin American groups, two in the United States, one in urban Mexico, and another in rural Guatemala. The authors identified representative samples of households at each location. Participants, mostly adult women, were informed that this was a study of attitudes and that there were no incorrect answers. The minimum sample size needed was calculated from a low expected minimum CC value of 0.50, a high CL (0.999), and an accuracy level of 0.95. The minimum number of subjects per group was estimated to be 29, although they interviewed a third more subjects than this to allow for incomplete returns, which would then have to be excluded. Questions were framed such that the answers were either "yes" or "no." If subjects could not commit to either of these, the answers were coded as unclassified and left out of the analysis. The number of unclassified answers was 5% or less among the two United States samples, and 11% and 19% for the urban Mexican and rural Guatemalan samples, respectively. CCM was then used to determine whether there was sufficient agreement in responses to warrant their aggregation according to a single set of beliefs with respect to diabetes, regardless of whether they were medically correct or not. All four groups met the goodness-of-fit criteria for using the model, with eigenvalue ratios exceeding 3:1 in all cases, and was 9.3 for the total sample of all four groups. The four groups therefore shared a core set of beliefs about diabetes (Table 23.2). CC was highest for the two United States samples, marginally lower for the urban Mexican sample, and lower again for the rural Guatemalan sample.

All four groups agreed that both men and women are susceptible to diabetes, as are old people of both genders. All groups also agreed that diabetes is not a consequence of aging but of uncontrolled sugar in the blood, eating sugar or sweets, and drinking sodas, but not from hot/cold imbalances or witchcraft. Concerning symptoms and treatment, all four groups identified the principal clinical signs in concordance with biomedical descriptions, including excessive thirst, frequent urination, sugar in the blood, craving for sweet things, dizziness, and headaches. With respect to treatment, all four groups viewed clinical treatment to be the best, and that consumption of a balanced diet was important. All four groups agreed that a lack of treatment could cause kidney problems, heart problems or heart attack, coma, and early death, and that diabetes gets worse if no biomedical treatment is sought. Three of the four groups showed an additional set of values, in relation to type 1, or heritable diabetes, as opposed to type 2, or maturity-onset diabetes. People in all sites apart from the rural Guatemalan one agreed that children could become diabetic, as could relatives of a diabetic individual. They also believed that one could be born with it and that it could be caused by a lack of insulin.

TABLE 23.2 Beliefs Regarding Diabetes among Latinos

Sample	Who is susceptible	Causes	Symptoms	Treatments	Consequences of lack of treatment
Guatemala, Mexico, Texas, Connecticut	Men, women, old people	Not from aging Uncontrolled sugar in blood Eating sugar or sweets; drinking sodas Not from hot/cold imbalances Not from witchcraft Not as a consequence of taking medicines Not from allergies, pollution, smoking Not from overexertion Not from spoiled or undercooked food	Excessive thirst Lack of animation; tired, no energy Affects kidneys Frequent urination Burns with urination Sugar in blood Craves sweet things Dizziness Headaches Crankiness, irritability Problem with blood circulation and increased blood pressure Eye problems, loss of vision More susceptible to other illnesses	Doctor is best Will not go away by itself Not pharmacist Must care for self No cure, only control Check blood pressure regularly Pills help to process sugar Eat balanced diet Lose weight, if overweight No liquid diet cure No sweets, no alcohol, no fat	Kidney problems Heart problems or heart attack Coma Early death Gets worse with no treatment
Mexico, Texas, Connecticut	Children Relatives of a diabetic individual	Hereditary Lack of insulin Not contagious; not from a parasite or virus Not from anemia Not from drinking too much alcohol	Wounds heal slowly Do not have to stay in bed		

Source: Adapted from Romney et al., 1986.

Similar methodology was undertaken by Chavez et al. (1995) to examine the extent to which knowledge and attitudes about breast cancer risk factors were concordant among women of Latin American origin in the United States, their Anglo-American counterparts, and physicians. The authors used ethnographic interviews to obtain their data. By using rank ordering of interview data, they could quantify their responses and use them in CCM. In their semistructured questionnaire, there were more than 300 closed- and open-ended enquiries regarding cancer in general, breast cancer, cervical cancer, general access to medical care, access to cancer screening and treatment services, and personal demographic characteristics. Bilingual investigators translated the questionnaire from English to Spanish and also back-translated it to ensure that nothing was lost in translation. Subjects were asked to rank order their responses to the questions. When determining the sample size needed, the researchers chose an even lower than expected minimum CC (0.36) but an accuracy (0.95) similar to the study of Weller et al. (1999). With this they determined that a minimum of 17 respondents were needed in each group. These sample sizes were exceeded with the authors interviewing 30 physicians, 26 Anglo-American women, 26 Chicanas, 31 Mexican immigrants, and 28 Salvadoran immigrants.

CCM was applied to the groups individually, then in combination with each other (Table 23.3). When all the groups were combined, they did not attain consensus with a ratio of eigenvalues of 1.2, and a CC value of 0.40. When separated into the five groups, physicians had far and away the greatest cultural consensus with respect to the values they shared concerning breast cancer risk. This is hardly surprising, since it is their job to know this, and they were defined in this study according to employment. Following the physicians, the Anglo-American and Chicana groups each had a high degree of cultural consensus, followed by the Mexican and the Salvadoran immigrant groups. When the data from the physicians and Anglo-Americans were combined in analysis, they were shown to have similar cultural consensus to those of the individual Mexican and Salvadoran groups. There was also high cultural consensus among Anglo-Americans and Chicanas when grouped together, but not among Chicanas and physicians grouped together. There was consensus among Chicanas, Mexicans, and Salvadorans when grouped together, whether paired (Chicanas/Mexicans, Chicanas/Salvadorans, Mexicans/Salvadorans) or all three as one group (ratio of eigenvalues between 3.0 and 3.4). Thus each group had its own cultural model of breast cancer risk, with great similarity among the cultural models of the Chicana, Mexican, and Salvadoran groups. Physicians and Anglo-Americans also had similar cultural models of breast cancer risk, presumably because most physicians in the study were Anglo-Americans. The authors thus demonstrate two broad cultural models regarding beliefs about breast cancer risk factors: a Latina one and a biomedical one. The Latina model incorporates beliefs that emphasize physical trauma to the breast and bad behavior such as drinking alcohol and using illegal drugs. The physicians and Anglo-American women share a biomedical model that differs considerably from the Latina one,

TABLE 23.3 Summary Statistics for Cultural Consensus Modeling of Breast Cancer Risk

Sample	Individual Samples		Combined Samples			
	Cultural competence	Cultural consensus (ratio of eigenvalues)	Mean competence	Cultural consensus (ratio of eigenvalues)	Mean competence	Cultural consensus (ratio of eigenvalues)
Physicians	0.73	8.8			0.61	3.0
Anglo–Americans	0.64	4.1	0.58	3.4		
Chicanas	0.58	4.2			0.48	3.4
Mexican immigrants	0.51	3.0	0.48	3.0		
Salvadoran immigrants	0.47	3.0				

Source: Adapted from Chavez et al., 1995.

in that it emphasizes epidemiologically determined risk factors such as age and family history.

The two examples given here show how CCM can help unpack similarities and differences in knowledge and values of different groups with respect to disease causation, risk, and management. The first study shows that so-called Latina groups largely share the same values with respect to understanding of diabetes, although one group, the Guatemalan one, differs in some important respects. The second example shows that physicians have a strong cultural consensus concerning breast cancer risk, and this differs in important ways from those of Latin American immigrant groups in the United States. It also confirms the expectation that Anglo-Americans share more values with physicians than with Latin American immigrants.

DISCUSSION

CCM is useful for identifying similarities within and across groups in knowledge and beliefs about almost anything and can be considered in part the quantification of common knowledge. With respect to health and disease, the ability to quantify common knowledge and how it differs between groups is useful for understanding why disease patterns may differ among seemingly similar groups, or - be homogeneous among seemingly different groups. It can also be useful in improving health care delivery.

The two examples, from the United States and Latin America, show that knowledge and attitudes about diabetes and breast cancer can vary between groups that might otherwise be considered homogeneous according to census classifications. The value of the method for health research can go beyond the identification of knowledge and attitudes about specific diseases. If questioned about more than one disease, for example, the extent to which CC and cultural consensus varies according to disease could be determined. If used longitudinally, it could measure changing competence and consensus, and therefore the efficacy of health services in bringing everyone "on-message" with respect to prevention and management of important diseases and disease categories. It could also reveal differences in the extent that health professionals of different kinds share the message, whatever it might be.

REFERENCES

Barcelo, A., Aedo, C., Rajpathak, S., Robles, S., 2003. The cost of diabetes in Latin America and the Caribbean. Bulletin W.H.O 81, 19–28.

Chavez, L.R., Hubbell, F.A., McCullin, J.M., Martinez, R.G., Mishra, S.I., 1995. Understanding knowledge and attitudes about breast cancer. A cultural analysis. Archives Family Medicine 4, 145–152.

Engelgau, M.M., Geiss, L.S., Saadine, J.B., Boyle, J.P., Benjamin, S.M., Gregg, E.W., Tierney, E.F., Rios-Burrows, N., Mokdad, A.H., Imperatore, G., Narayan, K.M.V., 2004. The evolving diabetes burden in the United States. Annals of Internal Medicine 140, 945–950.

Romney, A.K., 1999. Culture consensus as a statistical model. Current Anthropology 40 (Suppl.), S103–S115.

Romney, A.K., Weller, S.C., Batchelder, W.H., 1986. Culture as consensus: a theory of culture and informant accuracy. American Anthropology 88, 313–338.

Ruebush, T.K., Weller, S.C., Klein, R.E., 1992. Knowledge in beliefs about malaria on the Pacific coastal plain of Guatemala. The American Journal of Tropical Medicine and Hygiene 46, 450–459.

Smith, C.S., Morris, M., Hill, W., Francovich, C., McMullin, J., Chavez, L., Rhoads, C., 2004. Cultural consensus analysis as a tool for clinic improvements. Journal of general internal medicine: official journal of the Society for Research and Education in Primary Care Internal Medicine 19, 514–518.

Ulijaszek, S.J., 2007. Models of population obesity and cultural consensus modelling. Economics and Human Biology 5, 443–457.

United States Census Bureau, 2012. Hispanic Population of the United States. http://www.census.gov/population/www/socdemo/hispanic/about.html.

Weller, S.C., 1987. Shared knowledge, intracultural variation, and knowledge aggregation. American Behavioral Scientist 31, 178–193.

Weller, S.C., Baer, R.D., Pachter, L.M., Trotter, R.T., Glazer, M., de Alba Garcia, J.E.G., Klein, R.E., 1999. Latino beliefs about diabetes. Diab. Care 22, 722–728.

Weller, S.C., 2007. Cultural consensus theory: applications and frequently asked questions. Field Methods 19, 339–368.

Chapter 24

Reconsidering Meaning and Measurement: An Ethno-Epidemiology Study of Refugee Youth Settlement in Melbourne, Australia

Sandra M. Gifford

The Swinburne Institute for Social Research, Swinburne University of Technology, Victoria, Australia

INTRODUCTION

What are the methodological challenges that arise in conducting a longitudinal ethnographically informed study of settlement and well-being among a cohort of newly arrived youth with refugee backgrounds? Is it possible to achieve all of the objects of a study that uses both qualitative and quantitative methods, is informed by the disciplines of medical anthropology and social epidemiology, and must produce results that will inform policy and practice and contribute to a positive experience of settlement among participants in their first years in Australia? This was the aim of the Good Starts for Refugee Youth study (Gifford et al., 2009)—a project that grew out of an interdisciplinary mix of theory, method, and a practical need to better understand how to make life better for adolescents building a life in a new country. This chapter reflects on these challenges as they arose from the Good Starts for Refugee Youth Study, which followed 120 youth over a four-year period. The starting point for these reflections is the first paper published from the study, Meaning or Measurement? Researching the Social Contexts of Health and Settlement among Newly Arrived Refugee Youth in Melbourne, Australia (Gifford et al., 2007), which reported on the methods and their challenges in the Good Start study.

The paper (Gifford et al., 2007) has provided a point of reference for other researchers investigating refugee youth settlement (e.g., Schweitzer and Steel, 2008; Sturgess and Phillips, 2009, 2010; Svensson et al., 2009; Wilding, 2009; Nathan et al., 2010; Block et al., 2012), and this literature has generated some useful critiques of the research tools as they have been applied in other studies of refugee youth settlement. Part of that first paper (Gifford et al., 2007) is reproduced here, and with the benefit of hindsight, I reflect on some of the key challenges of that study and discuss what worked, what did not, and why. In this article, I reflect back on what might be done differently if we could start again, and what lessons might be learned for future studies of this nature. Importantly, I ask to what extent can a mixed method study truly do justice to both meaning and measurement?

BACKGROUND: IT ALL STARTED WHEN ...

In the late 1990s, I began working as a medical anthropologist, with a nongovernmental organization that provided a range of services for newly arrived refugees settling in Victoria, Australia. The organization provided services to support the psychosocial well-being of newly arrived refugees including intensive counseling for those suffering from the traumas of their past. A key question that kept arising among management and staff was, "Do our services make a difference to people's settlement in the longer term?" Answering this is not straightforward and it opened up a unique opportunity to design an innovative research project that might provide some answers while at the same time, contribute to a broader evidence base about what works best when it comes to refugee settlement. This question was particularly important because a large number of clients were young people who had their futures ahead of them. Thus began the Good Starts for Refugee Youth study.

Many different interests informed the Good Starts study, practically, theoretically, and methodologically. Practically, the research had to be nonintrusive and if possible, engage research participants in a positive experience. Theoretically, the research needed to bridge a range of disciplines including social work, psychology, anthropology, social epidemiology, and policy while being fundamentally framed by a social determinant of health approach. Methodologically, the study needed to gather empirical data using tools that were valid and yielded comparative data and strategies that were user friendly for newly arrived, ethnically diverse young people.

The study was also informed by a growing critique of the research on refugee settlement (see, e.g., the work of Marlowe, 2010, 2011), most of which approached the problem of refugee settlement with the glass half empty. By this I mean the research, both quantitative and qualitative, tended to focus on the trauma of the past and how this impacted on settlement in the present, but very little focused on the more positive aspects of making a new life in Australia despite a traumatic past. Thus, while we knew a lot about the difficulties of being a refugee in a settlement context, we understood very little about how people shed the refugee label or what services work best to support good settlement outcomes. Finally, most studies were cross sectional providing a snapshot at a particular point in time. Very few studies were longitudinal, so there was little information about how resettled refugees might fare over time.

These concerns framed the Good Starts for Refugee Youth study, the pilot of which was carried out from 2001 to 2002. The main study then followed a cohort of 120 newly arrived refugee youth over a four-year period between 2004 and 2008 (Gifford et al., 2009). In 2012, we received funding for a fifth round of follow up eight years after the first wave of data collection and at a stage in life where the participants have now transitioned into early adulthood.

CHALLENGES OF RESEARCHING REFUGEE SETTLEMENT AND WELL-BEING

A key element of Australia's commitment as a participant in the system of international protection for the plight of refugees is the Humanitarian Program, a regular and planned component of the country's Migration Program (Karlsen, 2011). At the time of this study, Australia's Humanitarian Program granted approximately 50,000 visas to refugees and other displaced persons between January 2001 and December 2005. Approximately 50% of the Program's intake were people under the age of 20 (DIMIA, 2005).

The challenges of researching the determinants of well-being and good settlement among newly arrived refugees include developing appropriate methods of sampling, recruitment, and informed consent, and appropriate data collection methods. There are additional logistical issues of conducting research with people who have many pressing health and settlement needs within their first few months of arrival. Furthermore research with refugee young people requires parental consent, which can be complex given the family history and settlement demands.

One of the key methodological challenges of developing an appropriate research approach is the difficulty associated with eliciting relevant information from a population with a range of literacy skills and languages, that is, unfamiliar with research, and has diverse pre-arrival experiences. In addition to the developmental challenges of being an adolescent in a new country, refugee young people are grappling with premigration experiences, which may include growing up in a context of war, violence, and protracted periods spent in refugee camps. Many of these young people have experienced displacement from one or more communities and homes, disrupted schooling, separation from close family and friends, and the trauma and loss associated with their refugee experiences (VFST, 1996; Rousseau et al., 2001; Coventry et al., 2002). Previous experiences of persecution, mistrust, and fear can continue to be played out in the resettlement country (Coventry et al., 2002). Many refugee youth find themselves faced with the often fraught process of negotiating conflicting cultural values of their families and of their host country (Hyman et al., 2000; Coventry et al., 2002; Brough et al., 2003). Given the immediate challenges facing young people in their first year, research with this population must, at a minimum, not add further to the burdens of settlement, and should ideally contribute to a positive experience of making a new home in Australia.

Researching health and well-being more specifically among young people with refugee backgrounds is both theoretically and methodologically fraught with difficulties (Ahearn, 2000). First, refugee studies are inherently multidisciplinary, drawing upon many different theoretical and methodological approaches (Black, 2001). While this provides a rich environment in which to approach research questions, it also presents many complexities, as there is no straightforward approach to theory, method, or design. Second, there is a tension between meaning and measurement. While qualitative studies of the refugee experience provide valuable insights into the meanings of transition and settlement (Ahearn, 2000), it is difficult to generalize these findings to the broader resettled population. And when it comes to measurement, there are at present very few quantitative instruments that demonstrate the validity and rigor required to assess constructs of psychosocial well-being, health, resilience, and other key variables that are associated with settlement outcomes (Hollifield et al., 2002; Gagnon and Tuck, 2004; Porter and Haslam, 2005). The methodological problems of carrying out survey research with refugee populations range from issues of cross-cultural translations and equivalency of concepts, through to the practical issues of sampling and negotiating with community gatekeepers (Bloch, 1999). Sensitive ethical issues (Jacobsen and Landau, 2003; Rogers, 2004) and the need to establish a sense of trust between researchers and refugee communities (Hynes, 2003), while at the same time ensuring methodological rigor (Kopinak, 1999), often give rise to competing demands. This has led to an increasing recognition of the value of participatory and action research approaches, focusing on research *with* rather than *on* refugee communities (Johannsen, 2001; Briant and Kennedy, 2004). Finally, there is a growing trend within the field that consists of combining different methodological approaches, thus allowing for both meaning and measurement. Research designs that combine qualitative approaches that give voice to the refugee experience (Powles, 2004), with quantitative approaches that can provide population-based evidence, are likely to prove as fruitful as they have in other areas of social science and health research (Hines, 1993; Maton, 1993).

Change is central to the refugee experience, yet surprisingly few studies with refugee populations have adopted a longitudinal approach, and the majority of designs (qualitative and quantitative) are cross sectional or conducted at one point in time. In a systematic review of longitudinal studies on refugee children and youth published between 1984 and 2004, only five studies could be identified, all with relatively small sample sizes, most with short follow-up periods, and all using only quantitative methods (Correa-Velez et al., 2005). In qualitative research follow-up studies are rare; however, the ethnographic approach of anthropology has much value for longitudinal investigation, due to its in-depth focus on both context and change over time (Barley, 1990; Alverson et al., 2000). Although no such studies on refugee youth were identified at the start of Good Starts, a number of studies had adopted longitudinal ethnographic designs to investigate teenage smoking (Bell et al., 1999), substance abuse (Alverson et al., 2000), injecting drug use (Sherman and Latkin, 1999), and school success (McLeod, 2000).

Several studies have highlighted the strengths of longitudinal ethnographic approaches for researching cultural diversity and change over time (Moerman, 1993; Sissons, 1999) and this approach has been shown to be especially appropriate for research with children and young people in contexts of cultural diversity (Boyden and Ennew, 1997). In sum, the majority of research with refugee populations has been cross sectional with few longitudinal or ethnographic studies, and it is rare to find a study that combines both qualitative and quantitative approaches (Loizos, 2000).

The strength of longitudinal designs in studies of refugee settlement is that they allow us to examine points in time and over time, which is especially important when investigating key transitions in people's lives. Retrospective studies are limited in that individuals are often unable to accurately recall the details of earlier experiences due to both memory effects and also the influence of later experiences on the recollection and interpretation of earlier events. When asking respondents about the past, events may be forgotten, partially remembered, or misplaced in time (Uncles, 1988). Past intentions may be recorded inaccurately as a result of *post hoc* rationalization of events that did not take place as originally expected (Uncles, 1988; Rose et al., 1991). An important advantage of a longitudinal (cohort) study is that it reduces the likelihood of inaccuracy by decreasing the time between the occurrence and the recording of an event (Robinson and Marsland, 1994). Another advantage of longitudinal studies is that they allow the analysis of change at both the individual and the aggregate levels (Uncles, 1988; Rose et al., 1991). Especially in the first years of settlement, a time fraught with emotions and pressing needs, documenting experience as it happens provides a richer picture of this process.

THE GOOD STARTS STUDY: AIMS AND STUDY DESIGN

The overall aim of Good Starts was twofold: (1) to identify the psychosocial factors that assist refugee young people in making a good start in their new country and (2) to describe in depth contexts, settings, and social processes that support, enhance, and facilitate settlement and well-being among this dislocated and often traumatized population of youth. A particular focus was on key transitions from pre-arrival to Australia, from the language school to mainstream school, and from mainstream school to higher education or to the workforce.

The specific objectives of the study were to (1) identify the psychosocial determinants at the individual and community level, which promote health and well-being of newly arrived refugee youth over time; (2) describe how young refugees build social capital; (3) describe how young refugees re-establish a sense of coherence and control over their lives and futures; (4) identify and describe the factors within specific settings (school, family, community) that young refugees regard as health enhancing; and (5) explain the ways in which specific settings act to support physical, mental, and social well-being.

Good Starts recruited a total of 120 newly arrived young people with refugee backgrounds into the study through three English Language Schools (ELS). Classes with students only from refugee backgrounds were selected. Participants were aged 12 to 19 with a mean age of 15.1, and they represented 10 different countries of birth and more than 20 different languages. The mean time since arriving in Australia was 5.3 months and they arrived with an average of six years of schooling. (Gifford et al., 2009, Correa-Velez et al., 2010). At the end of the fourth year of data collection, 80 (66%) of the participants remained in the study.

The methods of data collection were eclectic ranging from standardized questions to open-ended interviews with a mix of procedures in between. Quantitative measures were chosen to examine the relationship between psychosocial factors (which may act as risk or protective factors) and health and well-being outcomes. We selected specific questions and scales from instruments that had been used in large-scale studies of youth well-being, social determinants of health, and studies of migrant/ethnic health and social well-being (Correa-Velez et al., 2010). Qualitative methods were drawn from a range of disciplinary fields including social psychology, anthropology, sociology, and participatory/action/ evaluation research. Importantly, some of the visual methods were designed to count—for example, social status ladders where the rungs form a 10 point scale and social circles—and to elicit meaning where we could ask participants to explain their responses. Some of the visual methods including drawings and photographs were designed to anchor short interviews of participant's experiences as well as to gather more specific information about particular themes (Gifford et al., 2009). Thus, the mix of methods included some items that were purely quantitative, some only qualitative, and some that elicited both kinds of information. It was through this mix of methods that we aimed to achieve data that would enable an analysis of both meaning and measurement.

LOGISTICAL ISSUES WITH SAMPLING AND RECRUITMENT

One of the first challenges of the study was sampling. Participant recruitment and follow-up are key issues for any longitudinal study and particularly with refugee young people. Building a sense of trust and establishing relationships between participants and researchers is critical for short-term and longer term success. Thus, recruitment strategies focused on settings where potential participants already felt a sense of belonging, security, and trust. In the pilot, we trialed a range of recruitment strategies including through ELS, community, and family networks. However, recruiting through the latter networks did not prove successful mostly due to the restrictions placed on having to collect data in the home environment with family present. Thus, recruitment for the longitudinal study took place through ELS.

When refugee young people first arrive in Australia they are eligible to attend an ELS for up to one year before transiting to a mainstream school. Although young people frequently move from one residential location to another in the first 12 months of settlement, they usually remain in the same ELS. Thus, recruitment strategies focused on building partnerships with ELS that had high numbers of refugee students. This strategy proved advantageous for a number of reasons. Students enjoyed the school environment; they trusted their teachers and their parents also respected the school environment as a safe place that had their children's interests at heart. Thus, it was relatively easy to establish a relationship with participants through their school. Data collection was conducted within the school setting, and consent from parents was gained through the partnership with the school. By selecting ELS with high numbers of refugee students, we were able to achieve a sampling profile that was similar to Australia's overall humanitarian intake. Researchers then worked with the ELS to integrate the first year of data collection into the school curriculum, thereby allowing researchers to go into the classroom over a series of sessions. This enabled relationships to be established and for students to become more familiar with the concept of research over a number of weeks.

A key challenge for the longitudinal study was determining an adequate sample size—one that was large enough to generate valid quantitative associations (measurement) but small enough to generate in-depth qualitative data (meaning). The study aimed to involve a minimum of 10% ($n = 80$) of the 802 humanitarian arrivals in Melbourne in 2003 aged between 10 and 19 (DIMIA, 2004). At the end of the four years of data collection, the study had an attrition rate of 34%, with 80 of the 120 participants having completed the final year of data collection. This sample size has enabled statistical analysis of the quantitative data and the collection of qualitative data from all participants as well as providing opportunities for more in-depth nested case studies of young people's experiences. A range of strategies including telephone calls, newsletters, postcards, and brief personal contacts with youth in public venues (e.g., train stations) have been implemented to prevent and limit dropout.

Logistics of Gaining Informed Consent

The pilot stage was critical for developing a process of informed consent, as these refugee young people—in addition to being unfamiliar with this requirement for research—came from environments where human rights had been violated. Thus, the first step was to rethink the standard process for obtaining informed consent, beginning with the recognition that young people and their families needed to develop an awareness and trust of the research and consent process. Briefly, a process was developed that consent commenced with an initial session in the classroom setting discussing broader issues of autonomy and the voluntary nature of research participation. Particular attention was given to informing students about their right to say no to being part of a research project.

Second, an invitation was extended to parents/guardians to attend a briefing session to hear about the project. Students were given project fliers and consent letters translated in the appropriate languages. In cases where consent letters were not returned, interpreters/bicultural workers discussed the issue with participants and in some cases telephoned parents/guardians to further explain the study and respond to any of their concerns.

The same process of informed consent was incorporated into the longitudinal study, with even more time given to explain the project to young people and their families. Where difficulties or concerns arose, bicultural workers were again involved in discussions with young people and parents, and the project employed a community liaison worker to better facilitate this communication.

Logistical Issues with Follow-Up

Developing strategies for follow-up was limited within the scope of the pilot project, given the short time line and lack of resources. Two different strategies were piloted for students recruited from ELS settings including sending the follow-up instrument through the mail and organizing a data collection reunion party. The time between baseline and follow-up in the pilot was between 6 and 8 months during which time contact was maintained predominantly via post. Participants were sent first-year completion certificates, greeting cards, and a disposal camera so they could take photos for the second round of data collection. Fifteen follow-up journals were returned by the participants (i.e., 33% participant retention at follow-up). Many of the materials sent by post were returned due to incorrect addresses, indicating participants had moved. Letters were sent inviting participants to attend an after-school data gathering party during which group discussions were planned. However, only six attended this activity.

The information gained from the pilot follow-up highlighted the frequency with which families move in the first year of arrival and the importance of establishing relationships between participants and the Good Starts study. Strategies to assist young people to remain connected to the study despite changes in schools and home were critical. Applying this information from the pilot to the longitudinal study has resulted in a range of strategies that build a sense of connection to the Good Starts project. For example, given the turnover in research staff year by year, the focus is on building sense of belonging to the Good Starts study rather than building relationships with individual research staff. A strong and positive graphic design has been developed and used for all project materials. The Good Starts logo and themed design make all project products easily identifiable for participants. Data completion certificates incorporating a group photo are sent to participants at the end of year one. Postcards (thank you, change of address, season greetings, and invitations) are sent to the young people throughout each year reminding them of upcoming data collection and thanking them for their participation. Participants are sent an annual Good Starts newsletter designed using their own drawings and words and sharing some of the study findings.

Maintaining contact with schools has been an important follow-up strategy to build relationships with participants in a safe environment over time and to assist with tracking participants when they leave the ELS for a mainstream school. In year one, all participants attended one of three ELS. However, in year two participants collectively attended 29 different schools, one moved inter-state, two were in the tertiary sector, and several were not in school and working in paid employment.

In summary, follow-up strategies required explicit consideration of the impact of the refugee experience on participants. The building of trust and a sense of belonging were critical for these young people, and research with this potentially vulnerable group must be shaped by their unique characteristics and experiences. Research that puts "scientific objectivity" above social responsi-bility is both ethically and scientifically flawed. While it can be argued that the establishment of a relationship with the Good Starts study biases study out-comes, these relationships are crucial to the viability of the longitudinal study.

Logistical Issues with Data Collection

Developing and piloting methods of data collection involved the need to both count/measure as well as to elicit meaning and experience. Many of the young people had disrupted schooling, varying levels of literacy in their own language, and a limited comprehension of English and had no prior experience involved in research. They had no familiarity with research questions and scales or with qualitative approaches. Thus, we developed a strategy of collecting data in a way that complemented the school curriculum, was seen by teachers and young people as adding value to the classroom experience, and that engaged young people who had no familiarity with the research endeavor.

Both quantitative and qualitative methods of data collection were integrated and organized around the five theoretical themes of the study (identity and self, social support, connections to place, health and well-being, and aspirations for the future). Each of the data collection sessions focused on one of these themes with both standardized quantitative questions and a range of qualitative activi-ties all contained within the "Settlement Journal."

In the first year data were collected in 100-minute sessions in the classroom, over 8–10 weeks of the term. Each session had a particular theme (driven by the theory) and involved a range of activities (qualitative and quantitative) where information was recorded in a personal Settlement Journal. Activities included photo novellas (students were each given a disposable camera), drawing exer-cises, open-ended short-answer questions, and responding to some standardized health and well-being instruments (see Gifford et al., 2009). Given that students collectively spoke more than 20 different languages, the length of the data collection instrument, and the small amount of funding for the project, it was not feasible to translate the settlement journal into community languages. Instead, students were divided up by language group, with 3 to 10 students in each group who then worked with a bicultural worker, interpreter, or multicultural education aide to complete the activities. While there are obvious methodological limitations to this approach, it proved to be well accepted by both students and teachers as the study was seen to contribute to learning English and gaining new skills.

Finally, in order to give something back to participants, we designed the data collection to take place in the form of a Settlement Journal, which young people could keep as a document of their first five years in Australia. Questions and instruments within the Settlement Journal were not designed to be a self-administered survey; rather it was to be administered with the assistance of a bilingual interpreter or researcher. Training was provided to interpreters/research assistants on the administration of the data collection instruments and on the process for clarification of questions. Given the diversity of language and literacy skills among the participants and the limitation of resources, it was not feasible to translate the Settlement Journals into all languages and it was not possible to carry out cross-cultural validity of standardized instruments (Brown, 2003). However, method triangulation has been used to increase the rigor of the data (Patton, 2002). Many visual methods were used in the study to accommodate limited language and literacy, and also to provide other mediums by which young people could express and present their experiences. Data collection in years 2, 3, and 4 took place in a range of venues including schools, libraries, and homes.

Logistics of Analysis

Studies that combine qualitative and quantitative data present many challenges for analysis, particularly given that each requires a different set of skills and approaches. Added to these issues is the fact that this study has had to address issues of missing data, resulting from participants having different levels of confidence and skills. For example, the completion of qualitative exercises varied in the first year of data collection, with some young people choosing to use very simplistic sketches or a few words only. Some of the standardized questions eliciting quantitative information were equally challenging for some young people and so, while all participants completed their journals, some of the items in the journals were left blank. Experience in the second year of data collection indicates that participants were better able to complete all of the exercises and questions. The problem of missing data has been dealt with in a number of ways including follow up of participants for additional sessions and the use of specific statistical techniques. In sum, although every attempt has been made to ensure full completion of the journals, the problems of missing data have been an ongoing challenge for this study.

Quantitative data was analyzed using mixed effects models with a random intercept for each subject and an exchangeable correlation structure was used to model the effect of independent variables on outcome measures over time. The Generalized Estimating Equations model was used to run these longitudinal models (Diggle et al., 1996) as participants with incomplete data have not been excluded (Twisk and Vente, 2002).

Qualitative data including drawings, photo novellas, open-ended responses, field notes, and interview and focus group transcripts have been managed with the assistance of NVivo 7, a qualitative software package. Thematic, content, and narrative analysis (Patton, 2002) are the key strategies informing interpretation of qualitative data.

LOOKING BACK: WHAT DID WE LEARN?

Good Starts successfully completed four years of follow-up and it remains one of the few studies to explore settlement experiences and outcomes among young people with refugee backgrounds over time. Longitudinal studies require a substantial commitment of resources, such as time, money, and personal commitment of the research team and of the participants. Especially with mobile study populations such as refugee migrants, follow-up becomes a major hurdle. It is not only that the study population, in this case settled refugee migrant youth, remained mobile over time, but also the contexts in which they live are also changing. Vigh (2009) has described this as "motion squared" and is an important insight for social research into experiences of refugee displacement, flight, and settlement. In the case of the Good Starts study, participants moved houses, changed schools, and moved interstate. The social environment also changed over time—family and households became reconfigured as new members arrived from overseas or moved out to live with other family households. The Australian policy environment was and remains fluid as settlement and youth service models change and as the broader political context of Australia's humanitarian program and border control policies respond to the flux of irregular migration. An important lesson from Good Starts is that change lies not only at the heart of longitudinal study designs, but also at the heart of the refugee experience, and change does not stop with settlement. People and place remain ever-changing.

The realities of change have made it particularly difficult to produce policy-relevant results in a timely manner. We had to wait until the end of the four-year follow-up before we could analyze and report on quantitative findings and while qualitative insights were published along the way (see, e.g., McMichael et al., 2009; Sampson and Gifford, 2010), they could not be linked to the quantitative outcomes. This was especially difficult for the research partner settlement organization, which needed timely evidence to support their submissions for policy change and bids for program funding. It is difficult for longitudinal studies like Good Starts to produce policy-relevant evidence in the short term. A key lesson learned from this study is that the expectations about timing of study results need to be made clear to both funders and industry partners. Longitudinal studies may not fit their short-term interests, especially in a volatile policy environment.

A second key lesson had to do with the timing of recruitment into the study. Because we wanted to measure settlement from the time participants entered Australia, we aimed to begin data collection no longer than six months after arrival. While working through the ELS was a good strategy for recruiting participants and to administer the first round of data collection, we question the validity of some of the first-year data. Despite the efforts to acquaint participants with research tools and processes, they had difficulties responding to scales and to yes/no questions. We felt that there was a strong courtesy bias operating, with which participants were keen to please researchers perhaps in the same ways that they were keen to please their teachers and their settlement workers. We wonder if the task of trying to be "a good refugee settler" impacted their responses to some of the items. Additionally, some questions, for example, those that focused on social relationships and family, were answered differently in year one to year two. For example, in some cases a participant's mother in year one became her aunty in year two—a result of participant's reluctance to disclose relationships about family reunion for polygamous families. Finally, qualitative interviews and group discussions were especially difficult in year one because of the linguistic diversity between the cohort and their limited knowledge of English.

The second and subsequent years brought different challenges as participants moved into mainstream schools, took on jobs, had additional family responsibilities, and began to live life as a teenager in Australia (enjoying movies, recreational activities, hanging out with friends). Good Starts youth were no longer captive, they were increasingly mobile and life had begun to open up and they had other things to do besides Good Starts. However, because of the effort invested in making them feel part of something special, we managed to retain participants. Indeed, in interviews conducted at the end of the four years, many said they were sorry that Good Starts had ended. They explained that they appreciated the fact that the Good Starts researchers were interested in how they were faring and what they were doing (Gifford et al., 2009). For many, the Good Starts study provided ongoing relationships with Australian researchers and through this, a bridge to the wider Australian society.

The building of personal relationships with the Good Starts participants has proven particularly important for these youth. The Good Starts researchers were often the first people they got to know outside of their own ethic community who were not their teachers or from the settlement or youth welfare sector. Importantly, the Good Starts researchers were all young and provided a bridge to youth culture in Australia more broadly. These relationships can be criticized as an intervention possibility biasing the results. However, with potentially vulnerable groups like these youth, there is an ethical and moral obligation with intensive studies like Good Starts to ensure that the research contributes positively to the settlement experience in Australia. Indeed, Good Starts can be seen as a valuable resource for the participants in learning how to go about making their future in their new country.

In considering the mix of methods for data collection, we found that visual techniques (photographs, drawings, maps) worked well in the first two years, but not as well in the last two years. Participants grew up and learned English and many were no longer interested in the more artistic approaches we used for data collection. The fourth year of data collection proved especially challenging as many of the participants were either too busy to meet and/or they found doing the Settlement Journal yet again, too boring. Thus, we developed a minimum data tool, which we used for some of the participants over the phone. Once again we found that change was core to this longitudinal study with the methods having to be adapted as the cohort matured.

Good Starts aimed to gather high-quality, rich, and in-depth qualitative data throughout the four years. A key intention was that the quantitative and qualitative data would complement each other and together provide a more holistic picture of settlement over time. However, doing justice to the qualitative component of this study proved difficult. Each year, researchers conducted interviews on a particular theme with a subsample of the cohort. However, the interviews were not as rich as they could have been in part because an additional time commitment from participants was required, and they already had spent a considerable amount of time and effort in relation to the main data collection each year. All the researchers kept detailed field notes and these proved to be more useful in many ways than the qualitative interviews conducted with the youth. The field notes continued over the four years for each participant and thus provided greater insight than the once off in-depth interviews. Additionally, the field notes were important for recording the methodological issues that arose and for elaborating on the back stories to key life events of these youth over time.

Finally, The Settlement Journals and the production of high-quality materials proved a success. We employed a graphic designer so that the research tools were attractive and integrated year to year and in the themed research reports. I think that this let the youth know that we cared about their time and we were able to offer them a journal they could keep of their settlement journey over time.

MEANING OR MEASUREMENT?

The Good Starts Study is a mixed methods study, with the product attempting to marry two different approaches to researching well-being and refugee settlement over time. Through a combination of theory and methods from anthropology and social epidemiology, the aim was to design a study that produced both meaning and measurement. Has this been achieved? The answer to this question is yes and no. Yes, we have been able to measure the social determinants of well-being and settlement over time. Yes we have been able to gain important, in-depth understandings of how young people experience the circuitous settlement journey. Yes, we have been able to use all of the data yielded from this mixed method approach in building an evidence base for policy and practice. But we have not been able to obtain truly ethnographically thick descriptions of settlement experiences or what it means to young people navigating new settlement scapes. Although we have integrated both qualitative and quantitative findings in the full final study report (Gifford et al., 2009), it is a challenge to do justice to both kinds of data in shorter journal style manuscripts. In sum, mixed methods studies are always challenging and Good Starts was all the more so because of the explicit attempt to combine ethnography with epidemiology.

The Good Starts Study has been a methodological adventure and the ultimate challenge for someone like myself with training both in anthropology and epidemiology. Almost 30 years ago, when I was a Ph.D. student in medical anthropology, I co-chaired a panel titled Anthrodemiology at the annual meetings of the American Anthropology Association. The panel was composed of Ph.D. students who, like myself, also had degrees in epidemiology. We were trying to bridge the divide between the two disciplines recognizing that, in the world of public health and applied medical anthropology, both meaning and measurement were necessary. The reaction to our panel title was scoffed at by some of the senior anthropologists who commented on the silliness of trying to merge these two disciplines. As foolhardy as this may have been, I remain committed to the importance of multiple understandings that the mix of qualitative and quantitative methods brings. I remain no less idealistic about the strengths of both and no less blind to their weaknesses. Meaning and measurement are complementary and, if in reality, doing one a little bit better means doing the other a little bit less, it is still a worthy goal to set out to achieve a synthesis.

EPILOGUE

In 2011, the Department of Immigration and Citizenship secured significant funding to carry out a large-scale longitudinal study of humanitarian settlement. My colleague and co-investigator, Ignacio Correa-Velez, and I sit as members of the Technical Advisory Committee in our role as social scientists. We are both gratified that there is acknowledgment of the need for longitudinal research on refugee settlement and the need for mixed methods. There is a proposed nested qualitative study to sit alongside the quantitative component. And finally, a fifth follow-up of the Good Starts participants, now that they are in their mid-twenties, has been funded. Good Starts 2 will have a minimal quantitative data instrument with a more focused, in-depth qualitative component—a dialog, a conversation—with the Good Starts participants, reflecting on life in Australia, past, present, and future.

ACKNOWLEDGEMENTS

Funding for Good Starts (2) is being provided by the Australian Research Council–Discovery Grant and is being conducted by Dr. Celia McMichael, Dr Ignacio-Correa-Velez, and myself. I wish to acknowledge my co-authors Dr. Ignacio Correa-Velez, Christine Bakopanos, and Dr. Ida Kaplan, of the original paper "Meaning or Measurement? Researching the Social Contexts of Health and Settlement among Newly Arrived Refugee Youth in Melbourne, Australia," published in the *Journal of Refugee Studies* in 2007. Funding for Good Starts (1) was provided by VicHealth, Foundation House (VFST), and La Trobe University Faculty of Health Sciences. Thank you so very much to Dr. Cathy Banwell who urged me to write this chapter and began by giving the original paper a good edit. I am grateful to Annika Lems for assistance in chasing and tidying references.

REFERENCES

Ahearn, F.L. (Ed.), 2000. Psychosocial Wellness of Refugees: Issues in Qualitative and Quantitative Research, Berghahn Books, Oxford.

Alverson, H., Alverson, M., Drake, R.E., 2000. An ethnographic study of the longitudinal course of substance abuse among people with severe mental illness. Community Mental Health Journal 36 (6), 557–569.

Barley, S.R., 1990. Images of imaging: notes on doing longitudinal field work. Organization Science 1 (3), 220–247.

Bell, R., Pavis, S., Amos, A., Cunningham-Burley, S., 1999. Continuities and changes: teenage smoking and occupational transition. Journal of Adolescence 22, 683–694.

Black, R., 2001. Fifty years of refugee studies: from theory to policy. International Migration Review 35 (1), 57–78.

Bloch, A., 1999. Carrying out a survey of refugees: some methodological considerations and guidelines. Journal of Refugee Studies 12 (4), 367–383.

Block, K., Warr, D., Gibbs, L., Riggs, E., 2012. Addressing ethical and methodological challenges in research with refugee-background young people: reflections from the field. Journal of Refugee Studies First published online May 7, 2012.

Boyden, J., Ennew, J., 1997. Children in focus—a manual for participatory research with children. Radda Barnen-Swedish Save the Children, Stockholm.

Briant, N., Kennedy, A., 2004. An investigation of the perceived needs and priorities held by African refugees in an urban setting in a first country of asylum. Journal of Refugee Studies 17 (4), 437–459.

Brough, M., Gorman, D., Ramirez, E., Westoby, P., 2003. Young refugees talk about well-being: a qualitative analysis of refugee youth mental health from three states. Australian Journal of Social Issues 38 (2), 193–209.

Brown, K., 2003. A Critical Ethnography of the Cross-Cultural Adaptation of HRQoL Instruments. Doctor of Philosophy, Thesis entitled: Deakin University.

Correa-Velez, I., Gifford, S., Bisht, T., 2005. Systematic review of longitudinal studies of refugee youth well being. Unpublished. Refugee Health Research Centre. La Trobe University, Melbourne, Australia.

Correa-Velez, I., Gifford, S., Barnett, G., 2010. Longing to belong: social inclusion and wellbeing among youth with refugee backgrounds in the first three years in Melbourne, Australia. Social Science & Medicine 71 (8), 1399–1408.

Coventry, L., Guerra, C., Mackenzie, D., Pinkney, S., 2002. Wealth of all nations: Identification of strategies to assist refugee young people in transition to independence. National Youth Affairs Research Scheme, Hobart, Australia.

Diggle, P.J., Liang, K.Y., Zeger, S.L., 1996. Analysis of Longitudinal Data. Oxford University Press, Oxford.

Dimia Department of Immigration and Multicultural and Indigenous Affairs, 2004. Settlement Data Base. ACT, Australia.

Dimia Department of Immigration and Multicultural and Indigenous Affairs, 2005. Population Flows: Immigration Aspects 2004-2005 Edition. ACT: Department of Immigration and Multicultural and Indigenous Affairs, Belconnen.

Gagnon, A.J., Tuck, J., 2004. A systematic review of questionnaires measuring the health of resettling refugee women. Health Care for Women International 25 (2), 111–149.

Gifford, S.M., Bakopanos, C., Kaplan, I., Correa-Velez, I., 2007. Meaning or Measurement? Researching the social contexts of health and settlement among newly-arrived refugee youth in Melbourne, Australia. Journal of Refugee Studies 20 (3), 414–440.

Gifford, S.M., Correa-Velez, I., Sampson, R., 2009. Good starts for recently arrived youth with refugee backgrounds: promoting wellbeing in the first three years of settlement in Melbourne. La Trobe Refugee Research Centre, La Trobe University, Melbourne, Australia. 1–132.

Hines, A.M., 1993. Linking qualitative and quantitative methods in cross-cultural survey research: techniques from cognitive science. American Journal of Community Psychology 21 (6), 729–746.

Hollifield, M., Warner, T.D., Lian, N., Krakow, B., Jenkins, J.H., Kesler, J., Stevenson, J., Westemeyer, J., 2002. Measuring trauma and health status in refugees. Journal of the American Medical Association 288 (5), 611–621.

Hyman, I., Vu, N., Beiser, M., 2000. Post-migration stresses among southeast Asian refugee youth in Canada: a research note. Journal of Comparative Family Studies 31 (2), 281–293.

Hynes, T., 2003. The issue of 'trust' or 'mistrust' in research with refugees: Choices, caveats and considerations for researchers. New Issues in Refugee Research, Working Paper No. 98, Geneva: UNHCR.

Jacobsen, K., Landau, L., 2003. Researching refugees: Some methodological and ethical considerations in social science and forced migration. New Issues in Refugee Research, Working Paper No. 90, Geneva: UNHCR.

Johannsen, A.M., 2001. 'Participatory action-research in post-conflict situation: The example of the war-torn societies project,' Berghof Handbook for Conflict Transformation. Berghof Research Center for Constructive Conflict Management, Berlin.

Karlsen, E., 2011. 'Refugee resettlement to Australia: what are the facts?' Background Note, 6 December 2011. Parliamentary Library, Parliament of Australia, Department of Parliamentary Services, Canberra.

Kopinak, J.K., 1999. The use of triangulation in a study of refugee well-being. Quality and Quantity 33, 169–183.

Loizos, P., 2000. Are refugees social capitalists? In: Baron, S., Field, J., Schuller, T. (Eds.), Social Capital: Critical Perspectives, Oxford University Press, Oxford.

Marlowe, J., 2010. Beyond the discourse of trauma: shifting the focus on Sudanese refugees. Journal of Refugee Studies 23 (2), 183–198.

Marlowe, J., 2011. Walking the line: Southern Sudanese masculinities and reconciling one's past with the present. Ethnicities 12 (1), 50–66.

Maton, K.I., 1993. A bridge between cultures: linked ethnographic-empirical methodology for culture anchored research. American Journal of Community Psychology 21 (6), 747–775.

Mcleod, J., 2000. Subjectivity and schooling in a longitudinal study of secondary students. British Journal of Sociology of Education 21 (4), 501–521.

McMichael, C., Gifford, S.M., Correa-Velez, I., 2009. Negotiating family, navigating resettlement: family connectedness amongst resettled youth with refugee backgrounds living in Melbourne, Australia. Journal of Youth Studies 14 (2), 179–195.

Moerman, M., 1993. Ariadne's thread and Indra's net: reflections on ethnography, ethnicity, identity, culture and interaction. Research on Language and Social Interaction 26 (1), 85–98.

Nathan, S., Bunde-Birouste, A., et al., 2010. Social cohesion through football: a quasi-experimental mixed methods design to evaluate a complex health promotion program. BMC Public Health 10, 587.

Patton, M.Q., 2002. Qualitative Research and Evaluation Methods. Sage, Thousand Oaks.

Porter, M., Haslam, N., 2005. Predisplacement and postdisplacement factors associated with mental health of refugees and internally displaced persons. Journal of American Medical Association 294 (5), 602–612.

Powles, J., 2004. Life history and personal narrative: theoretical and methodological issues relevant to research and evaluation in refugee contexts. New Issues in Refugee Research: Working paper no. 106, Geneva: UNHCR.

Robinson, S., Marsland, L., 1994. Approaches to the problem of respondent attrition in a longitudinal panel study of nurses' careers. Journal of Advanced Nursing 20, 729–741.

Rogers, G., 2004. 'Hanging out' with forced migrants: methodological and ethical challenges. Forced Migration Review 21, 48–49.

Rose, D., Buck, N., Corti, L., 1991. Design issues in the British Household Panel Study. Working Papers of ESRC Research Centre on micro-social change. University of Essex, Colchester.

Rousseau, C., Mekki-Berrada, A., Moreau, S., 2001. Trauma and extended separation from family among Latin American and African refugees in Montreal. Psychiatry 64 (1), 40–59.

Sampson, R., Gifford, S., 2010. Place-making, settlement and well-being: the therapeutic landscapes of recently arrived youth with refugee backgrounds. Health & Place 16 (1), 116–131.

Schweitzer, R., Steel, Z., 2008. Researching Refugees: Methodological and Ethical Considerations. Doing Cross-Cultural Research, P. Liamputtong, Springer Netherlands 34: 87–101.

Sherman, S., Latkin, C., 1999. A qualitative exploratory study of injection drug users' participation in a long-term epidemiological study of HIV. AIDS and Behavior 3 (4), 289–299.

Sissons, J., 1999. Siteless ethnography: possibilities and limits. Social Analysis 43 (2), 88–95.

Sturgess, P., Phillips, C., 2010. Google, email and Facebook: Internet literacy to improve the health and well-being of newly arrived refugees and migrants. A Pilot Study. MSJA Research Papers 2(2), http://eview.anu.edu.au/medical_journal/vol2_10_12/pdf/whole04.pdf#page=11.

Sturgess, P., Philips, C., 2009. Enhancing Internet literacy as a health promotion strategy for refugees and migrants. Health Promotion Journal of Australia 20 (3), 247.

Svensson, M., Ekblad, S., et al., 2009. Making meaningful space for oneself: photo-based dialogue with siblings of refugee children with severe withdrawal symptoms. Children's Geographies 7 (2), 209–228.

Svensson, M., Ekblad, S., et al., 2009. Making meaningful space for oneself: photo-based dialogue with siblings of refugee children with severe withdrawal symptoms. Children's Geographies 7 (2), 209–228.

Twisk, J., Vente, W., 2002. Attrition in longitudinal studies: How to deal with missing data. Journal of Clinical Epidemiology 55, 329–337.

Uncles, M.D., 1988. Issues in longitudinal data analysis. In: Uncles, M.D. (Ed.), Longitudinal Data Analysis: Methods and Applications, Pion/Methuen, London.

VFST, 1996. Guide to Working with Young People who are Refugees. Victorian Foundation for Survivors of Torture, Melbourne.

Vigh, H., 2009. Motion squared: a second look at the concept of social navigation. Anthropological Theory 9 (4), 419–438.

Wilding, R., 2009. Refugee youth, social inclusion, and ICTs: can good intentions go bad? Journal of Information, Communication and Ethics in Society 7 (2/3), 159–174.

Chapter 25

The Cultural Economy Approach to Studying Chronic Disease Risks, with Application to Illicit Drug Use

Jane Dixon and Cathy Banwell

The Australian National University, Canberra, Australia

DISEASES OF MODERNITY AND CONSUMPTION

Over the same period in which the epidemiologic transition described in Chapter 1 has been taking hold, sociologists have been describing the greater sophistication in commodity production and marketing, and the importance of new modes of niche production and consumption (Allen, 1992). Producers strategically use price (market) and brand (cultural) symbols to communicate to different socioeconomic groups. They use consumer research and flexible production systems to refine product qualities—taste, appearance, and any number of emotional associations—and mass, specialized, and viral media are used to target and communicate with consumers.

Consumption-related practices can cause harm for different reasons:

- The nature of the commodity itself (tobacco, some illicit drugs)
- Excessive consumption of the commodity (alcohol, saturated fat foods, car use entailing unsafe speed)
- The hazards of the practices that facilitate commodity consumption (violent crime to obtain money for gambling and drugs, sharing needles for drug use)

In some of these instances, less affluent groups pay a disproportionate amount of their income to be able to participate in these forms of consumption, which in turn denies them income to repair any damage done by the commodities (Froud et al., 2002). This vicious cycle contributes in part to the unequal distribution of modern diseases.

While consumption behavior risks generally begin in affluent subpopulations, the social gradients of most risk behaviors reverse as more advantaged populations adjust their consumption practices in line with health-promoting

When Culture Impacts Health. http://dx.doi.org/10.1016/B978-0-12-415921-1.00025-7

principles and as lower socioeconomic status groups become sufficiently afflu-ent to adopt the harmful commodities and practices. As a result, poorer groups in modernizing and modern nations are subject to a "double burden" of disease: they experience diseases of poverty and affluence simultaneously and synergis-tically (Prentice, 2006).

Consumption plays a leading role in governing and facilitating socially acceptable ways of living and is enshrined in what we call the "consumptogenic environment." The conditions underpinning the consumptogenic environment involve the routine yet unscrutinized encouragement and enabling of the con-sumption of a range of goods and services. The concept of the consumptogenic environment usefully highlights the structural forces that underpin what are considered to be an individual's "choice" to smoke, use harmful drugs, and eat fatty foods. As we gradually acquire empirical evidence and understanding of how many of the causes of modern disease and disability are based in danger-ous consumptions, there is a particular urgency to better understand the reasons behind the consumption choices that people make.

STUDYING THE CULTURAL ECONOMY OF CONSUMPTION

The consumptogenic environment is the outcome of social action occurring at two levels. At the societal level, it reflects efforts from cultural actors working alongside economic actors to encourage market transactions. At the subpopula-tion level, routines and practices are forged around consumption as individuals go about their daily lives: moving about in physical and social space, paying money for goods, and adorning themselves with the symbols appropriate to their status group.

To find out how the consumptogenic environment shapes healthy and unhealthy practices, we have applied a byproduct of more than two centuries of interdisciplinary endeavor that goes by the name "cultural economy" theory. Cultural economy theory (Harvey, 1989; Lash and Urry, 1994) contends that the supply and demand of goods, services, and experiences are not innocent or freely chosen; instead they are contingent upon the conscious acceptance of various ideas associated with the good life, a healthy life, a moral life, and a disciplined life. This view accommodates people's "pursuit of many goals at once: from meeting material needs and accumulating riches to seeking symbolic satisfaction and satisfying fleeting pleasures" (Amin and Thrift, 2004, p. xiv). Understanding consumption involves exploring the sources of gratification and esteem that surround a commodity or a social practice, as well as its material costs and benefits.

This perspective has been applied in exploring the way products and services are increasingly identified on the basis of perceptions of their qualities, and how the value adding of quality takes place (Callon et al., 2004). It has also been used to identify how commercial pressures can promote the circulation of some ideas and limit the circulation of unorthodox or oppositional ideas (Negus, 2002).

Cultural economy theory focuses attention on how commodities and practices are bestowed with social uses and prized qualities. In asking why people consume what they do, cultural economy research attends to people's expectations and conventions, and who produces these expectations and conventions (Shove, 2003, p. 9).

Theory about cultural economy has been accreting for centuries. Amin and Thrift (2004) dated its origins to Adam Smith and *The Theory of Moral Sentiments* written 250 years ago. Smith was explicit about the appropriateness of moral judgments guiding economic behavior. In the mid-nineteenth century, Karl Marx provided evidence of a rich convergence between the Protestant Reformation and the emergence of capitalism, and half a century later, Max Weber (1947) showed how capitalism's consolidation was due to Calvinist values.

Pierre Bourdieu (1984), who has been ordained the father of cultural economy (Lash, 1990), brought to the fore the importance of cultural and economic actors in shaping what is deemed acceptable to consumers, thereby maximizing the likelihood of consumption. He highlighted the powerful role of cultural intermediaries, actors who imbue products and services with their acceptable and desirable qualities, by appealing to (and indeed, influencing) the values and expectations of particular groups. These might include government regulators who issue dietary guidelines and product safety guidelines, advertisers and marketers who symbolically represent the capital gains from using products in certain ways, and academics who benchmark standards like cost-benefit and efficiency.

We have incorporated these insights into an approach for analyzing a range of consumption domains pertinent to health. In the following section we lay out the approach before applying it to illicit drug use.

THE CULTURAL ECONOMY APPROACH TO UNDERSTANDING SOCIAL PRACTICES

The method that we have developed is based on the "4 As" model illustrated in Figure 25.1. The model places emphasis on both culture and economy in explaining the "adoption" of commodities or practices by subpopulations.

"Availability" refers to the production and distribution of a commodity or practice. Data on availability can include aspects of production (e.g., sales rates); changes in price and factors that have influenced price; the extent of distribution (e.g., ownership rates or descriptions of accessibility); the presence (or lack) and quality of supporting infrastructure; and, importantly, the availability of alternatives.

"Acceptability" describes the ways in which a commodity or practice is rendered known, esteemed, or normal. Descriptions of acceptability require a historical account of the invention, its development and diffusion; common discourses pertaining to the commodity (including values, meanings, the extent of its normalization); symbolism of both the commodity itself and its industry; the

The Cultural Economy of Goods and Practices

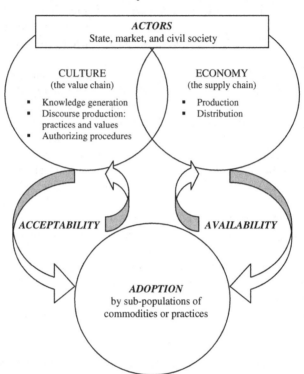

FIGURE 25.1   The cultural economy of goods and practices.

impacts of the commodity and practice on everyday life and experiences; the function of the commodity or practice in the performance of roles (e.g., gender roles); impacts on society and the environment; and, once again, the acceptability of alternatives.

Availability and acceptability are represented as overlapping because both processes are interdependent and essential in influencing the extent and character of the commodity or practice's "adoption," or consumption.

The adoption part of the cultural economy model (see Figure 25.1) represents the point at which processes of availability and acceptability are differentially acted upon by subpopulation groups. In describing adoption, we utilize Bourdieu's explanations of how structure shapes cultural practices and behaviors.

Bourdieu (1988) theorized that social life consists of individuals who are constantly competing for multiple kinds of capital. Competition for capital is hardly ever conducted openly or consciously. He asserted that individuals and social groups compete for capital through social practices, and in particular the ownership and uses of goods.

The adoption of a commodity or practice must be examined using group- and individual-level data for subpopulation groups. Adoption of the consumption trend can be informed by survey data, ideally augmented by in-depth interviews or focus groups to ascertain socioeconomic variations in motivations and justifications for adopting or eschewing a particular consumption practice. Comparing the reasons given by social groups for consuming dangerously or healthy provides not only practical insights for health promotion agencies but allows for a more complete rendering of the class-ridden nature of disease.

Finally, the cultural economy model highlights the overarching role of "actors," some of whom benefit from promoting the commodity or practice while others benefit from resisting its production, distribution, and consumption. Actors operate at the collective unit, such as the firm, the union, and transnational body like the World Trade Organization, and at the individual level, such as the worker, housewife, and student. Actors operate within the spheres of the market, the State, and also civil society and may include political parties, government departments, private companies, community group, citizens, and consumers.

Through using key informant interviews (see Chapter 26) the method is capable of exploring the complex motivations and inter-relationships that encourage particular consuming practices. Using in-depth interviews and participant observation allows for the analysis of changing, contradictory, and even self-defeating aspects of various actors' involvement in consumption. Textual analysis of company and government documents, marketing campaigns, and other devices to transmit the cultural normalization of the practice is highly relevant also.

Data Sources

It is clear from the previous sections, that the data sources utilized in cultural economy studies are many and varied. They include academic literature, government reports, datasets from government surveys (e.g., census) and nonacademic or "gray literature" such as market research reports, details of government programs and spending, company performance (through annual reports), and advocacy and lobby group policy positions. Moreover, gray literature may become the subject of documentary analysis to show how the producers of these sources are involved in the processes of availability and acceptability.

Sources are searched strategically rather than completely in a way that is analogous to the nonrandom, theoretical, and purposive recruitment often used in theoretical or purposive sampling. Purposive or "information-rich" sampling can be refined throughout data collection to seek incidents, time periods, or people on the basis of important insights and emerging theoretical constructs (Patton, 1990). For example, in a cultural economy audit, documents pertaining to the defining moments in the social life of a commodity or practice are sought, along with those by or about "key informants." From these, subsidiary documents are followed up in a manner analogous to snowball sampling.

The data collection proves to be much more holistic than the model in Figure 25.1 might suggest: the emphasis on actors allows for a concurrent assessment of the processes of availability and acceptability. For example, the government may simultaneously provide subsidies for a commodity, while extolling the economic virtues of the industry, as has happened with Australia's car industry. Indeed actors may act in contradictory ways, simultaneously supporting availability of a commodity, while resisting its acceptability, or vice versa. It may resist taxations and other regulations making the products cheaper and easier to access as is happening with calls for the volumetric taxation of alcoholic beverages and restrictions of opening hours of licensed premises.

The 4 As framework offers a way for the researcher to organize, think about, and present the resulting complex and broad sweep of data. With the exception of adoption, the cultural economy method brings together mostly descriptive secondary data within a framework that enables comparisons. Rather than employ statistical comparisons, it compares and contrasts various historical events, deeds, and outcomes. The data are juxtaposed to enable the detection of complementary, reinforcing, and contradictory events; trends; and decisions.

Applying the Model to Illicit Drug Use

In terms of the adoption of illicit drug use, the 2004 National Drug Strategy Household Survey (NDSHS) (Australian Institute of Health and Welfare, 2005) estimates that more than 6 million Australians over the age of 14 have used illicit drugs in their lifetime. However, among subsections of the population, such as 20- to 29-year-old males, and for drugs, such as marijuana, the proportion of users is higher (29.3%).

The economic and health outcomes are not insignificant, with mortality and morbidity from drug use estimated to cost $6 billion annually (Department of Health and Ageing, 2006). The elements that make up this estimate include the costs of policing, prevention, and treatment, and the costs of lives abbreviated or lost through mental and physical illnesses and overdoses.

There were a total of 357 deaths attributed to opioids in 2004 (Degenhardt et al., 2006), but illicit drugs, particularly when administered via injection, are also implicated in the transmission of public health epidemics, including HIV/AIDS and Hepatitis C (HCV). By December 2004, 9,618 cases of AIDS and 6,590 deaths had been reported and 14,840 people were living with HIV/AIDS in Australia (National Centre for HIV Epidemiology and Clinical Research, 2005). An estimated 194,260 people were living with HCV (National Centre for HIV Epidemiology and Clinical Research, 2005). A small proportion of newly acquired HIV infections (2.4%) were attributed to injecting drug use, but this route was responsible for more than 73% of newly acquired HCV cases (National Centre for HIV Epidemiology and Clinical Research, 2005).

In Western societies psychotropic drugs are deemed socially unacceptable and made illegal, thereby curtailing their availability. However, the cultural economy model is highly applicable because it encourages investigation into the cultural and economic values that illicit drugs have for the individuals and organizations who both promote and oppose them.

Elements of the 4 As model have already been used in drug research, although rarely have the different strands been assembled in a theoretically informed model as we are proposing. To date, government agency research attention has focused primarily on the production and distribution of drugs and their availability in the Australian marketplace. For example, police seizure data are routinely used in modeling studies to produce estimates of the economic costs of illicit drug use, and the international and regional drug markets are analyzed for their impact on the availability of drugs on the street (Farrell and Thorne, 2005; Gibson et al., 2005). Academic researchers have investigated actors implicated in production and regulation in, for example, histories of drug use and drug policy (Berridge and Edwards, 1981; Ensor and Cooper, 2004), while others are concerned with the acceptability dimension of lifestyle choice or pleasure that illicit drugs hold. Often these accounts depict illicit drug users as pathological, deviant, and/or criminal with, for example, an addictive personality or poor coping skills (Brook and Stringer, 2005; Nurco et al., 1998).

Beyond the obvious producers, distributors, and consumers of illicit drugs, an audit of other actors involved in their regulation reveals a host of very different institutions whose very mission and identity are tied up with drug use: police forces, customs and other government departments occupied with their regulation, legislators, and drug education agencies, as well as church organizations, charities, and health care professionals that play a role managing the drug using population and attempting to prevent illicit drug use.

So who encourages drug use? While comparatively underdocumented thus far, illicit drugs make a contribution to the income of legitimate as well as illegitimate businesses. Cultural intermediaries, including recording companies and musicians, benefit from producing material that contains drug references, as do the companies that produce drug technologies, and promote and amplify the cultural meanings of illicit drugs among subgroups of the population. Research with young heroin users argues that music industry products coupled with musicians' behavior provides an incitement or excuse to use heroin. Drug use, some argue, has been normalized by the actions of cultural intermediaries creating a market of consumers "already predisposed to the chemical management of mood and behavior as means to the end of adapting to their world" (Agar and Reisinger, 2004). Australian research is more ambivalent about the influence of drug references in popular culture on the acceptability of illicit drugs to young people (Dance et al., 2006).

Irrespective of whether drug references in popular culture influence drug use, drugs are imbued by their promoters and users with subtle distinctions that are loaded with cultural meanings and have important, if not mortal, health consequences. Such distinctions can be found between the social meanings of cocaine rather than heroin, between injection and other routes of administration, or between using one brand of Ecstasy marked by a certain color or logo as opposed to another (Moore, 2004) or one form of heroin rather than another (Ciccarone and Bourgois, 2003). Just like the distinctions that legitimate products reveal, distinctions within the illicit drug world are socially meaningful and crucially important to those who understand the differences. They facilitate a process of social stratification that provides an alternative to that taking place in the "straight" world.

Despite higher socioeconomic status (SES) groups consuming illicit drugs at higher risk levels than lower SES people, Australian burden of disease data from 1999 show that low SES men and women are at greater risk of years of life lost due to disability from their consumption of these particular commodities (Mathers et al., 1999, p. 59). From a cultural perspective this finding is of little surprise. Commodities are rarely inherently dangerous, but it is their excessive consumption that is dangerous, and the hazardous contexts in which they are consumed. Low SES users are more exposed to disability and injury because of how/where they consume. They do not have access to the purer forms of the drugs, the safe equipment, or the safe injecting spaces. Instead of using in the household or exclusive club environment, they are consuming down dark alleys and in fight-prone hotels and clubs. As commodities become known as dangerous, high SES people do not shun the commodity altogether, rather they seek out the quality end of the range, such as party-use cocaine over low grade material.

These are the types of insights that are required by governments if they are to act on the data of who uses illicit drugs. Adopting a systematizing approach to the analysis of consumption of commodities and practices yields more complex, and potentially more useful, insights for those wanting to intervene on public health issues. Table 25.1 summarizes some of the elements of a cultural economy model of illicit drug use.

The cultural economy approach to illicit drugs reveals the often contradictory roles played by social actors. While governments trumpet their generosity in the funding of prevention and treatment programs, illicit drug users receive relatively little financial and moral support from government, particularly if the less visible forms of organizational supports and subsidies are considered. For drug users, government attention often comes in the form of penalties, incarceration, and treatment regimes that can be financially crippling because workforce participation may be curtailed. In the Australian context, despite the relatively lower health care costs of drug use than car use, governments use considerable resources to reduce their availability through law enforcement activity (Gibson et al., 2005), and to diminish their acceptability via government campaigns such as the National Illicit Drugs Campaign called Tough on Drugs. Since its launch, the Australian Government has committed more than $1.5 billion to the strategy for measures to reduce the supply of, demand for, and harm caused by, drugs

TABLE 25.1 Cultural Economy Audit of Illicit Drugs

The 3 As		Promotion	Resistance
Availability		"Backyard" producers Australian geographical proximity to producer countries Climate that encourages household marijuana production	Government criminal legislation and deterrent policies International treaties attempt to limit production and affect price changes
Acceptability		Images of needles, freedom, rebellion, pleasure, piercings, tattoos promoted through subcultures, in print media, film, clothes, music	Discourses of disease, sickness, Stigma, disciplinary sanctions, penal codes, moral high ground
Actors	State (a)	Indirectly through harm reduction policies and funding of safe injecting places	Public health policies Policing and criminal justice system
	Market (b)	Black market producing illicit drugs, e.g., new "designer" drugs Drug user technologies, e.g., new injecting methods	Private treatment clinics and jails Self-help literature Production of methadone, naltrexone
	Civil Society	Expectations of a medicinal quick fix Supporters of decriminalization, user groups	Religious groups, not-in-my-backyard movements

(Department of Health and Ageing, 2006). The practical necessities of controlling disease associated with injecting drug use has forced the government to adopt harm minimization policies like needle and syringe programs, which could be seen as a muted form of government support for illicit drug use, although this would be strongly denied (Ministerial Council on Drug Strategy, 1998).

Applied to illicit drug use, the cultural economy approach acknowledges that injecting drugs and related practices have cultural value for users, thereby contradicting orthodox economic assessments that drug use is irrational behavior because its use value is outweighed by social, health, and economic costs. Under the fourth "A," adoption, this approach encourages the investigation of individual responses to particular drugs through empirical research with subgroups, allowing the interrogation of terms such as "addiction" and "pleasure" (Keane, 2002; Brook and Stringer, 2005).

CONCLUSION

This paper addresses the roles of cultural and economic factors in the generation and transmission of disease. We argue that because consumption is based in culture as much as in economics, a method that can examine both fields simultaneously is required. The cultural economy approach provides a constructive way to address the availability and acceptability of what people eat, smoke, how they travel, and what they do for fun, and whose interests are being advanced from the uptake of a commodity or practice. It invites researchers to name and question "who" and "what" are responsible for the diseases of modernity. The approach we outline above has the capacity to contribute to the "epidemiology of ideas" (Audy and Dunn, 1974; Trostle, 2005), which concerns itself with the ways in which discourses and values circulate and encourage, or inhibit, health-related behaviors.

By revealing the complexities and interlinking processes behind a popular practice, researchers and policy makers may be better informed in making judgments about interventions or the "high leverage" aspects of the trend, and also in identifying the actors who will be supportive or resistant to such interventions. It also surfaces a number of possibilities regarding causation and associations, to better equip the epidemiologist or economist to include all the pertinent variables in their statistical models.

The cultural economy approach has another benefit. It operates at a sufficiently appropriate scale for governments and other institutional actors. One of the impediments to evidence-based policy is a lack of evidence at a scale deemed suitable for policy formulation (Lin and Gibson, 2003). Our proposed approach augments the many cross-sectional, longitudinal, and administrative datasets by explaining the social conditions that generate what is found in those data (for other examples see Hinde and Dixon, 2005; Dixon and Banwell, 2009).

REFERENCES

Agar, M., Reisinger, H.S., 2004. Ecstasy: commodity or disease? Journal of Psychoactive Drugs 36, 253–264.

Allen, J., 1992. Post-industrialism and post-Fordism. In: Hall, S., Held, D., McGrew, T. (Eds.), Modernity and its Futures. Polity Press, Cambridge, pp. 169–220.

Amin, A., Thrift, N., 2004. Blackwell Cultural Economy Reader. Blackwell Publishing, Malden.

Audy, J., Dunn, F., 1974. Community Health. In: Sargent, F. (Ed.), Human Ecology, North-Holland, Amsterdam.

Australian Institute of Health and Welfare, 2005. National drug strategy household survey: Detailed Findings. Australian Institute of Health and Welfare, Canberra.

Berridge, V., Edwards, G., 1981. Opium and the people. Opiate use in nineteenth-century England. St. Martin's Press, London.

Bourdieu, P., 1984. Distinction: A Social Critique of the Judgement of Taste. Routledge, London.

Bourdieu, P., 1998. Practical Reason. Polity Press, Cambridge.

Brook, H., Stringer, R., 2005. Users, using, used: a beginner's guide to deconstructing drugs discourse. The International Journal of Drug Policy 16, 316–325.

Callon, M., Meadel, C., Rabeharisoa, V., 2004. The economy of qualities. In: Amin, A., Thrift, N. (Eds.), The Blackwell Cultural Economy Reader. Blackwell Publishing, Malden, pp. 58–80.

Ciccarone, D., Bourgois, P., 2003. Explaining the geographical variation of IIIV among injection drug users in the United States. Substance Use and Misuse 38, 2049–2063.

Dance, P., Strachan, A., Deane, P., Bammer, G., 2006. Popular culture and the prevention of illicit drug use: A pilot study of popular music and the acceptability of drugs. Drug Policy Modelling Project NCEPH.

Degenhardt, L., Roxburgh, A., Black, E., Dunn, M., 2006. Accidental drug-induced deaths due to opioids in Australia. 2004. National Drug and Alcohol Research Centre, Sydney 2006.

Department of Health and Ageing, 2006. Tough on Drugs. Fact Sheet 4. http://www.health. gov.au/internet/main/publishing.nsf/Content/health-pubs-budget99-fact-hfact4.htm (accessed 20.10.12.).

Dixon, J., Banwell, C., 2009. Theoretically-driven research for explaining health risk transitions: the case of smoking. Social Science & Medicine 68, 2206–2214.

Ensor, T., Cooper, S., 2004. Overcoming barriers to health service access: influencing the demand side. Health Policy and Planning 19, 69–79.

Farrell, G., Thorne, J., 2005. Where have all the flowers gone? Evaluation of the Taliban crackdown against opium poppy cultivation in Afghanistan. International Journal of Drug Policy 16, 81–91.

Froud, J., Johal, S., Leaver, A., Williams, K., 2002. Not enough money: the resources and choices of the motoring poor. Competition & Change 6, 776–797.

Gibson, A., Degenhardt, L., Day, C., McKetin, R., 2005. Recent trends in heroin supply to markets in Australia, the United States, and Western Europe. The International Journal of Drug Policy 16, 293–299.

Harvey, D., 1989. The condition of postmodernity. Basil Blackwell, Oxford.

Hinde, S., Dixon, J., 2005. Changing the obesogenic environment: insights from a cultural economy of car-reliance. Transportation Research Part D - Transport and the Environment 10, 31–53.

Keane, H., 2002. What's wrong with addiction? Melbourne University Press, Melbourne.

Lash, S., 1990. The sociology of postmodernism. Routledge, London.

Lash, S., Urry, J., 1994. Economies of signs and space. Sage, London.

Lin, V., Gibson, B., 2003. Evidence-based health policy. Oxford University Press, Melbourne.

Mathers, C., Al, E., 1999. Burden of Disease and Injury in Australia. AIHW, Canberra.

Mathers, C., Vos, T., Stevenson, C., 1999. The Burden of Disease and Injury in Australia. AIHW, Canberra.

Ministerial Council on Drug Strategy Strategy, 1998. National Drug Strategic Framework 1998-99 to 2002-03: Building Partnerships. Commonwealth of Australia. Canberra.

Moore, D., 2004. Beyond "subculture" in the ethnography of illicit drug use. Contemporary Drug Problems 31, 181–212.

National Centre for HIV Epidemiology and Clinical Research, 2005. HIV/AIDS, viral hepatitis and sexually transmissible infections in Australia annual surveillance report 2005. AIHW, Canberra.

Negus, K., 2002. Identities and industries: the cultural formation of aesthetic economies. In: du Gay, P., Pryke, M. (Eds.), Cultural economy: cultural analysis and commercial life, Sage, London, pp. 115–131.

Nurco, D., Kinlock, T., O'Grady, K., Hanlon, T., 1998. Differential contributions of family and peer factors to the etiology of narcotic addiction. Drug and Alcohol Dependence 512, 229–237.

Patton, M.Q., 1990. Qualitative Evaluation and Research Methods. Sage, Newbury Park.

Prentice, A., 2006. The emerging epidemic of obesity in developing countries. International Journal of Epidemiology 35, 93–99.

Shove, E., 2003. Comfort, cleanliness and convenience. Berg, Oxford.

Trostle, J., 2005. Epidemiology and Culture. Cambridge University Press, Cambridge.

Weber, M., 1947. The theory of social and economic organization Free Press, New York.

Chapter 26

Doing Health Policy Research: How to Interview Policy Elites

Phillip Baker

National Centre for Epidemiology and Population Health, Australian National University

INTRODUCTION

Many studies in the domain of public health policy source their data from interviews with policy elites. Yet understanding, designing, and conducting "elite interviews" can pose a challenge for researchers. Some scholars have noted the considerable difficulties with, and offer practical guidance on gaining access to, planning and conducting interviews (Zuckerman, 1972; Aberbach and Rockman, 2002; Goldstein, 2002; Harvey, 2010, 2011), while ensuring validity and reliability in doing so (Berry, 2002). Others note the epistemological implications of interviewing elites (Bygnes, 2008; Morris, 2009; Neal and McLaughlin, 2009), while others reflect on the social dynamics and micro-power relations between highly empowered, intelligent, and knowledgeable informants and the less-empowered researcher (Herod, 1999; Smith, 2006; Walt et al., 2008). These are some of the most common problems inherent to "studying up," and researchers should familiarize themselves with them (Smith, 2006).

But first, what meaningful intersection is there between culture and this subset of societal actors? What or who, for that matter, are policy elites? From the health policy perspective, elites are the individuals who exercise considerable influence in the development of health policy. They are often considered "norm entrepreneurs"—those who actively shape beliefs, values, and expected behaviors important to policy and institutional decision making. In essence, they shape "governance culture." Understanding this level and type of culture is an important part of health policy analysis (Hoppe, 2007).

Key informant interviewing is a qualitative method for data collection commonly used in the social and political sciences. Interviews may be used in conjunction with other forms of qualitative method (e.g., document analysis) or with quantitative methods (often determined by a range of factors, including what might best answer the research questions, the study design, and the researchers' own preferences). It is a method used when one wishes to: learn what a group of people think about the concepts proposed by the research questions and aims;

When Culture Impacts Health. http://dx.doi.org/10.1016/B978-0-12-415921-1.00026-9

how they interpret certain events, people, or topics; how and why they have
made decisions in response to certain events; or to attain a particular document
or piece of information (Aberbach and Rockman, 2002; Goldstein, 2002).

In this chapter, I provide a step-by-step guide to designing and conducting
interviews with policy elites, drawn from reflections by other scholars (primarily Hertz and Imber, 1995; Aberbach and Rockman, 2002; Berry, 2002; Goldstein, 2002), but also from my own experience interviewing almost 50 elites
in Australia and internationally during my Ph.D. research. How interviews are
designed and conducted will depend, first and foremost, on the research questions and study objectives.

RESEARCH QUESTIONS AND STUDY OBJECTIVES

The first and most important step in interviewing is to formulate the research
questions and study objectives: what is to be generalized (Aberbach and Rockman, 2002; Goldstein, 2002)? Almost always, there will be a leading academic
(or set of academics) with an in-depth understanding of the research topic in
hand and the policy domain of interest. Such a person may be recruited for
an initial "exploratory" interview to critique the study and methodology, and
to map the general policy domain of interest. A literature review of the specific policy domain or a workshop with colleagues will also help to define and
articulate the research questions. Another recommended step is to review the
policy sciences literature in search of a theoretical framework that may be most
applicable to the topic.[1] Such frameworks may be thought of as "intellectual
scaffolding" on which the research questions are constructed.

The second step is to define who to interview by asking: Who will have
valid answers to these questions? This can be a tricky process, because unlike
in epidemiology, political elites are not always bound by shared and definite
population characteristics such as age, gender, income level, and so on. In policy terms, elites can be defined by membership within groups, referred to by
policy scholars in terms of epistemic communities (Haas, 1992), issue networks
(Heclo, 1978), policy communities (Miller and Demir, 2007), and policy networks. The latter, for example, can be defined as the groups of individuals or
organizations that are known to one another by reputation and have the capacity
to influence policy within a specific domain (Rhodes, 1997; Lewis, 2005). The
characteristics of members of networks will change depending on what policy
issue, or "domain" is under consideration (Wilks and Wright, 1987; Howlett
and Ramesh, 1995). Policy domains are often nested within other, mutually
inclusive, higher order domains. For example, within "health policy" there are
subdomains of health care, preventive health, indigenous health, and so on.

---

1. Two useful texts for students are Parsons, W., 1995. *Public Policy*. Edward Elgar, Cheltenham
and Sabatier, P.A., 2007. *Theories of the Policy Process*. Westview, Boulder.

SAMPLING STRATEGY AND REPRESENTATIVENESS

The next step is to design a sampling strategy—the process of selecting a set of individuals for a study, so that they are broadly representative of the larger group from which they were selected. The method I have used in my own research is peer-nomination snowball sampling (Goodman, 1961; Ostrander, 1995). This process involves identifying a number of initial elites within the domain of interest and asking each to nominate others based on specific criteria. For example, members of the elite may be asked to nominate other informants who may have an interesting point of view, or one that might conflict with their own, or to simply nominate others that they consider "influential." The sampling frame thereby snowballs as new informants are asked in turn to nominate others. Eventually (depending on the size of the network), few additional nominations are made and a robust sampling frame is approached.

The next question is how to increase the likelihood that the set of key informants being interviewed is broadly representative of the stakeholders within the policy domain under investigation (Berry, 2002; Goldstein, 2002). One way to understand this is to prepare a table listing stakeholder groupings (e.g., civil society, private sector, public sector, professions, and academics) and determine the proportion of respondents and nonrespondents in each group. This will determine what groupings of informants are under- or over-represented in the sample. The most common problem here is nonresponse: what proportion of the sampled population cannot be contacted and does not respond (and therefore participate) in the research? For example, the policy domain under investigation may include a diversity of stakeholders, and nonrespondents may be concentrated within a particular group (e.g., civil society or industry). Taking the above into account, adjust the sampling and recruitment process as the study proceeds in order to achieve representativeness.

RECRUITMENT AND PARTICIPANT MANAGEMENT

As Goldstein states, rigorous preparation is meaningless unless one "gets in the door" (Goldstein, 2002). Policy elites are often very busy individuals with many people competing for their time and attention. Although recruiting elites to a study is more art than science, a systematic recruitment strategy is very helpful. The first step in securing the interview involves sending a letter on an official letterhead (Goldstein, 2002). This should outline the basic aims of the research and clearly state the amount of time participating will involve—between 30 and 60 minutes should be appropriate (although interviews may run longer). It should also include answers that the elite might ask. Why were they selected? How will confidentiality be ensured? In what format will the information be published? Outlining next steps are also important. Indicate that the letter will be followed up with an e-mail or phone call. Thank them for their time. Include with the letter information and consent forms to provide more detail. If it is intended that particular information may be attributed to an individual, outline some options for their preferred level of anonymity. Alternatively, it may be easier to report on the interview results in aggregate form. The next step is to phone the potential informant, to discuss his or her participation, and ideally, to schedule an interview time.

If there is a low response rate, it is possible to change tactics. Faxing the letter can sometimes be a more effective way to get the person's attention—e-mail can be obsolete in this regard. Furthermore, the letter can be faxed straight to the person at the top of the organization of interest. Although one might not secure an interview with this individual, protocol usually ensures that the next most senior executive will be assigned to the interview (Drahos, 2010).

To streamline the management of the recruitment process a practical step is to design a participant management spreadsheet. This might include as column headings each elite member's study number, first and last name, position and organization, e-mail address and phone number, mailing address (for your letters), and also notes specific to the process (Has a letter been sent to him or her? Has a reply been received? When? And so on). Updating this as the study proceeds will save considerable time in the long term.

STRUCTURING THE INTERVIEWS

Interviews should be structured in a way that best informs the research questions and study objectives. Utilizing the appropriate interview structure will determine to what extent the answers inform the research questions (Kvale, 2009). There are three common forms of interviews: structured, unstructured, and semistructured. When deciding on structure (Aberbach and Rockman, 2002), it is important to know what is already known about the research topic. If the investigation is of a topic that has already had considerable investigation, it will be easier to define both the questions and possible responses. In this case, a structured interview might be appropriate. If the research topic is relatively new or an exploratory investigation is being undertaken, a semistructured or unstructured interview may be more suitable. This allows for maximum coverage of the subject area, and may generate interesting leads or new ideas. However, policy elites and other highly educated and empowered individuals may not react favorably to "being put in the straight-jacket of close-ended questions" (Aberbach and Rockman, 2002). On this basis, the rest of this chapter assumes the use of semistructured or unstructured interview formats that use open-ended questions.

VALIDITY AND RELIABILITY IN INTERVIEWING

Two important methodological issues in elite interviewing are validity or "how appropriate is the measuring instrument to the task at hand," and reliability or "how consistent are the results of repeated tests with the chosen measuring instrument?"

This, however, presents a paradox—the attainment of validity and reliability of structured interviewing is offset against the flexibility and responsiveness of open-ended questioning (Berry, 2002). The reliability of the interview questions might be tested by comparing the consistencies or inconsistencies of answers between similar informants included in your study, asking, does a question produce similar responses from similar informants (Goldstein, 2002)? Another test of validity and reliability is to determine the point (if any) at which data saturation is achieved—the point at which ongoing responses generate little to no further information.

WHAT QUESTIONS SHOULD BE ASKED?

Now it is time to generate the interview questions, yet there is a diversity of question types one might ask (Leech, 2002). Are the questions closed or open? The abstract nature and complexity of politics and policy necessitates that questions should be open, allowing informants to be probed for new informa-tion and allowing "maximum flexibility" as to how the informants shape their answers (Aberbach and Rockman, 2002). It may not be clear at this stage what is important and not important, and informants should be given flexibility in asserting exactly that. Open-ended questions in such a context also provide bet-ter response validity because informants can shape their answers through their own world views, rather than those imposed by closed questions (Aberbach and Rockman, 2002). And most simply, it is the opinions of respondents that are of primary interest—those from intelligent, experienced policy actors, and not their answers to a preconceived questionnaire placed within a constrict-ing framework. There are, however, risks to using open-ended questions; infor-mants might wander or go off topic, which means that a strategy must be in place to refocus their answers. Generally speaking, questions should be avoided when the answers can be found elsewhere (e.g., in documents).

In the formulation of specific interview questions, the intellectual scaffold-ing referred to earlier (policy science framework applicable to the work in hand) can be used as a guide. In my own work, for example, I have used the Multiple Streams (Zahariadis, 2007), the Advocacy Coalition (Sabatier and Jenkins-Smith, 1999), and Shiffman (Shiffman and Smith, 2007) frameworks. Each of these provides a set of hypotheses that can inform the development of interview questions.

New material will emerge in the interviews, and the researcher must take the opportunity to ask probing questions to explore particular points of inter-est. There can be verbal and nonverbal probes. Verbal probes might include, for example, "that is particularly interesting; please tell me more" or "and how does the Minister perceive that?" Nonverbal probes include remaining silent and appearing expectant, waiting for the informant to continue (Berry, 2002). Probe notes can also be written into the interview protocol for key areas of inter-est. If it is perceived that more information could be gained on a subject, or if no further information is arising from new questions, it is possible to double back by asking a "bridging question." For example, "You made a very interesting comment earlier about <insert subject here>. Do you mind elaborating on how that came about?" (Berry, 2002).

Before the Interview

It is important to research the individual or organization of interest before attending the interview. This will help to conceptualize the challenges and opportunities that the interview might present. Second, it is important to know the subject area to the extent that the interviewer knows what to talk about but never appears more knowledgeable than the informant on the subject. The informant is the expert, and should be treated as one (Leech, 2002). Third, it is important to dress and act professionally. The informant is less likely to respect the interviewer if he or she arrives in shabby garb. It is important to turn up early, and be polite to assistants. It is also important to make sure that a study consent form is prepared for interviewees to sign, with an additional copy for them to keep.

Technical Considerations

Unless an interviewer has an outstanding memory, it is worth recording the interview in some way. Notes can be made of key themes and quotes. This approach is less time-consuming than other methods, but it leaves less data to work with during analysis. There is also the risk of inadequately noting important points. Alternatively, a recording device may be used. Digital voice recorders are commonly used and some smartphones also have "apps" that serve this function. Some informants might find a recording device intimidating, however, and permission will be needed from them to record the interview. The benefit to using a recording device is that a record of the interviews can be stored and used as reference during analysis. Recordings can also be used to prepare text transcripts that can be uploaded into qualitative analysis software. A word of caution—every hour of interview time requires between three and four hours of transcription.

During the Interview

The opening dialog should be an informal one to build rapport with the informant, making him or her laugh if possible, discussing current events, the weather, etc. The point is to make him or her feel relaxed and receptive. If possible, a lead sentence should be placed in to the next section—for example, "X, thank you kindly for talking with me today as I know you must be busy" (Drahos, 2010). Ask, "How much time do you have?" This question should be used to ascertain how long the interview might go and to allow prioritization of questions accordingly. It is important for the interviewer to ask for the informant's business card and to be prepared with his or her own. The business card is important for keeping a record of informants' contact details, but also for ascertaining the nature of their occupation and position.

The next question is where best to interview? It is best to interview key informants in their office in their usual environment. They may, if asked correctly, provide key documents including memos, e-mails, and so on, that are useful to informing the research (Woliver, 2002; Drahos, 2010). It is sometimes necessary to interview participants "on-the-fly," such as in their car as they are driving, over lunch, or as they walk to a meeting. It is important to be prepared for these situations.

Taking notes will also allow quick identification of what the key points in the interview were, and to quickly search for these in the interview transcripts. Notes, in this sense, may allow the analysis of huge volumes of data more quickly. If it is not possible to take notes during the interview, it is important to rely on taking "mental notes" and transcribing them following the interview.

Before beginning any interview, the research topic should be verbally conceptualized, the "rules" of the interview outlined, and the consent form made available. For example;

I will begin by telling you about the research I have under way as a part of my research at <your place of employment>. My research aims are to <insert your research aims>. Today I would very much like to hear your thoughts on these topics as I know you are familiar with them. I have prepared a list of open-ended questions that will help to guide the interview today. I will protect your confidentiality completely whenever you express your desire for me to do so <explain the rules of the attribution here>. I will also ask you to sign this form, which constitutes your consent to be interviewed—please take your time to read it.

The rules of the interview are the journalistic rules of attribution (see Goldstein, 2002). Outlining these are important because the informant can confuse the meaning of "off the record" with "not for attribution" and valuable information may be lost (Goldstein, 2002). A good way to start is to ask harmless questions about the informant's background. For many informants, this will make them amenable to more probing questions (Aberbach and Rockman, 2002). It is then acceptable to refer to the list of questions or interview guide as appropriate, making sure that questions and question order are adapted to the responses of the informant. In relation to open-ended questioning, "the riskiest but potentially most valuable type of elite interviewing," it is important to "know when to probe and how to formulate follow-up questions on the fly" (Berry, 2002). The informant should be asked to clarify points that are unclear, and the informant's own language used by the interviewer to summarize what they have just said. Besides enhancing the validity of the responses, this will also communicate to the informant that you are listening. It is important not to reinterpret what has been said in the interviewer's own words (Leech, 2002; Kvale, 2009).

After the Interview

Once the interview is over, the informants should be thanked, directly, as well as later by letter or e-mail. They may not reply, but are likely to understand your appreciation. At this stage, the informants can be provided with a summary of the interview, or a copy of the transcript, providing them the opportunity to review their comments, and to ensure that their views have been accurately recorded and not misconstrued. This is known as "member-checking," which is an important part of any rigorous case study design (Yin, 1993).

CONCLUSION

This chapter has provided a how-to guide for designing and conducting interviews with health policy elites. My intention was to provide practical advice for those embarking on research that applies this method and to save researchers considerable time in the process. This chapter does not provide a comprehensive review of scholarship on this subject. To build further rigor into the interview method, I recommend a very detailed introduction to the subject including theoretical and other methodological issues in the book *Interviews: An Introduction to Qualitative Research Interviewing* by Kvale. The journal issue of *Political Science* 35(4) also provides a series of useful articles. Interviewing is, as others have described, "a high-wire act" (Berry, 2002). Nothing can replace learning through the process of "doing" interviews. An interviewer's skill set improves with practice and the validity and utility of interviewing will also improve with time. It can also become a pleasurable undertaking.

REFERENCES

Aberbach, J.D., Rockman, B.A., 2002. Conducting and coding elite interviews. PS: Political Science and Politics 35, 673–676.

Berry, J.M., 2002. Validity and reliability issues in elite interviewing. PS: Political Science and Politics 35, 679–682.

Bygnes, S., 2008. Interviewing people-oriented elites, Eurosphere online working paper series: Online Working Paper No. 10.

Drahos, P., 2010. Personal communication. Meeting at ANU, Canberra; April 23.

Goldstein, K., 2002. Getting in the door: sampling and completing elite interviews. PS: Political Science & Politics 35, 669–672.

Goodman, L., 1961. Snowball sampling. Annals of Mathematical Statistics 32, 148–170.

Haas, P.M., 1992. Introduction: epistemic communities and International Policy coordination. International Organization 46, 1–35.

Harvey, W.S., 2010. Methodological approaches for interviewing elites. Geography Compass 4, 193–205.

Harvey, W.S., 2011. Strategies for conducting elite interviews. Qualitative Research 11, 431–441.

Heclo, H., 1978. Issue networks and the executive establishment. In: King, A. (Ed.), The New American Political System, American Enterprise Institute for Public Policy Research, Washington, DC, pp. 87–124.

Herod, A., 1999. Reflections on interviewing foreign elites: praxis, positionality, validity, and the cult of the insider. Geoforum 30, 313–327.

Hertz, R., Imber, J.B., 1995. Studying elites using qualitative methods. Sage Publications, Thousand Oaks, Calif.

Hoppe, R., 2007. Applied cultural theory: Tool for Policy Analysis. In: Fischer, F., Miller, G., Sidney, M.S. (Eds.), Handbook of public policy analysis: theory, politics, and methods, CRC/Taylor & Francis, Boca Raton, pp. 289–308.

Howlett, M., Ramesh, M., 1995. Studying public policy. Oxford University Press, Oxford.

Kvale, S., 2009. Interviews: an introduction to qualitative research interviewing. Sage Publications, Thousand Oaks.

Leech, B.L., 2002. Asking questions: techniques for semistructured interviews. PS: Political Science & Politics 35, 665–668.

Lewis, J., 2005. Health Policy and Politics: networks ideas and power. IP Communications, Melbourne.

Miller, H., Demir, T., 2007. Policy communities. CRC Press, Boca Raton.

Morris, Z.S., 2009. The truth about interviewing elites. Politics 29, 209–217.

Neal, S., McLaughlin, E., 2009. Researching up? Interviews, emotionality and policy-making elites. Journal of Social Policy 38, 689–707.

Ostrander, S.A., 1995. 'Surely you're not in this just to be helpful': Access, rapport and interviews in three studies of elites. In: Imber, J.D. (Ed.), Studying elites using qualitative methods. Sage, Thousand Oaks.

Rhodes, R.W., 1997. Understanding governance: policy networks, governance, reflexivity and accountability. Open University Press, Buckingham.

Sabatier, P., Jenkins-Smith, H., 1999. The advocacy coalition framework: an Assessment. In: Sabatier, P. (Ed.), Theories of the policy process, Westview Press, Boulder, Colo., pp. 177–166.

Shiffman, J., Smith, S., 2007. Generation of political priority for global health initiatives: a framework and case study of maternal mortality. The Lancet 370, 1370–1379.

Smith, K., 2006. Problematising power relations in 'elite' interviews. Geoforum 37, 643–653.

Walt, G., Shiffman, J., Schneider, H., Murray, S.F., Brugha, R., Gilson, L., 2008. 'Doing' health policy analysis: methodological and conceptual reflections and challenges. Health Policy Plan 23, 308–317.

Wilks, S., Wright, M., 1987. Conclusion: Comparing Government-Industry Relations: States, Sectors, and Networks. In: Wilks, S., Wright, M. (Eds.), Comparative Government-Industry Relations: Western Europe, the United States, and Japan, Clarendon Press, Oxford, p. 301.

Woliver, L.R., 2002. Ethical Dilemmas in Personal Interviewing. PS: Political Science & Politics 35, 677–678.

Yin, R., 1993. Applications of case study research. Sage, London.

Zahariadis, N., 2007. The multiple streams framework: structures, limitations, prospects. In: Sabatier, P. (Ed.), Theories of the Policy Process, Westview Press, Cambridge, pp. 65–92.

Zuckerman, H., 1972. Interviewing an ultra-elite. Public Opinion Quarterly 36, 159–175.

Chapter 27

Thai Food Culture in Transition: A Mixed Methods Study on the Role of Food Retailing

Matthew Kelly, Cathy Banwell, Jane Dixon, Sam-ang Seubsman, and Adrian Sleigh

The Australian National University, Canberra, Australia

INTRODUCTION

In the modern world, urbanization, industrialization, and technological change have transformed food systems, affecting food production, processing, distribution, and retailing. A new globalized food environment has been created with transnational food corporations increasingly controlling all four of these aspects of the food system. Accompanying the changes have been profound changes in diet for much of the world's population. Traditional diets, particularly in urban areas, are being replaced by diets higher in fats, salts, sugar, and animal products and often with lower intakes of fresh fruits and vegetables—a nutrition transition. Such fundamental changes to the food system, along with increasing food availability and diversity, have helped countries worldwide reduce their levels of malnutrition and produce healthier populations in the short term. But in recent decades countries around the world, even the poorest countries, have begun to experience an epidemic of obesity and diet-related disease (Drenowski and Popkin, 1997; Chopra, 2002).

Thailand is a country with a strong food culture that is intimately connected to local agriculture and retail markets, which provide affordable sources of healthy fresh foods. It is important in this context to examine ways in which changes to this food culture may impact the health status of the Thai people. The ways in which local food cultures and diets react to these upstream influences in the global food system are complex and difficult to characterize. Teasing apart the positive and negative influences of a modernizing food system in developing country contexts is particularly problematic. However, the task is researchable and in this chapter we describe one approach adopted by a contemporary study in Thailand. This research assesses the interaction between the

When Culture Impacts Health. http://dx.doi.org/10.1016/B978-0-12-415921-1.00027-0
319

rapid modernization of food retailing in Thailand, Thai food culture and food preferences, and nutrition and health outcomes for Thai people in a context of rapidly rising obesity and diet-related diseases. To accomplish this, building on an overarching longitudinal study of the health-risk transition in Thailand (The Thai Cohort Study; TCS), an innovative mix of quantitative and qualitative methods is employed, as detailed below in the section Thai Food Culture Transition Study.

THAI TRANSITIONS

Economic Growth, Poverty Reduction, and Health Transitions

Thailand is a Southeast Asian country that has achieved a rapid and fundamental transformational economic growth and development over the past four decades. This has been achieved from a very low economic base; after World War II Thailand was considered one of the world's poorest countries and had not been observed to have experienced substantive economic growth for a century before this time. Since the 1960s, however, and accelerating in the 1980s, industrial development, as well as the commercialization of agriculture, resulted in 40 years of GDP growth (Warr, 2005). Thailand is now an upper middle income country with an annual GDP per capita of $4600 (World Bank, 2011). Economic growth in Thailand has occurred in a period of globalization and has involved profound social, cultural, and lifestyle changes for the Thai population. In 1960 over 80% of the Thai workforce was agricultural, and by the late 2000s this figure had fallen to around 35% (Kelly et al., 2010b). The changes in employment have also been accompanied by a process of urbanization; nearly half of all Thais now live in urban areas (Webster, 2005). These workforce changes and moves toward more modern urban lifestyles have repercussions for the health behaviors and nutrition profiles of Thai people.

Health and Nutrition Transitions in Thailand

In Thailand the major health challenges of poverty—malnutrition, high mortality, and infectious disease—are being replaced by increased longevity, lower mortality, and an increasing prevalence of chronic disease. Between 1964 and 2006 Thai life expectancy increased from 56 to 70 for males and from 62 to 78 for females; the maternal mortality ratio fell from 374.3 to 9.8 per 100,000 live births and the infant mortality rate from 49 to 21 per 1000 live births (Wilbulpolprasert, 2008). However, recent decades have seen increases in cardiovascular disorders, diabetes, obesity, cancers, and traffic injuries. Eight of the top ten causes of death in Thailand can now be related to modern lifestyles (ESCAP, 2008).

An important factor in this change in health profile is the rapid change in the diet of the Thai population. Traditional Thai diets can be considered to be protective against chronic diseases, being rich in cereals, legumes, and fresh fruit, vegetables, and herbs, with the majority of protein coming from fish. Urbanization and modernization have meant an increasing demand for both more convenient foods and more modern foods, which are more processed and higher in fats, animal proteins, and sugars (Kosulwat, 2002). Indeed while per capita sugar consumption in Thailand was estimated at about 7 kg/year by 1983, this figure was 33.2 kg by 2006 (Wilbulpolprasert, 2008) and between 1969 and 2003 the estimated intake of kilocalories in Thailand increased from 2110 to 2400 (Food and Agriculture Organization, 2006). In addition to increases in the amount of fat and animal protein consumed, just as concerning may be decreases in fresh fruit and vegetable consumption, with only around one-quarter of adult Thais meeting recommended intakes (Satheannoppakao et al., 2009).

Through this period severe malnutrition has been virtually eliminated in Thailand while in the last 20 years obesity has rapidly developed as a new problem with prevalence growing four times in the last two decades. By 2009 obesity (body mass index ≥ 25) affected 40.7% of women and 28.4% of men. This is now an important public health concern in Thailand (Kosulwat, 2002; Aekplakorn et al., 2007; Wilbulpolprasert, 2008). In addition to obesity, related health problems of diabetes, gallbladder disease, and some cancers are expected to become significant problems for the Thai population in coming years.

Changes in the Food Retailing Sector in Thailand

In Thailand the fresh market (*talad sot*) has for centuries been a center of Thai communities. Marketplaces are part of the ritual, symbolic, and cultural life of Thai people and function as repositories of local food culture and ingredients, regionally and nationally. Importantly, markets in Thailand also function as social centers maintaining social capital for Thai communities and a source of livelihood for large numbers of poorer Thais, especially women, who predominate as stall holders in fresh markets (Jaibun, 2006). In recent decades these traditional formats have been joined by modern food retailing outlets including convenience stores (especially 7-11 stores), supermarkets, and hypermarkets. This process began in the 1980s with the opening of the first supermarkets in Bangkok. Retail change accelerated after the 1997 Asian Financial Crisis and resulting deregulation of foreign investment in food retailing with transnational food corporations (TFCs) including Tesco and Carrefour increasing their store numbers, store sizes, and spreading the reach of modern food retailing into provincial centers outside Bangkok for the first time (Kelly et al., 2010a). Since 1997 the number of modern food retail outlets in Thailand has increased from 1290 to 6654 with the largest growth occurring at the two ends of the food retail spectrum in hypermarkets and convenience stores. Perhaps even more striking is the growth of market share of modern food retail, which was only around 5% in 1980 but grew to nearly 50% by 2006 (AC Nielsen, 2006; Shannon, 2009).

As supermarkets control more of the food supply and diet-related diseases escalate it is important to consider the links between supermarkets and nutrition outcomes. Supermarkets respond to consumer demand to some extent (in Western countries they are starting to respond to health concerns), but they also create consumer preference (Hawkes, 2008). Supermarkets also have differing influences on nutrition in developing and already developed countries. In most Western developed countries supermarkets are an essential source of dietary diversity and affordable fresh foods. They achieve this position through their economies of scale and vertical supply chain efficiencies including subcontracting farmers to grow food directly for them. In developing countries, however, supermarkets may have a more ambiguous effect on public health. Supermarkets often first concentrate on the processed, packaged foods that they can deliver cheaply and where they receive the highest profit margin, allowing aggressive price discounts and promotions. The processed packaged foods offered through modern retail outlets are also often new novel foods that attract customers; however, these are often the very foods associated with negative outcomes of the nutrition transition (Hawkes, 2008; Hattersley and Dixon, 2010). At the international level, studies, including a joint World Health Organization/ Food and Agriculture Organization (WHO/FAO) expert consultation, implicate the spread of food outlets selling energy-dense foods in population weight gain (Joint WHO/FAO Expert Consultation, 2003; Burns and Inglis, 2006).

The increasing market share of modern retail in Thailand now is beginning to impact traditional food retail outlets. Consequently, making obesogenic foods more available and affordable as described above may also make affordable fresh healthy foods more expensive and harder to access. Prices for fresh fruits and vegetables have also been shown to be consistently lower at traditional fresh markets in Thailand than in modern retail formats (Schaffner et al., 2005; Vandergeest, 2006). Thai hypermarkets sell processed products 12% cheaper and fresh foods 10% cheaper than traditional retailers (Minten and Reardon, 2008).

In Thailand public health policy responses to the rapidly growing problem of diet-related chronic disease are well under way. Programs target physical activity, healthy body size, and appropriate diet particularly for school-age Thais. However, economic change, foreign investment laws, and international trade agreements mean that the Thai food environment is now fundamentally linked to the globalized trade in food and modern retail outlets that now control around half of the Thai food retail sector. It is important therefore for Thailand to understand, in a more holistic manner, the factors influencing nutritional outcomes for its people.

There have been few studies to date that investigate how changes in the food environment, and particularly changes in the food retailing sector, impact population nutrition in developing countries. Here we discuss a collaborative study conducted by the Australian National University and Sukhothai Thammathirat Open University (STOU) in Bangkok, which tackles this topic.

THAI FOOD CULTURE TRANSITION STUDY

Research Question

The aim of the collaborative food culture transition study is to understand how changes in the food system in Thailand, particularly in food retailing and provisioning behavior, interact with changes in diet and health outcomes. The objective is to analyze the interaction between the food environment in Thailand and individual- and household-level food provisioning behavior and links between this food provisioning and health and nutritional outcomes.

The research question posed to answer this objective was what effect has the rapid growth in modern food retailing in Thailand had on individual food provisioning behavior and nutritional outcomes? We hypothesize that persons who mainly shop at modern food retailers will make distinctive food choices and these will be reflected in their nutritional outcomes.

Difficulties in Measuring Food Environments and Connecting with Health Outcomes

Measuring the influence of environmental factors on health is complex. The physical design of a person's environment, the socioeconomic structure, or even the dominant culture can all influence how an individual interacts with his or her environment and the health implications of that interaction (Lake and Townshend, 2006). These observations also apply to individuals' food environments. The influence on health outcomes of supermarket presence depends on the range of goods sold at the supermarket, the relative prices of food types, and the mix of food retail outlets that are available within that food environment. Importantly, although studies have been carried out on the relationship between food environments and health, very few have been able to establish a causative relationship, that is, low availability of fresh foods in poorer areas may be due to low demand from those societal groups rather than low supply causing unhealthy diets (Cummins and Macintyre, 2006). What is clear, however, is that individual health behaviors including food intake are influenced by many factors at multiple levels, and frameworks now exist for empirically describing food environments with factors including availability, accessibility, and relative pricing of different food types all contributing to the obesogenicity of a given food environment (Ford and Dzewaltowski, 2008).

Methodology for Thai Food Culture Transition Study

The Thai setting is significantly different from those described in much of the existing literature on food environments, food retailing, and nutrition. Indeed, there are very few examples of this type of study in developing nations where the modernization of food retailing is more recent and traditional food retail outlets persist and perhaps a greater variety of food sources are available. In the study described here we attempt to address this issue of the links between food retail environment, food provisioning choices, and nutritional outcomes in Thailand. Rather than attempting, as the studies discussed above, to measure objectively the constitution of particular food environments, we have chosen to use people's own perceptions of what constitutes their local food environment and what food retail choices they have available to them and to link those perceptions to these individuals' food shopping and dietary patterns.

The Thai food culture transition study adopts a mixed quantitative and qualitative approach and connects to a long running study of health transitions in Thailand, the TCS. The TCS involves researchers based at the Australian National University in Canberra and STOU in Bangkok. The study involves a large multidisciplinary team consisting of epidemiologists, anthropologists, sociologists, demographers, and nutritionists in both Australia and Thailand who are bringing their combined expertise to bear on understanding the changes that are occurring in the health of the Thai population. The varied expertise involved in the team allows a unique analysis of the sociocultural as well as medical determinants of these health transitions. The team has been conducting joint research for nearly eight years and has produced much new information with nearly 60 publications so far addressing varied aspects of the health status of the Thai population.

In 2005 the TCS sent a 20-page questionnaire to all 200,000 registered STOU students. Completed questionnaires were received from 87,134 people who then formed the baseline cohort for the study. Topics covered in the baseline questionnaire included sociodemographic and economic details, height and weight, injury and disease history, food and physical activity, tobacco and alcohol use, and transport behavior. In 2009 a four-year follow-up was conducted with a response rate of around 70% (60,000 respondents). The follow-up questionnaire covered broadly similar topics to the baseline.

The members of the TCS have a similar geographic and demographic distribution to the general Thai population but are somewhat more urbanized and more highly educated. Urbanization and tertiary education are important mediators in the adoption of modern ideas and behaviors and thus this Thai Cohort will be an ideal group in which to study the effects of the transitions under way in Thailand, perhaps indicating future trajectories in the general Thai population (Sleigh et al., 2008).

Quantitative Study

The quantitative part of the research on food culture transition will utilize data derived from the TCS. A subsample of 3,500 members of the Thai Cohort living in the four distinct regions of Thailand and Bangkok also will be sent a supplementary questionnaire covering various aspects of their food environment and food provisioning behavior. The questions asked are divided into the following sections:

A. Personal information on the respondent: household size, rural/urban residence, household income, and body size (height and weight).

B. Local food environment of respondent: mix of stores available now and in the past and relative accessibility of different food store types.

C. Food shopping behavior: frequency of visiting different food store types, types of food purchased at each store, time and money spent on food shopping.

D. Food consumption behavior of respondent: frequency of eating certain types of foods, fruit and vegetable consumption, and a 24-hour food diary.

Data derived from these supplementary questionnaires will then be linked to the other information already provided by respondents in the 2005 and 2009 whole cohort questionnaires and informative associations analyzed. Information from these previous questionnaires will include sociodemographic information, physical and mental health indicators (including disease history and self-rated health), health risk behaviors (including smoking and alcohol), and family history. It will then be possible to characterize respondents as using modern, traditional, or mixed venues and describe these groups in terms of socioeconomic status, urban rural residence, demographic characteristics, health indicators, and importantly, terms of dietary differences. Implied will be the assessment of whether shoppers who favor modern food retail outlets have progressed further along the nutrition transition by comparing the quality of their diets with traditional shoppers.

Qualitative Research on Food Purchasing Patterns

Mail-based quantitative questionnaires can only produce data within the limits of the questions and answers offered. A qualitative study will therefore be conducted to gather in-depth information. A subsample of respondents to the mailed food environment questionnaire will be asked whether they are willing to host a researcher for a short period to accompany them on their usual shopping trips. From among those who respond positively, a random selection of six participants from each region of Thailand (enough to achieve information saturation; Guest et al., 2006) will be selected to participate in a brief study consisting of "accompanied shopping trip(s)" (Jackson et al., 2006), providing an opportunity to discuss their activities.

These qualitative insights on influences on food provisioning and consumption behavior will help to flesh out the findings from the quantitative study, allowing us to understand in a deeper manner how Thai food culture is being experienced by modern Thais and how values and personal preferences are formed, which is information that is difficult to derive quantitatively. Observing actual shopping behavior as it occurs will help us to understand the various factors that influence food purchasing decisions beyond the economic and enable us to understand the values associated with various retail formats including cultural predilections and preferences.

CONCLUSIONS

There are few existing studies of the links between food environments, food retail options, and health outcomes in developing countries. Existing studies in such settings often describe the situation from an economic perspective, rather than considering impacts on food culture and nutrition. Most studies have been conducted in developed Western countries that have fundamentally different food retail sectors from countries such as Thailand, where the modernizing of food retailing and the globalization of diets are much more recent.

The qualitative and quantitative information that the current study produces will be valuable in helping determine to what extent changes in Thai food retailing are producing positive and negative impacts on the diets of Thai consumers, and also how these impacts are being experienced differentially depending on socioeconomic status, gender, area of residence, and other relevant factors. Our use of the existing TCS gives us access to an extensive database of information on the group being studied and the benefit of a long running research partnership with a strong multidisciplinary team of Thai and Australian researchers.

Resulting information will potentially be of use to Thai policy makers who are currently considering approaches to addressing the rapid rise in obesity and diet-related disease in Thailand. Current approaches are primarily focusing on individual behavior modification through public education campaigns on diet and exercise and improved food nutrition labeling. These approaches have experienced some past success in Western countries. By the late 1990s, however, it was becoming clear that a combination of medical intervention and consumer education on risky eating behaviors was not enough. A new approach to addressing consumption-related disease is now being adopted by many national and international bodies, which focuses on the broader "obesogenic" environment (Chopra, 2002). Quantifying and qualifying the role of different food retail formats in fostering an obesogenic environment in Thailand will assist in developing policies that support the access of Thai consumers to affordable healthy food options and help in identifying ways in which upstream and downstream factors influence food provisioning and dietary choice.

REFERENCES

Aekplakorn, W., Hogan, M.C., Chongsuvivatwong, V., Tatsanavivat, P., Chariyalertsak, S., Boonthum, A., Tiptaradol, S., Lim, S.S., 2007. Trends in Obesity and Associations with Education and Urban or Rural Residence in Thailand. Obesity 15, 3113–3121.

Burns, C., Inglis, A., 2006. The relationships between the availability of healthy and fast food and neighbourhood level socio-economic deprivation: a case study from Melbourne, Victoria. Obesity Reviews 7, 39.

Chopra, M., 2002. "Globalisation and food: implications for the promotion of healthy diets. Globalisation, diets and non-communicable disease". World Health Organization, Geneva.

Cummins, S., Macintyre, S., 2006. Food environments and obesity—neighbourhood or nation? International Journal of Epidemiology 35, 100–104.

Drenowski, A., Popkin, B.M., 1997. The nutrition transition: new trends in the global diet. Nutrition Reviews 55, 31–43.

ESCAP, 2008. "Improving vital statistics and cause of death statistics: The experience of Thailand". Economic and Social Commission for Asia and the Pacific, Bangkok.

Food and Agriculture Organization, 2006. Dietary energy consumption of countries. FAO, Rome.

Ford, P.B., Dzewaltowski, D.A., 2008. Disparities in obesity prevalence due to variation in the retail food environment: three testable hypotheses. Nutrition Reviews 66, 216–228.

Guest, G., Bunce, A., Johnson, L., 2006. How many interviews are enough? An experiment with data saturation and variability. Field Methods 18, 59–82.

Hattersley, L., Dixon, J., 2010. Supermarkets, food systems and Public Health: facing the challenges. In: Lawrence, G., Lyons, K., Wallington, T. (Eds.), Food security, nutrition and sustainability, Earthscan, London.

Hawkes, C., 2008. Dietary implications of supermarket development: a global perspective. Development Policy Review 26, 657–692.

Jackson, P., Perez del Aguila, R., Clarke, I., Hallsworth, A., De Kervenoael, R., Kirkup, M., 2006. Retail restructuring and consumer choice 2. Understanding consumer choice at the household level. Environment and Planning A 38, 47–67.

Jaibun, K., 2006. Markets and ways of life: an intital investigation into research on markets and the Thai way of life. In: Chaisingkanon, S. (Ed.), Markets in life and life in markets, Centre for the Study of the Humanities, Bangkok.

Joint WHO/FAO Expert Consultation, 2003. "Diet, nutrition and the prevention of chronic diseases." Report of a joint WHO/FAO expert consultation. WHO Technical report series 916, 34–38.

Kelly, M., Banwell, C., Dixon, J., Seubsman, S., Yiengprugsawan, V., Sleigh, A., 2010a. Nutrition transition, food retailing and health equity in Thailand. Australasian Epidemiologist 17, 4–7.

Kelly, M., Strazdins, L., Dellora, T., Khamman, S., Seubsman, S., Sleigh, A., 2010b. Thailand's work and health transition. International Labour Review 149, 373–386.

Kosulwat, V., 2002. The nutrition and health transition in Thailand. Public Health Nutrition 5, 183–189.

Lake, A., Townshend, T., 2006. Obesogenic environments: exploring the built and food environments. The Journal of the Royal Society for the Promotion of Health 126, 262–267.

Minten, B., Reardon, T., 2008. Food Prices, Quality, and Quality's Pricing in Supermarkets versus Traditional Markets in Developing Countries. Applied Economic Perspectives and Policy 30, 480–490.

Nielsen, A.C, 2006. "Asia Pacific Retail and Shopper Trends". Available at: <http://au.nielsen.com/site/documents/AP_2006_ShopperTrends.pdf> (accessed March 2012).

Satheannoppakao, W., Aekplakorn, W., Pradipasen, M., 2009. Fruit and vegetable consumption and its recommended intake associated with sociodemographic factors: Thailand National Health Examination Survey III. Public Health Nutrition 12, 2192–2198.

Schaffner, D., Bokal, B., Fink, S., Rawls, K., Scweiger, J., 2005. Food retail-price comparison in Thailand. Journal of Food Distribution Research 36, 167–171.

Shannon, R., 2009. The transformation of food retailing in Thailand 1997-2007. Asia Pacific Business Review 15, 79–92.

Sleigh, A., Seubsman, S., Bain, C., and the TCS team., 2008. Cohort profile: the Thai cohort of 87,134 Open University students. International Journal of Epidemiology 37, 266–272.

Vandergeest, P., 2006. "Natural markets: remaking food and agriculture in Southeast Asia". Paper presented at the 2006 Annual Meeting of the Association of American Geographers, March 7–11, Chicago, IL.

Warr, P., 2005. "Thailand: Beyond the crisis". Routledge, Oxon.

Webster, D., 2005. Urbanization: new drivers, new outcomes. In: Warr, P. (Ed.), Thailand Beyond the Crisis, Routledge, Oxon.

Wilbulpolprasert, S. (Ed.), 2008. "Thailand Health Profile 2005–2007". Ministry of Public Health, Bangkok.

World Bank, 2011. Thailand Now an Upper Middle Income Economy. Available at: < http://go.worldbank.org/OQV5D81040> (accessed March 2012).

Chapter 28

Developing Culturally Appropriate Interventions to Prevent Person-to-Person Transmission of Nipah Virus in Bangladesh: Cultural Epidemiology in Action

M. Saiful Islam,[1] Stephen P. Luby,[1,2] and Emily S. Gurley[1]

[1]*International Centre for Diarrheal Disease Research, Bangladesh (ICDDR,B), Dhaka, Bangladesh,*
[2]*Director of Research, Centre for Innovation and Global Health, Stanford University, USA*

INTRODUCTION

To respond to and control epidemics, the technical guideline of the World Health Organization (WHO) stated that, "Special attention must be given to the actual perception of the outbreak by the community…. In particular, specific cultural elements and local beliefs must be taken into account to ensure proper messages, confidence, and close cooperation of the community" (World Health Organization, 1997; Leach and Hewlett, 2010). Over the past decades, the collaboration between anthropology and epidemiology has helped us to better understand public health crises and to design disease prevention interventions. For many infectious disease prevention interventions, there is a gap between biomedical and local understanding of disease transmission, a gap which reduces community uptake of preventative behaviors (Cargo and Mercer, 2008). As epidemiology explicates biomedical pathways of disease transmission, and anthropology explicates local explanatory models, combined efforts can contribute to the improved response to infectious disease outbreaks and control. By understanding the context in which the intervention will be implemented, and considering the target community's culture and resources, successful behavior change interventions can be developed (Wallerstein and Duran, 2008). In this chapter, we will provide an example of the complementary process of combining an

When Culture Impacts Health. http://dx.doi.org/10.1016/B978-0-12-415921-1.00028-2

epidemiological and anthropological approach to develop a public response to an emerging infectious disease, Nipah virus (NiV).

UNDERSTANDING EPIDEMIOLOGY OF NIPAH ENCEPHALITIS

Collaboration with epidemiologists and thorough reviews of up-to-date related epidemiological literature are important to understand the magnitude and nature of a specific disease. The magnitude of the illness helps public health professionals to prioritize responses for prevention and control. For anthropologists who are involved in developing interventions, it is the key to identify the exposures that increase the risk of illness. Epidemiological risk factor studies permit focusing interventions on reducing those exposures that will prevent disease.

NiV was first identified in Malaysia and Singapore in 1999 and caused severe febrile encephalitis in 276 humans and 106 (38%) deaths (Chew et al., 2000; Lam and Chua, 2002). Since then outbreaks have been reported in India in 2001 and 2007, and in Bangladesh from 2001 to 2011 (Kumar, 2003; Hsu et al., 2004; Chadha et al., 2006; Luby et al., 2006, 2009a,b; Gurley et al., 2007; Homaira et al., 2007a,b; Hossain et al., 2008; ICDDRB, 2011). There is no vaccine for this usually fatal infectious disease.

NiV is a zoonotic virus and fruit bats of the genus *Pteropus* are the host reservoir. The prominent modes of NiV transmission in Bangladesh are from bats to humans through drinking raw date palm sap and person to person (Luby, 2006, 2009b; Gurley et al., 2007). The largest known person-to-person NiV outbreak occurred in 2001 in hospitals in Siliguri, an Indian province adjacent to the Bangladesh border, where 66 cases of encephalitis were identified. The case–fatality ratio was 74%. The outbreak began at a single hospital, and cases were subsequently detected at three other hospitals. Forty-five people infected with NiV were either hospital staff or had attended to or visited patients in those hospitals. During the 2004 outbreak in Faridpur, Bangladesh, NiV spread through five generations from person-to-person transmission (Gurley et al., 2007). Among the 36 case patients, 33 had a history of close contact with NiV patients prior to their illness. In this outbreak, one person was apparently responsible for transmitting the virus to 22 persons (Gurley et al., 2007). From 2001 through 2007, almost 50% of NiV infections were due to person-to-person transmission in Bangladesh (Luby et al., 2009b). In a review analysis, 62 persons were infected with NiV while caring for 9 NiV case patients (Luby et al., 2009a).

Epidemiological Understanding of Risk Exposures

Our research group identified exposures that were associated with NiV infection using data collected during the 2004 Faridpur outbreak. Through a case-control study, the epidemiologists found that touching an NiV patient or having received a cough or sneeze in the face from an NiV patient was significantly associated with acquiring NiV infection. Maintaining a certain distance from a person infected with NiV and washing hands with soap after contact were protective (Gurley et al., 2007). Lab investigators also found NiV RNA in saliva collected from patients during the 2004 outbreak (Harcourt et al., 2005). Based on this evidence, the epidemiologists then built a likely transmission model where exposure to a NiV patient's respiratory secretions were an important risk factor for person-to-person transmission of NiV (Gurley et al., 2007; Luby et al., 2009a). The epidemiology team reasoned that when an NiV-infected person was coughing and sneezing due to respiratory distress, the large respiratory droplets expressed from the patients' mouth and nose likely transmitted NiV from an infected patient to an uninfected care provider (Gurley et al., 2007).

Anthropological Understanding of the 2004 Faridpur Outbreak

In May 2004, at the end of the Faridpur outbreak, Lauren Blum (2009), an anthropologist, and her team conducted an explorative study of this public health crisis through a social and cultural lens. They identified that close personal care giving for Nipah patients by family members was the social norm. They found that family members provided hands-on care through feeding the patient, cleaning a patient's body fluids (including secretions of frothy discharge from the mouth), disposing of body fluids, and administering medications (Blum et al., 2009). While caregiving, family members continued to share food and utensils of sick patients, and several family caregivers also slept in the same bed with NiV patients. Family members maintained close physical contact while comforting patients or whispering *Koranic* verses into the sick person's ear (Blum et al., 2009). These behaviors corresponded with the risk factors associated with NiV transmission identified by the epidemiological outbreak investigation team.

SELECT POSSIBLE BEHAVIOR CHANGE MESSAGES

Based on the findings of Blum and Gurley, a multidisciplinary team including medical epidemiologists, anthropologists, and clinicians who had several years of experience of responding to NiV outbreaks convened to examine how the epidemiological transmission model and the identified cultural practices could inform a behavior change intervention that was both acceptable and practicable. This team decided on four behavior change messages to limit caregivers' exposures to NiV patients' respiratory secretions. The messages included (1) washing hands with soap during key times, such as before eating, after feeding patients, and after cleaning patient's saliva, vomit, cough, urine, or feces; (2) keeping caregivers' food and the patient's food in separate bowls, and avoiding sharing patient's leftovers; (3) sleeping in a separate bed, or on the floor, or with the back to the patient or holding child patient's head to caregiver's chest; and (4) keeping one's face more than one hand's length from the patient's face. The team developed two sets of pictorial cards showing these four messages: one for caregivers of adult patients and one for caregivers of child patients.

Assessing Feasibility and Acceptability of the Messages

To assess the acceptability and practicality of the pictorial messages, the anthropologists carried out a number of qualitative research activities at Rangpur Medical College Hospital in northern Bangladesh and in adjacent communities where ICDDR,B has ongoing encephalitis surveillance. With approximately 350 beds, this hospital annually admitted around 300 encephalitis patients, including Nipah cases. This hospital was typically crowded; patients were cared for on the floor when no beds were available. Family members stayed in the hospital wards with the patients and provided hands-on care. The anthropologists reviewed the line list of patients who were admitted in the hospital from June to December 2008 and met the clinical case definition of meningoencephalitis. We purposively selected family caregivers of these patients, and a total of 38 caregivers of adult and child patients participated in this research. We also conducted in-depth interviews with five recovered encephalitis patients in their residence and asked how they would react if the caregiver began practicing these suggested behaviors. We conducted 23 in-depth interviews with family caregivers who had each cared for a relative with encephalitis: patients with encephalitis included 13 adults and 10 children of both sexes. We included these caregivers because cultural expectations and practicability of adopting behavior varied among patients of different sexes and ages. Some of these 23 patients had died (30%), which also could influence caregiver perceptions about changing their behavior. In the in-depth interviews, we requested feedback on the basic understanding of the pictorial messages, feasibility of the behavior changes suggested, and the likelihood of using the suggested behaviors when caring for a sick person in hospital in the future. We also asked caregivers to describe in detail the barriers to behavior change and feasible ways to overcome these barriers based on their experience.

To get some insight into the feasibility of adopting these four behaviors, we conducted two focus group discussions (FGD) with 15 purposively selected family caregivers at the hospital who were currently providing care to either meningoencephalitis or pneumonia patients (since NiV can also present as a pneumonia-like illness) (Hossain et al., 2008). We presented the pictorial messages to them and probed about how those behaviors compared with their current caring practices. We specifically asked them to rank each of the proposed behaviors on its acceptability and its practicability. We expected that the responses of these current hospital-based participants would differ from the community participants.

Feedback from Participants

We found no notable differences between patients and caregivers, or with those with either past or current hospital experience, in the acceptability of adopting the four suggested behaviors as shown in the pictorial cards. Many respondents related these messages with cleanliness.

Washing Hands with Soap during Key Times: Before Eating, after Feeding Patients, and after Cleaning Patient's Saliva, Vomit, Cough, Urine, or Feces

Among the four proposed behavior change messages, all focus group discussion participants ranked hand washing as number 1 on a scale of acceptability and feasibility. This could be because washing hands with soap was already part of their existing practice. One of the participants in the focus group discussion said:

When we eat meat or any type of oily food we wash our hands with soap (after eating). So it is already a normal practice.

Participants raised the concern that this recommended behavior might not be practical for people with lower incomes who might not be able to afford soap. They suggested that we should provide soap to the caregivers. One of the participants from the focus group discussion said:

There are many people who cannot afford even their food, how could they buy soap for hand washing? If you provide them with soap, it will be possible for them to practice the advice . . . . Moreover if a caregiver forgets to wash his/her hands, the provided soap will remind them about hand washing.

The hand washing station was located outside the patient's area and frequent hand washing would require the caregiver to spend more time away from the patient. Caregivers might not leave their severely ill patients unattended during hand washing. Some of the respondents said that patients might be offended if their caregivers frequently wash their hands with soap. They said that the patient's concern can be addressed by discussing the intervention messages with the patient. Some of the respondents talked about the hospital infrastructure and mentioned the unavailability of water and the dirty environment in the toilet area might discourage them to adopt this behavior. One adult patient said:

But if you really want that all of our people to perform this behaviour, you have to take necessary steps to create the suitable environment in the hospital. Like keeping the toilet clean, ensuring availability of water supply and keeping the hospital clean. If you can do that, our people will perform this enthusiastically. But if they have to perform this behavior in the current situation, it will be difficult to do for them.

Keeping Caregivers' Food and Patient's Food In Separate Bowls, and Avoiding Sharing Patient's Leftovers

The FGD participants ranked keeping caregiver's food and the patient's food in separate bowls and avoiding sharing patient's leftover as number 2 on a scale of acceptability and feasibility. Sharing food with family and friends is a cultural practice in Bangladesh and therefore caregivers believed any intervention to limit this practice will be difficult unless the benefits could be explained clearly. The hospital provided food for patients three times a day, but the caregiver needed to bring the plate to serve it on, which then tended to encourage sharing. They said that all the caregivers will not have separate dishes for caregivers and patients. Some people, especially poorer patients, may only have one plate or bowl in the hospital. However, all of the respondents said that they either had these items with them or would have been able to get them from home for the hospital stay, even if at first day they do not bring them. Some participants mentioned that poorer families will be reluctant to throw away food not eaten by the patient.

Sleeping in a Separate Bed or on the Floor, or with the Back to the Patient or Holding Child Patient's Head to Caregiver's Chest

The FGD participants ranked this behavior as number 3 on a scale of acceptability and feasibility. They mentioned that sleeping on the floor was often unpleasant because there usually is a bad smell on the floor, in addition to a lot of patients already sharing that space. When a critical patient needed constant care, the participants suggested preference for sleeping head to foot with the patient in the same bed and mentioned that it was more comfortable this way. A female caregiver said that,

There are patients everywhere in the hospital, also on the floor. So how can caregivers sleep on the floor? It is easy to sleep facing opposite in the same bed or in opposite direction, instead of sleeping on the floor.

An adult patient said:

We didn't face any problem sleeping in one bed. My father kept his legs directed at my head and I kept my legs directed at my father's face.

Keeping One's Face More Than One Hand's Distance from the Patient's Face

The FGD participants ranked keeping their face more than one hand's distance from the patient's face as the least feasible and acceptable of the four messages. One mother who cared for her child who died said that keeping a distance from him would not have been possible. She knows now that it was medically advisable, but would not have heeded our advice when she was caring for her son. She said:

My child is my heart; would I not come close to my child, not comfort him touching his face? I didn't follow these. But we should maintain these messages.

The patients' cultural expectations of close physical contact from caregivers and their severely ill conditions were pointed out as barriers to maintain the proposed distance from their patients. The participants said that this could be addressed by discussing the social ("clean" people will be praised by other caregivers), economic (another illness costs more money to treat), and health benefit of intervention messages with the patient as well as the caregiver. Both the caregivers and the patients emphasized that the delivery of these messages should be done in such a way that everyone can understand the proposed behaviors and their benefits, including social, economic, and health benefit. They suggested delivering the messages by the intervention group (anthropologists).

LESSON LEARNED AND NEXT STEPS

The collaboration between epidemiology and anthropology has been labeled as cultural epidemiology (Trostle and Sommerfeld, 1996). This study provides an example of how cultural epidemiology can contribute to developing an infectious disease prevention program. This comprehensive approach considered not only the scientific and medical perspectives, but also the indigenous understanding of the intervention by the community along with their cultural, psychological, and economic context (de Zoysa et al., 1998).

The indigenous understanding of the target community helped us to select the context appropriate behaviors and provided clues to overcome barriers to making these behaviors practicable. For example, when the multidisciplinary team suggested that caregivers might be able to sleep on the floor to avoid patients' respiratory secretions, they pointed out that there is no space to do this, as other patients are sleeping on the floor. Therefore, this intervention would provide no reduced risk. An alternative suggested by the caregivers was that they could sleep head to foot with the patient in the same bed, which was appropriate in this context, and from a biomedical perspective it could also be effective in reducing exposures to patient's respiratory secretions.

Our next steps are to pilot the messages in practice. Based on the formative qualitative research findings, we finalized the pictorial cards depicting the four behaviors and laminated them onto an easily handheld card. Although the behavior of keeping one's face more than one hand's distance from the patient's face was not seen as totally acceptable or feasible in every situation, we incorporated this behavior in the piloting to explore the barriers and opportunities in practice.

Overall, since many public health interventions do not incorporate the target audiences' cultural context and lived reality, these individuals or communities often do not follow the recommendations and are then blamed for their irresponsibility and incompetence (Douglas, 1992). Cultural epidemiology can minimize this misunderstanding and improve the overall response (Walker, 1998).

CONCLUSION

In this chapter, we aimed to show how collaboration between epidemiology and anthropology can be helpful in designing a public health intervention. The epidemiological study of Nipah provided important clues to causal mechanisms and served to identify the groups at greater risk, which also helped us to prioritize which related practices or behaviors should be targeted in the intervention. The anthropological study helped us to understand the cultural context of these exposures, and to design interventions based upon people's own perceptions and motivators. The formative qualitative research helped us to explore the intervention in a specific cultural, social, and economic context that may facilitate or constrain behavior change, and suggested ways to improve the behavior change messages. Due to the complexity of human behavior and the different mode of transmission of emerging infectious diseases, epidemiologists and social researchers, including anthropologists, need to consistently work together to develop interventions in public health research that are more time and resource efficient.

ACKNOWLEDGMENT

This study was supported by the Centers for Disease Control and Prevention through cooperative award number I-U01-C1000298 and by the Government of the People's Republic of Bangladesh. We thank the study participants for their time and respect and Dorothy Southern for her support in guiding and editing this manuscript. The International Center for Diarrheal Disease Research, Bangladesh, acknowledges with gratitude the commitment of the Centers for Disease Control and Prevention and the Government of the People's Republic of Bangladesh to our research efforts.

REFERENCES

Blum, L.S., Khan, R., Nahar, N., Breiman, R.F., 2009. In-depth assessment of an outbreak of Nipah encephalitis with person-to-person transmission in Bangladesh: implications for prevention and control strategies. The American Journal of Tropical Medicine and Hygiene 80, 96–102.

Cargo, M., Mercer, S.L., 2008. The value and challenges of participatory research: strengthening its practice. Annual Review of Public Health 29, 325–350.

Chadha, M.S., Comer, J.A., Lowe, L., Rota, P.A., Rollin, P.E., Bellini, W.J., Ksiazek, T.G., Mishra, A., 2006. Nipah virus-associated encephalitis outbreak, Siliguri, India. Emerging Infectious Diseases 12, 235–240.

Chew, M.H., Arguin, P.M., Shay, D.K., Goh, K.T., Rollin, P.E., Shieh, W.J., et al., 2000. Risk factors for Nipah virus infection among abattoir workers in Singapore. The Journal of Infectious Diseases 181, 1760–1763.

de Zoysa, I., Habicht, J.P., Pelto, G., Martines, J., 1998. Research steps in the development and evaluation of public health interventions. Bulletin of the World Health Organization 76, 127–133.

Douglas, M., 1992. Risk and Blame: Essays in Cultural Theory. Routledge, London.

Gurley, E.S., Montgomery, J.M., Hossain, M.J., Bell, M., Azad, A.K., Islam, M.R., Molla, M.A., et al., 2007. Person-to-person transmission of Nipah virus in a Bangladeshi community. Emerging Infectious Diseases 13, 1031–1037.

Harcourt, B.H., Lowe, L., Tamin, A., Liu, X., Bankamp, B., Boweden, N., Rollin, P.E., et al., 2005. Genetic characterization of Nipah virus, Bangladesh, 2004. Emerging Infectious Diseases 11, 1594–1597.

Homaira, N., Rahman, M., Hossain, M.J., Epstein, J.H., Sultana, R., Khan, M.S., et al., 2007a. Nipah virus outbreak with person-to-person transmission in a district of Bangladesh. Epidemiology and Infection 138, 1630–1636.

Homaira, N., Rahman, M., Hossain, M.J., Nahar, N., Khan, R., Rahman, M., Podder, G., et al., 2007b. Cluster of Nipah virus infection, Kushtia District, Bangladesh. PLoS One 5, e13570.

Hossain, M.J., Gurley, E.S., Montgomery, J.M., Bell, M., Carroll, D.S., Hsu, V.P., et al., 2008. Clinical presentation of Nipah virus infection in Bangladesh. Clinical infectious diseases: an official publication of the Infectious Diseases Society of America 46, 977–984.

Hsu, V.P., Hossain, M.J., Parashar, U.D., Ali, M.M., Ksiazek, T.G., Kuzmin, I., et al., 2004. Nipah virus encephalitis reemergence. Bangladesh. Emerging Infectious Diseases 10, 2082–2087.

ICDDRB, 2011. Nipah Outbreak in Lalmonirhat district, 2001. Health and Science Bulletin 9.

Kumar, S., 2003. Inadequate research facilities fail to tackle mystery disease. BMJ (Clinical research ed.) 326, 12.

Lam, S.K., Chua, K.B., 2002. Nipah virus encephalitis outbreak in Malaysia. Clinical infectious diseases: an official publication of the Infectious Diseases Society of America 34 (Suppl. 2), S48–S51.

Leach, M., Hewlett, B.S., 2010. Haemorrhagic Fevers: Narratives, Politics and Pathways. In: Dry, S., Leach, M. (Eds.), Epidemics: Science, Governance and Social Justice, Earthscan, London.

Luby, S.P., Gurley, E.S., Hossain, M.J., 2009a. Transmission of human infection with Nipah virus. Clinical infectious diseases: an official publication of the Infectious Diseases Society of America 49, 1743–1748.

Luby, S.P., Hossain, M.J., Gurley, E.S., Ahmed, B.N., Banu, S., Khan, S.U., Homaira, N., et al., 2009b. Recurrent zoonotic transmission of Nipah virus into humans, Bangladesh, 2001-2007. Emerging Infectious Diseases 15, 1229–1235.

Luby, S.P., Rahman, M., Hossain, M.J., Blum, L.S., Husain, M.M., Gurley, E., Khan, R., et al., 2006. Foodborne transmission of Nipah virus. Bangladesh. Emerging Infectious Diseases 12, 1888–1894.

Trostle, J.A., Sommerfeld, J., 1996. Medical Anthropology And Epidemiology. Annual Review of Anthropology 25, 253–274.

Walker, S., 1998. Health interventions: a focus for applied medical anthropology theory. NEXUS 13, 74–88.

Wallerstein, N., Duran, B., 2008. The Theoretical, Historical and Practical Roots of CBPR. In: Minkler, M., Wallerstein, N. (Eds.), Community Based Participatory Research for Health, Jossey Bass, San Francisco, pp. 25–46.

World Health Organization, 1997. WHO recommended guidelines for epidemic preparedness and response: Ebola haemorrhagic fever (EHF). WHO, Geneva.

Conclusion

Chapter 29

From Local Tales to Global Lessons

Jane Dixon,[1] Cathy Banwell,[1] and Stanley Ulijaszek[2]

[1]National Centre for Epidemiology and Population Health, Australian National University, Canberra, Australia, [2]Institute for Social and Cultural Anthropology, University of Oxford, UK

This book illustrates the breadth and diversity of culture-in-health research. Our studies span the distal to proximal determinants of health from the global, national, national subpopulation, and village to the individual body. They range from small but temporally extensive ethnographic studies in the highlands of New Guinea to desktop, or secondary data, analyses of national cultural trends. Geographically, the book's contents traverse southeast Asia to islands in the mid Pacific Ocean, and they encompass enormous demographic variety from millions of people to hundreds.

A similar breadth is shown in the types of societies analyzed from those transitioning away from subsistence and agrarian economies in countries like Papua New Guinea, Malaysia, and Bangladesh through to the industrial and service economies of South Korea, Australia, and New Zealand. The nature of the health problems addressed is also diverse: old and new infections diseases, chronic conditions, and the impact of professional discourses and health system operations on health-seeking behaviors and understandings of health risks. The question becomes what general lessons can be learned about a culture-in-health approach from this array of studies.

Returning to our discussion in Chapter 1, we see culture as operationalized in three main ways: as a noun (referring to a collectivity who see themselves as sharing something in common); as an adjective (when distinguishing cultural from other forms of social action); and as an adverb (the processes by which cultural factors come to be shared, contested, and transformed). The following section summarizes how various chapters reflect this variety. Together the studies confirm the utility of applying cultural perspectives in the identification of health risks. We then turn to summarizing the breadth of methods that appear throughout the chapters, before highlighting some of the lessons for intervention that stand out. We do not attempt to be exhaustive, but try to move forward the discussion about research and intervention designs.

When Culture Impacts Health. http://dx.doi.org/10.1016/B978-0-12-415921-1.00029-4

APPLYING CULTURAL CONCEPTS WHEN IDENTIFYING HEALTH RISKS: SECTION B

Industrial and Postindustrial Societies

Several of our studies illustrated that medical anthropology is not confined to the ethnographic method at village or subpopulation level. The critical and reflexive modes of anthropology are still useful when researchers take other cultural approaches, often placing epidemiological and other large datasets in sociocultural, historical, and political context. For example, Keane, in Chapter 6, used a literature synthesis refracted through sociology and anthropology theory to examine the *cultural process* of medicalization of attention deficit hyperactivity disorder (ADHD). Medicalization has implications for disease diagnoses and patient experiences, with possibilities for additional health risks as exposure to the formal medical system intensifies. In an era of biological citizenship, ADHD constitutes an assemblage of ideas, practices, and institutions, which cross many state and societal borders. In this sense, she illustrated how culture operates at the *global/cross-national/national levels.*

Using a different methodology—in-depth interviews interpreted through a cultural risk transmission theory lens—Olsen and colleagues (Chapter 8) also discussed the mismatch between epidemiologically based expert discourses of risk and disease in contrast to what they described as lay epidemiology, or public understandings of *the transmission of hepatitis C and risk.* Within a growing subpopulation or *culture*, their study illustrated the behavioral outcomes of a specific assemblage of attitudes and practices toward health and well-being shared via a particular *cultural transmission mode—normalization through peer group influence.* In this case, *gender is deployed as a cultural factor* signifying embodied power relations, influencing women's views of their roles and what is imaginable in terms of behaviors.

Hogan (Chapter 9) used a theoretical "testing" of epidemiological data to reflect on a social model of disability to reassess the pathways that link hearing loss to poor health outcomes. Hearing-impaired individuals, living in *a culture* that has a fixed view of acceptable hearing capacity, experience a range of stressful situations, which set up physiological stress responses. While Australian data are used, the argument is more generally applicable to situations where hearing loss is a low status condition leading to social isolation and everyday problems of access to resources and support. In this case, *national cultures*, which practice hearing discrimination, pose a risk to particular *subpopulations.*

Economically Transitioning Societies

In a case study involving Papua New Guinea, Maddocks (Chapter 15) detailed a tale of rapid cultural and health transition in a village close to Port Moresby. He used clinical data and field-based participant observation conducted over many years. Like Chapters 13, 14, and 16, he demonstrated the importance of historical viewpoints and approaches to managing social and environmental relationships. In this case, the erosion of meaningful *cultural practices* and the intrusion of new cultural practices are colliding with poor economic prospects for households leading to *a village-wide culture* of despair with poor health consequences.

In an ethnographic study among Orang Asli, an indigenous *minority* of Malaysia, Bedford (Chapter 17) examined the perceptions of leprosy patients and their *health-seeking behaviors and management approaches*. She concluded, like Olsen (Chapter 8) in the modern scientific context of people with hepatitis C in Australia, that Orang Asli approach their health from a standpoint as social outsiders, marginalized within the wider society. Their marginal status is reinforced by health care professionals.

Using in-depth interviews and observations in rural Bangladesh to explore issues identified via epidemiological surveys, Arman (Chapter 18) sought to understand the *cultural barriers* to people changing their water source behaviors. She demonstrated how the possibilities of invisible and distant illness, via arsenic-contaminated water, is regarded by consumers as less important than water that is conveniently located, pleasant to drink, and less likely to transmit diarrheal diseases.

UNIFYING THREADS IN SECTION B

Within this spread, can we discern unifying themes? This is an activity fraught with danger when a key feature of the culture concept is its reference to uniqueness, difference, and otherness. However, there is great value in looking beyond a specific culture, people, or disease for a critical analysis of shared and common beliefs and approaches to risk management. The search for cross-culturally shared characteristics that highlight what makes humans human has always been of interest to anthropology but, as we point out in Chapter 2, this approach has fallen out of favor in the last half century. Nevertheless, in this era of globalization—the movement of peoples, ideas, and technologies referred to in Chapter 1, not to mention the transfer of products, germs, toxins, and practices directly injurious to health—there is an imperative to return to studies that emphasize the interaction between the global and the local, and how global forces are given cultural meanings that make them local again.

Five lessons from this section stand out.

1. Despite the spread of globalization, cultures as assemblages of norms, beliefs, and practices, remain spatially, socially, environmentally, and historically located.

The difficulty for health researchers is in disentangling what is shared and what is specific, what is newly arrived, and what is temporally embedded.

An example is provided by Schwekendiek and colleagues (Chapter 13) who approached body-slimming behavior among the current cohort of South Korean men and women from a social and bio-anthropology perspective. They show how the *corporeal culture* has *changed rapidly* in the last 50 years with the attendant rise in health risks from popular approaches to slimming by reporting on national survey data contextualized and explained through social histories and theories of *biosocial transmission of risk*. The authors argue that it is important to undertake studies of the origins of biosocial stress and the importance of cultural history in understanding current health risks.

2. Cultural change can be slow or swift.

Reminiscent of Levi-Strauss it can be observed that some (hot) societies embrace change and innovation while others (cold) value tradition and continuity. Cultural change can be generated from within, as in recognition of women's rights for education or political expression, and other times it can be imposed by an outside force including calamity, migrants and missionaries, globalizing, and hegemonic discourses. In a dynamic world cultural change is usually a mix of both. Cultural change can be resisted, sometimes with beneficial effects and at other times with poor results. In all countries rapid cultural change generally comes about through technological innovation, which has usually benefited a few and had mixed effects on the population as a whole. Sociocultural trends, such as increasing car reliance and the increasing availability of mass-produced foods, have made life more comfortable and convenient for numerous subpopulations but are contributing to a rising prevalence of obesity. Methodologically, such change is difficult to study as it operates differently at different levels of the population. Large datasets are required to see where the effects are felt (i.e., the poorer in Western societies and the richer in poorer countries are more likely to be obese), and then ethnographically informed studies can be used to explore how these trends "get under the skin" (Ulijaszek, 2007; Banwell et al., 2012).

3. Culture and hence cultural risks or benefits are transmitted through a range of rather opaque mechanisms: copying, socialization, normalization, distinction, mimetic playing with, and regulation.

Some transmission mechanisms are generated from the ground up through the communicative activities of individuals and groups, while others are imposed through legislation and official regulation. Usually though, a dialectic comes into play. Tobacco control and smoking behavior demonstrates how government regulation, sparked by the activities of lobby groups, has led to a cultural change in countries where it is now frowned upon to smoke in public spaces like restaurants. However, as John Glover (Chapter 12) demonstrated, subgroups with their own cultural norms continue to transmit their own attitudes to smoking over generations (see also Dixon and Banwell, 2009).

4. Health relevant cultural processes, or modes of shaping practices, can be widespread. However, they play out or are manifested differently according to "local" historical and social contexts and environmental conditions.

Here we endeavor to isolate four important cultural processes that appear in numerous case studies.

Transnationalism: While this process has been under way since people could cross national boundaries, it often remains unexplored. Park and Littleton (Chapter 14) described the process beginning with a *cross-national comparison* of the epidemiology of tuberculosis (TB) in New Zealand, the Cook Islands, and Tuvalu before moving on to explain the trends in "migrant TB" within New Zealand. Using historical and ethnographic research among Cook Islanders resident in the Cook Islands and New Zealand and among Islanders resident in New Zealand, they offered cultural explanations for the effectiveness of various approaches to tackling TB risk environments and behaviors. Their chapter identified *sociocultural transmission routes* and the importance of a syndemic where conditions for one disease contribute to the spread of another, explaining the aggregation of ill health in some populations. *Transnationalism* is present in many guises. In the Fanany case (Chapter 20) international aid agencies tried to deliver a particular form of health intervention that had grown out of experiences in other places. It is also present in all of the chapters that use the universalizing discourse of risk, which has displaced meaning systems based on fate, destiny, and luck to assist in the interpretation of sickness, health, and dying.

Medicalization: This is a transnational process of enculturating (making a set of ideas, beliefs, and practices stable or durable) the supremacy and sanctity of diagnoses and interventions that emanate from the multipronged biomedicine institution. This process positions "medical" wisdom as superior to lay/folk wisdom and pits itself against "untrained" and "untested" approaches to health and illness. The process is in evidence in Chapter 6 by Keane in relation to ADHD, Chapter 15 by Maddocks, and the delegitimation of village approaches to health and well-being, such as the application of a WHO protocol for post-traumatic stress disorder in Chapter 20 on post-tsunami Aceh. It is present in Schwekendiek's account of contemporary approaches to slimming in South Korea in Chapter 13. Slimming is a bodily practice that rises and falls in popularity according to the broader social conditions reifying a particular body aesthetic. Within a context when more than one half of many national populations are medically classified as overweight and obese, the normal and underweight body has become a valuable state of being. It is considered to have high cultural capital and the epidemiology shows that it often coexists with higher socioeconomic status in modern societies. How to attain the

desired body shape is practiced differently according to local conditions, as the South Korea study illustrates: while medical elements
of the approach to slimming are found elsewhere (diets, surgery, and
pills), the way the practice is justified in terms of national identity can
be unique.

Adapting to environmental change: This is an individual and collective practice that can by highly stressful, and Chapters 14–20, concerning
transitioning societies, revealed significant interactions between the natural environment and health practices and beliefs going back indefinitely.
What is being asked of many people in rapidly transitioning societies
is that they make profound adjustments to their preferences, ideas, and
beliefs including those relating to health, health seeking, and compliance,
often as major changes are being inflicted on their physical environment
by outside forces. Mining, deforestation, tourism, and development processes are just a few examples, or those imposed by disasters such as
the 2004 tsunami. The dialectical process is the persistent observance
of social norms: consensus, conformity, and strong religious or village
attachment. This approach to everyday life will rub up against the pressures to adjust to environmental and social change. Chapter 20 illustrated
the tensions between the two within the context of a calamity, with a
people possibly being better off for not changing their attachments. In
contrast, Chapter 15 indicated the poor health consequences for a people
who are unable to continue with the same conviction their observance of
taken-for-granted attachments to village, income generation, and sharing.

Stigmatization, marginalization: This is a process of enculturating
discrimination against people judged to be "abnormal," thereby creating
insider and outsider social status. This process may go by the name of
social exclusion, and it may encompass those who refuse to, or cannot,
adapt to new social and environmental conditions. The process is evidenced in Chapter 9 about hearing impairment, Chapter 8 about women
who use illicit drugs, Chapter 17 about leprosy patients, and Chapter 14
about TB's association with "new migrants." While in Chapter 7, Crosbie
noted that the process is often applied to people who give off highly visual
cues (through their appearance and their behaviors), Chapters 8 and 9
indicated that the cues, which trigger the process, can be less obvious: in
the case of the hearing impaired, not fully engaging in social interactions;
and as in Chapter 8, bearing the demeanor of a poor person or drug user.

5. Building from the preceding points, a cultural perspective is essential to
understanding the nature, persistence, and mutability of health risks.

We cannot explain the reasons for country and individual health profiles without recourse to the historical cultural dimension. While social epidemiologists
argue that socioeconomic variables such as race, ethnicity, gender, education, and

socioeconomic position can explain the distribution of disease in populations, there are often inexplicable elements. Social epidemiologists usually do not attempt to explain them, but sometimes attribute them to culture. Through attempting to understand what these unexplained cultural factors are, as well as investigating the meaning of the socioeconomic factors to those who are labeled by them and how these features are manifest in practices, they gain greater explanatory power. To arrive at this point would require a mixed method approach as outlined variously in Chapters 11, 14–16, 17, and 20, and Chapter 24 found in Section C.

METHODS FOR DOING CULTURE-IN-HEALTH RESEARCH: SECTIONS B AND C

One task for contributors was to make their methodological approach more transparent. Most explicitly, Section B illustrated how culture-in-health research takes numerous forms because of the wide variety of contexts in which it is important to understand how culture is implicated in health profiles. While there are specific appropriate techniques according to scale—global to individual—there is a wealth of relevant methods using widely accepted qualitative and quantitative research techniques. As those who have written extensively on culture-in-health have pointed out, the basic building blocks are ethnography (long-term fieldwork, involving observation, participation, and discussion) and surveys (predetermined sets of questions used among representative populations).

However, as the cultural process of transnationalism becomes ever more intrusive, the traditional ethnographic method of anthropology becomes more difficult to practice when considering the global, supranational, and national levels: rarely are distinct groups easily defined within fieldwork settings, although they are discernible in demographic and epidemiological data as risk groups. Furthermore, populations and places map onto each other less now than they did in the past. In such situations researchers take other approaches, often placing epidemiological and other large datasets in sociocultural, historical, and political context. Large datasets are useful for capturing population-wide trends, whereas a range of critical reflective methods is necessary for gaining an understanding of subgroup norms, values, and practices.

Luby, Arman, Islam, and Parveen (Chapters 5, 18, 19, and 28), who have all worked at the International Centre for Diarrheal Disease Research in Bangladesh (ICDDR,B), discussed the value of working in multimethod teams where epidemiology is used to identify population-level disease patterns and ethnographic fieldwork is used to explore subjective experience placed in local context. Parveen (Chapter 19), for example, illustrated the value of detailed anthropological fieldwork, following epidemiological research. For two disease outbreaks, she and her co-authors demonstrated how an anthropological understanding of the everyday interactions with the natural world enhanced the work of a multidisciplinary team in discovering the cause and transmission routes of the outbreaks and led to identifying appropriate preventive measures.

Kelly's study (Chapter 27) is unusual because of its relationship with a national cohort study, which is one of the most powerful epidemiological tools available. To understand transitions in food practices, he used a geographically based subsample of cohort members selected to conform to epidemiological methodology. The subsample has completed a culturally informed questionnaire about food purchasing and consumption that will be analyzed in light of health outcome data collected through the standard cohort questionnaires. Ethnographic approaches will be used to understand the food purchasing locations from which the sample is drawn. Kelly has a background in Thai language and culture, and is working with Thai and Australian epidemiologists, food sociologists, and anthropologists to undertake this study.

Like Kelly's chapter, Gifford (Chapter 24) described a mixed methods approach, although the genesis of her approach is markedly different. She took an anthropological approach to drawing her sample through relevant community organizations working with recent African immigrants, and followed them longitudinally. Gifford's chapter provided an insight into an innovative mix of methods such as standardized questionnaires used in combination with techniques from visual anthropology. Qualitative longitudinal studies are extremely rare, but they illuminate the interplay between key events in time and transitions in people's lives: how people adapt their behaviors to new and changing environments and why.

Dixon and Banwell (Chapter 25) tried to achieve what Gifford did and track key events and processes in time and place that plausibly foster particular ideas and practices. A key difference is that they used a cultural economy approach that relies on secondary sources to determine how cultural and economic forces operating at a national level influence the acceptance and adoption of particular ideas and practices. The utility of the approach is enhanced if there is a primary data collection phase to "test" the hunches that arise from the secondary data.

Much social epidemiology is interested in associations between health status and socioeconomic indicators, including wealth. In Chapter 22, Ivory and colleagues problematized "wealth," using Bourdieu's conceptualization of multiple forms of capital. They developed a heuristic of the "wealthy environment" operating at multiple levels: the household, family, locality, and community. Drawing on data from a new longitudinal study under way in New Zealand, they were able to provide very concrete indicators for measuring what constitutes a wealthy environment in terms of childhood development. This is an excellent example of reinterpreting socioeconomic factors with a cultural lens.

Ulijaszek (Chapter 23) outlined a technique for estimating the extent to which people share common understandings and beliefs. He applied the Cultural Consensus Model to knowledge and attitudes toward diabetes and breast cancer in the United States and Latin America. This approach uncovers dissensus as well as consensus, which is most important when targeting health interventions. As was noted, it could be used with different health professional "camps" to identify barriers to consistent approaches to intervention.

Given that so many imposed cultural practices emanate in the public policy domain, it is important to understand what policy makers believe they are attempting to change and what new social orders they are wishing to engineer. In Chapter 26, Baker described the nuts and bolts of key informant interviewing as a basis for social network analysis. Knowing whether key networks are disposed toward action is fundamental in designing any intervention advocacy. Key informant interviewing is a key feature of studying those in power, whereas so much of public health research concentrates on studying the powerless.

FIVE METHODOLOGICAL ISSUES THAT TRAVERSE THE CASE STUDIES

1. How to best account for and "capture" ethnicity as a marker/factor that is sensitive enough to represent shared cultural beliefs and practices.

From Chapters 10–12, 14, 21, and 24, it seems that the specificities of the health risk context and/or health condition was key, and that it was not sufficient in all situations to use self-rated ethnic status adopted in surveys. Indeed, the imposition of an ethnic or race descriptor on people is unlikely to reflect insider cultural understandings and is often associated with openly racist practices.

Based on New Zealand "ethnic" *subpopulations*, and from within a broadly biocultural perspective, Callister and Galtry (Chapter 10) illustrated the health intervention dilemmas that follow from lack of clarity as to whether the key risk factor for melanoma incidence is "race," *culturally constructed ethnicity*, ancestry, or skin color. They highlighted how ethnic status is not easily measurable, and by being a cultural construct it has variable meanings that can change over time and can be unstable.

This is also the message from Chapter 21: people may identify as Aboriginal and Torres Strait Islander for some purposes but not for others. This does not matter as much as deciding whether identity, as self-reported in response to predetermined categories in a questionnaire, for example, is sensitive enough to explain what needs explaining. The issue unsettles the collection of large datasets where these descriptors are used. It is clear that there have been large-scale shifts in ethnic identity over time that cannot be explained by new births. These shifts throw into doubt any explanation of health outcomes on this basis and call for small-scale ethnographic studies to understand how people use these identity markers and what they mean in health statistics, as seen in Chapter 21.

Operating across a national population and undertaking *subpopulation* comparison, in Chapter 12 Glover and colleagues used age and ethnicity as cultural factors on the assumption that particular age groups and ethnic cohorts "inherit" and "inhabit" a shared time period and sociocultural and environmental conditions, and hence may be disposed to act in similar ways. This work applies epidemiological approaches to sociocultural data. Chapter 12 indicated that self-reported ethnic status can help describe variations, but that additional factors need to be introduced to move the description toward explanation. Other researchers have used socioeconomic status alongside ethnic status to good effect to explain that there is something about deprivation that makes smoking persistence more likely. Chapter 12 also took life stage and time period into account to see if new patterns emerged. Life stage can be classed as a cultural variable as it captures a cultural interpretation of biosocial facts/events/experiences; for example, being a teenager is generally a phase of separating from family-based established identities and early adulthood is a time for establishing a family and livelihood regime. However, Chapter 12 concluded, as so many other papers on the topic have, that the use of routine data only goes so far, and that without in-depth, qualitative data satisfactory explanations for variable smoking behaviors remain elusive. To this end, having the tools developed from a deep cultural understanding as demonstrated by Marewa Glover in Chapter 11 is critical.

These same issues arise for the variable/factor of gender and for religion. In Chapter 20 the Fananys examined the *cultural responses* to disaster relief in Aceh, Indonesia, following the 2004 tsunami. In the case of religion, they questioned whether the Acehnese response to the tsunami was due to their Malay character/ethnicity/race, their Muslim religion, or their history of living in their socioecological environment for many centuries having evolved abiding and durable customs and beliefs that are not amenable to rapid change. Like Park and Littleton in Chapter 14, the Fananys used a synthesis of multiple theoretical lenses traversing anthropology, history, environmental science, and public health to explain the responses.

2. Studying power by examining the history of ideas, practices, and beliefs; past and present trends in social inequalities and their causes; and points of consensus and dissent

This book contains several approaches to understanding why people believe and act as they do. We summarize those approaches next.

In Chapter 6 Keane used a Foucauldian approach to examine literature describing the dynamics of institutionalized cultural forces or processes associated with the entrenched power of the medical profession to define health and ill health and to suppress alternative approaches to health problems. In contrast, in Chapters 14 and 20, Park and Fanany employed deep immersion in a community to understand the potency of ideas, beliefs, and practices interpreted through a historical lens of power hierarchies—both ideational and social—and a theoretical lens of key anthropology constructs. Another approach is offered in Chapter 25 by Dixon, relying largely on secondary sources to determine how cultural and economic forces operating at a national level influence the acceptance and adoption of particular ideas and practices. In Chapter 26, Baker went directly to powerful figures (key informants) operating internationally to gain useful data. However, as he pointed out, it requires care and time to access these people who are certainly experienced enough to censor the information they supply.

Ivory's approach in Chapter 22 was different again in that it describes in detail a heuristic device for measuring various forms of resource allocation. By making explicit different forms of resource capital and how to access them, the power differential becomes more visible and comprehensible.

3. Capturing human–environmental factor interplay—another form of power

As we described earlier, within the transitioning or modernizing society case studies, the importance of people's relationships with their natural and physical environments is present. In the postindustrial society case studies, the emphasis becomes the social environment of signs and representations.

Environmental epidemiology has multilevel tools designed to find associations between social, physical, and man-made environments and population health outcomes. They are used when the factors take measurable form, but epidemiologic-based designs cannot help when there is a need to understand what such factors actually represent to people. The difficulties are most clearly borne out in Chapter 10 in relation to ethnicity and sun exposure, and in Chapter 8 with Olsen's problematizing of the gender and health behavior interplay. That chapter raises the question about how being a woman affects health behaviors and outcomes: Is it her biological status, her social status, her roles and responsibilities, or her relative poverty?

Chapter 27 examined the transition in the man-made physical environment toward supermarketization driven by large national and international companies in Thailand. Chapters 16, 18, and 19 dwelled on the cultural interpretation of the apparently "natural" world. In Chapter 16 Gardner brings together the *distribution of practices* and the Mian's history and environmental conditions with a survey of malaria prevalence and severity undertaken by his co-author Attenborough. They demonstrated that the presence of malaria is influenced by an interplay of *cultural as well as environmental factors*. Another example of this interplay is demonstrated by Parveen and colleagues (Chapter 19) who described the contributions of anthropological investigations to two outbreaks of environmentally related disease: the transmission of Nipah virus from bats to humans via palm sap and the pufferfish poisoning. In all of these chapters, close attention was paid to the human–environmental interplay within micro-settings.

4. The utility of cultural epidemiology versus the tacking approach

Chapter 2 described the antecedents to culture-in-health research, with one contemporary manifestation, cultural epidemiology. For Helman, the author of five editions of *Culture, Health and Illness*, cultural epidemiology is a multidisciplinary approach that has arisen to deal with "problems of comparing disorders [e.g., depression] across cultures." Most work has been done on patterns of social stress and suffering within communities, meanings attributed to illnesses (including by epidemiologists), and help-seeking behaviors. Several contributors in this volume find the current formulation of cultural epidemiology to be insufficient. In Chapter 14, Park and Littleton described it as an "add and stir" approach based on epidemiology and anthropology; and in Chapter 4, Brough argued that public health research as it is usually practiced is dominated by positivism, expressed through epidemiological research methods that apply complex quantitative and statistical methods to describe the distribution of disease and health risk. As we have observed in Chapter 2, it is this formulation of cultural epidemiology that satisfies neither epidemiologists nor anthropologists due to the inability and inappropriateness of trying to reduce cultural forces to quantifiable variables.

However, in the context of interventions that are based on measurable associations between the physical environment and health status, Luby supports the cultural epidemiology approach, which is endorsed by the Centers for Disease Control beyond the Bangladesh office. In Chapter 5, Luby affirmed the point made by Park and Kelly that within any one team, the anthropologists and other social scientists and epidemiologists play distinctive roles, and for Luby the social scientist perspective is invaluable for generating hypotheses about why interventions are succeeding or not.

Instead of confining culture-in-health research to the disciplines of anthropology and epidemiology, in Chapter 14, Park and Littleton encouraged public health researchers to draw on distinctive disciplines, acknowledging and utilizing their differing and sometimes conflicting logics. They argued that rather than trying to blend anthropological and epidemiological methods it is better to "tack between" different methods, alternating between one for explanation and the next for hypothesis generation and so on. Their case study is based on many years of work in the Pacific Islands by an experienced group of anthropologists.

5. Deploying theory—one theory or many

In Chapters 22, 23, and 25, a unitary theory or theoretical field informed the design of protocols, data collection, and analysis approaches and in Hogan's use of social theory in Chapter 9 to explain a society's stigmatization of the hearing impaired. Park, Gardner, Fanany, and Schwekendiek (Chapters 13, 14, 16, and 20) came at their studies from a broader ecological perspective. They embraced complexity in explanations, which incorporate observable phenomena that may or may not be measurable. Park and Littleton (Chapter 14) adopted the term *syndemic* to explain the synergistic interaction between "afflictions" to explain clusters of epidemics. In a similar fashion there may be a synergistic interaction of theoretical explanations, which may operate at the level of multiple diseases and/or social conditions that is somewhat akin to a web of influences or political ecology approach.

APPLYING A CULTURAL PERSPECTIVE TO INTERVENTIONS

Many of these chapters contain lessons for interventions. The primary lesson from Marewa Glover, Gifford, Crosbie, Olsen, Arman, Fanany, Parveen (Chapters 7, 10, 11, 18–20, and 24) and others is that it is necessary to understand the perspective of people in the context of their everyday lives if an intervention is to be successful. Sometimes these perspectives are described as "lay," "irrational," or "traditional"; all words that immediately display power relations and biases. Whatever the language used, the basic message from many chapters in this book remains: people do not easily relinquish their beliefs and practices, which are often sensible and functional, because they are told to do so for health reasons. Indeed, the continuing concerns about obesity and smoking in so-called "advanced" societies illustrates that "modern" citizens are as wedded to their unhealthy practices and beliefs as those from "traditional" societies.

In societies dominated by a scientific discourse of cause and effect, health risks, illness, and disease remain highly emotive topics and experiences, which are subject to lay beliefs, nonscientific interpretations, and perhaps unhelpful behaviors. In Chapter 7, Crosbie and colleagues described *beliefs about illness transmission* including magic, contagion, familiarity, and shared values operating in modern, complex *cultures*. Crosbie takes seriously people's nonscientific approaches to health, acknowledging that formal health education campaigns in Australia may not work if the irrational has a strong hold by performing valuable functions for people.

In a resource-poor environment, Arman showed in Chapter 18 that to make broad environmental change, like improving water infrastructure, we need to understand and appreciate the daily pressures on people's behavioral repertoires, because even if new behaviors have positive connotations they will not be adopted if they are too onerous or disruptive (quite apart from being financially onerous). Often understanding women's social position and work demands is the key to success as women are usually responsible for family health and well-being. In a similar setting and applying a similar approach in Chapter 28, Islam described how he and others developed culturally appropriate and acceptable interventions for the prevention of Nipah virus transmission in rural Bangladesh. Based on fieldwork and focus group discussions he identified four intervention strategies and ranked them on the basis of acceptability to their target population.

In Chapter 20, Fanany demonstrated that widely accepted health assessment protocols, even those from the global World Health Organization, are not universally applicable. Religious, ethnic, and cultural factors are unique and will influence people's experiences and responses to catastrophe, life, and death and will condition their responses to outside interventions. In this regard, people's past experiences of outside interventions are key (e.g., by missionaries).

A slightly different version of this argument is exemplified in Chapters 10 and 21 where Callister and Guthrie argued that before an intervention can be embarked upon there is a need to be able to specify whether the key factor is self-determined identity, race, ethnically influenced behaviors, ancestry, or skin color. In Callister's example, he would then target all interventions coherently, and consistently use the one factor as a basis for messages. In Chapter 28, Islam and his team took earlier anthropological work that identified a causal pathway between care giving and disease transmission to then pilot test alternative behavior change messages. By placing any intervention within a thorough understanding of the cultural context of people's perceptions, fears, and motivators, behavior change is more likely to result.

In Chapter 11, Marewa Glover took a holistic approach. She offered an example of an intervention to promote smoking cessation that uses a Maori paradigm of health called Te Whare Tapa Wha. She argued that for Maori the approach to quitting should build upon the physical, the spiritual, the psychological, and the familial and social context in a balanced way. Her example is a theoretically and culturally sophisticated approach to embracing cultural understandings to promote population health improvement.

While the embedded long-term ethnographic experience of anthropologists like Gardner and Attenborough is difficult to replicate in postindustrial societies, researchers like Maddocks, Guthrie, and Marewa Glover, Gifford, Olsen, and Hogan maintain long-term relationships with the organizations through which they have recruited participants. On occasion, they may act as advocates or advisors, helping to refine the advice being given to agencies keen to intervene.

CONCLUSION

Worldwide there is great diversity and divergence in health issues, mainly related to the extent of modernization, subpopulation diversity, cultural histories, and environmental conditions. These upstream determinants of health produce a variety of health problems: old and new infectious diseases, chronic conditions, medicalized conditions, and diffuse states of well-being not yet medicalized but deserving of social policy attention. This book offers a matching diversity of innovative approaches by which to improve public health that takes into account the cultural nature of health risks: environmental–cultural, biocultural, cultural economic, and political–cultural.

While providing some straightforward lessons, we note that many of these chapters lean toward embracing complex analyses, through the layering of multiple theories, epistemologies, disciplines, and methods. We also note that multifaceted research approaches are often difficult to achieve because of practical constraints, such as funding models, institutional silos, time limits, and researcher exhaustion. However, the evidence is piling up; health risks and problems in poor and rich countries alike are becoming increasingly complex, demanding sophisticated and novel research approaches and interventions.

REFERENCES

Ulijaszek, S., 2007. Obesity: a disorder of convenience. Obesity Reviews 8, 183–187.

Banwell, C., Broom, D., Davies, A., Dixon, J. (Eds.), Weight of Modernity: An intergenerational study of the rise of obesity. Springer, in press.

Dixon, J., Banwell, C., 2010. Theoretical integration for explaining the health inequalities risk transition. Social Science and Medicine. 68 (12), 2206–2214.

Chapter 30

Complementary Readings

1. Scope of the field: medical anthropology, culture in epidemiology, social epidemiology, biocultural anthropology, sociology of health, and social medicine

Cassel, J., 1962. Cultural factors in the interpretation of illness. In: Kark, S.L., Steuart, G.W. (Eds.), A practice of social medicine: A South African team's experiences in different African communities. Edinburgh, E., S. Livingstone LTD.

DiGiacomo, S.M., 1999. Can there be a "cultural epidemiology"? Medical Anthropology Quarterly 13, 436–57.

Dunn, F.L., Janes, C.R., 1986. Introduction: Medical anthropology and epidemiology. In: Janes, C.R., Stall, R., Gifford, S. (Eds.), Anthropology and epidemiology, Dordrecht, D. Reidel Publishing Company.

Durkheim, E., 1951. Suicide: A study in sociology. The Free Press, Glencoe.

Hruschka, D.J., Hadley, C., 2008. A glossary of culture in epidemiology. Journal of Epidemiology and Community Health 62, 947–951.

Krieger, N., 2001. A glossary for social epidemiology. Journal of Epidemiology and Community Health 55, 693–700.

Trostle, J.A., Sommerfeld, J., 1996. Medical anthropology and epidemiology. Annual Review of Anthropology 25, 253–274.

Weiss, M.G., 2001. Cultural epidemiology: an introduction and overview. Anthropology & Medicine 8, 5–29.

Worthman, C.M., Costello, E.J., 2009. Tracking biocultural pathways in population health: the value of biomarkers. Annals of Human Biology 36, 281–97.

2. Theories of culture: the contested terrain

Boyden, S., 2004. Some Useful Concepts. In: Boyden, S. (Ed.), The biology of civilisation: Understanding human culture as a force in nature, UNSW Press, Sydney, pp. 23–33.

3. Examples of the cultural epidemiology field

3.1 Inclusion of socio-cultural factors in epidemiology analyses of health risks:

Blakely, T., Fawcett, J., Hunt, D., Wilson, N., 2006. What is the contribution of smoking and socioeconomic position to ethnic inequalities in mortality in New Zealand? Lancet 368, 44–52.

3.2   Ethnographic analyses of health patterns and risks:
Gifford, S., 1986. The meaning of lumps: a case study of the ambiguities of risk. In: Janes, C.R., Stall, R., Gifford, S. (Eds.), Anthropology and epidemiology: Interdisciplinary approaches to the study of health and disease, D. Reidel Publishing Company, Dordrecht, 213–246.
Koch, E., 2006. Beyond suspicion: evidence, (un)certainty, and tuberculosis in Georgian prisons. American Ethnologist 33, 50–62.

3.3   Twinning of epidemiology and ethnography methods:
Janes, C.R., Ames, G.M., 1992. Ethnographic explanations for the clustering of attendance, injury, and health problems in a heavy machinery assembly plant. Journal of Occupational Medicine 34, 993–1003.

3.4   Cultural process interpretations of national / cross-national health transitions and health risks:
Dixon, J., Banwell, C., 2009. Theory driven research designs for explaining behavioural health risk transitions: the case of smoking. Social Science & Medicine 68, 2206–2214.
Eckersley, R., 2006. Is modern Western culture a health hazard? International Journal of Epidemiology 35, 252–258. (including commentaries by Dressler, Glass & Janes)
Ulijaszek, S.J., 2007. Obesity: a disorder of convenience. Obesity Reviews 8, 183–187.

3.5   Cultural process interpretations of subpopulation health transitions and health risks:
Kaufman, L., Karpati, A., 2007. Understanding the sociocultural roots of childhood obesity: food practices among latino families of bushwick, brooklyn. Social Science & Medicine 64, 2177–2188.
King, M., Smith, A., Gracey, M., 2009. Indigenous health part 2: the underlying causes of the health gap. The Lancet 374, 76–85.
Olsen, A., Banwell, C., Dance, P., 2009. Internal or infernal devices: experiences of contraception among Australian women living with hepatitis C. Health Care for Women Int. 30, 456–74.
Park, J., Littleton, J., 2007. 'Ethnography plus' in tuberculosis research. SITES, New Series 4 (1), 3–23.

3.6   Health services contact, and other cultural contexts, as a mediator of health outcomes:
Broom, D., Whittaker, A., 2004. Controlling diabetes, controlling diabetics: moral language in the management of diabetes type 2. Social Science & Medicine 58, 2371–2382.
Korda, R.J., Banks, E., Clements, M.S., Young, A.F., 2009. Is inequity undermining Australia's 'universal' health care system? Socio-economic inequalities in the use of specialist medical and non-medical ambulatory health care. Australian and New Zealand Journal of Public Health 33, 458–65.

Morgan, D.L., Slade, M.D., Morgan, C.M.A., 1997. Aboriginal philosophy and its impact on health care outcomes. Australian and New Zealand Journal of Public Health 21, 597–601.

4. Methodological approaches and insights

    4.1   Overview:

Hahn, R., 1995. Anthropology and epidemiology: one logic or two? In: Hahn, R. (Ed.), Sickness and Healing: An anthropological perspective, Yale University Press, New Haven, pp. 99–128.

    4.2   Epidemiology and sociocultural factor research:

Brown, R.A., Kuzara, J., Copeland, W.E., Costello, E.J., Angold, A., Worthman, C.M., 2009. Moving from ethnography to epidemiology: lessons learned in Appalachia. Annals of Human Biology 36, 248–60.

Christakis, N.A., Fowler, J.H., 2007. The Spread of obesity in a large social network over 32 years. The New England Journal of Medicine 357, 370–379.

    4.3   Ethnographic research:

Atkinson, P., Hammersley, M., 1994. Ethnography and participant observation. In: Denzin, N.K., Lincoln, Y.S. (Eds.), Handbook of Qualitative Research, Sage Publications, Thousand Oakes, pp. 248–261.

    4.4   Political economy / cultural economy analysis of the production of health behaviors:

Farmer, P.E., 2000. The Consumption of the poor: tuberculosis in the 21st century. Ethnography 1, 183–216.

Parker, R. 2001. Sexuality, Culture, and Power in HIV/AIDS Research. Annual Review of Anthropology 30, 163–179.

    4.5   Phenomenological research of experience and meaning:

Wray, N., Markovic, M., Manderson, L., 2007. Discourses of normality and difference: Responses to diagnosis and treatment of gynaecological cancer of Australian women. Social Science & Medicine 64, 2260–2271.

5. Doing culture-in-health research

Bourgois, P., 2002. Anthropology and epidemiology on drugs: the challenges of cross-methodological and theoretical dialogue. International Journal of Drug Policy 13, 259–269.

Dressler, W.W., Bindon, J.R., 2000. The health consequences of cultural consonance: Cultural dimensions of lifestyle, social support, and arterial blood pressure in an African American community. American Anthropologist 102, 244–260.

Helman, C., 2007. New research methods in medical anthropology. In: Helman, C. (Ed.), Culture, health and illness, fifth ed. Hodder Arnold, London, pp. 456–466.

Inglehart, R., (Ed.), 2005. The worldviews of Islamic publics in global perspective. In: Moaddel, M. (Ed.), Worldviews of Islamic publics, University of Michigan.

Mhurchu, C.N., Blakely, T., Funaki-Tahifote, M., McKerchar, C., Wilton, J., Chua, S., Jiang, Y., 2009. Inclusion of indigenous and ethnic minority populations in intervention trials: challenges and strategies in a New Zealand supermarket study. Journal of Epidemiology and Community Health 63, 850–855.

Trostle, J.A., 2005. Cultural issues in measurement and bias. In: Trostle, J.A. (Ed.), Epidemiology and culture. Cambridge University Press, pp. 74–95.

6. Intervening in culture for health improvement: possibilities, actors and pitfalls

Gracey, M., King, M., 2009. Indigenous health part 1: determinants and disease patterns. Lancet 374, 65–75.

Renne, E.P., 2009. Anthropological and public health perspectives on the Global Polio Eradication Initiative in Northern Nigeria. In: Hahn, R Inhorn, M.C. (Eds.), Anthropology and public health: Bridging differences in culture and society, second ed. Oxford University Press, pp. 512–538.

Person, B., Sy, F., Holton, K., Govert, B., Liang, A., 2004. Fear and stigma: the epidemic within the SARS outbreak. Emerging Infectious Diseases 10, 358–63.

Peace, A., 2008. Beauty and the beef. Anthropology Today 24, 5–10.

Index

Page numbers followed by *f,* indicate figure and *t,* indicate table.

Printed in the United States
By Bookmasters